ME/CFS: Causes, Clinical Features and Diagnosis

Editors

Derek F. H. Pheby
Kenneth J. Friedman
Modra Murovska
Pawel Zalewski

MDPI • Basel • Beijing • Wuhan • Barcelona • Belgrade • Manchester • Tokyo • Cluj • Tianjin

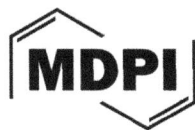

Editors

Derek F. H. Pheby
Society and Health
Buckinghamshire New
University
High Wycombe
UK

Kenneth J. Friedman
School of Osteopathic Medicine
Rowan University
Stratford, NJ
USA

Modra Murovska
Institute of Microbiology and
Virology
Riga Stradins University
Riga
Latvia

Pawel Zalewski
Department of Exercise
Physiology and Functional
Anatomy, Ludwik Rydygier
Collegium Medicum in
Bydgoszcz
Nicolaus Copernicus University
Torun
Poland

Editorial Office
MDPI
St. Alban-Anlage 66
4052 Basel, Switzerland

This is a reprint of articles from the Special Issue published online in the open access journal *Medicina* (ISSN 1648-9144) (available at: https://www.mdpi.com/journal/medicina/special_issues/myalgic_encephalomyelitis_chronic_fatigue_syndrome).

For citation purposes, cite each article independently as indicated on the article page online and as indicated below:

LastName, A.A.; LastName, B.B.; LastName, C.C. Article Title. *Journal Name* **Year**, *Volume Number*, Page Range.

ISBN 978-3-0365-2439-9 (Hbk)
ISBN 978-3-0365-2438-2 (PDF)

© 2022 by the authors. Articles in this book are Open Access and distributed under the Creative Commons Attribution (CC BY) license, which allows users to download, copy and build upon published articles, as long as the author and publisher are properly credited, which ensures maximum dissemination and a wider impact of our publications.

The book as a whole is distributed by MDPI under the terms and conditions of the Creative Commons license CC BY-NC-ND.

Contents

About the Editors vii

Preface to "ME/CFS: Causes, Clinical Features and Diagnosis" ix

Derek F. H. Pheby, Kenneth J. Friedman, Modra Murovska and Pawel Zalewski
Turning a Corner in ME/CFS Research
Reprinted from: *Medicina* 2021, 57, 1012, doi:10.3390/medicina57101012 1

Rosemary Underhill and Rosemarie Baillod
Myalgic Encephalomyelitis/Chronic Fatigue Syndrome: Organic Disease or Psychosomatic Illness? A Re-Examination of the Royal Free Epidemic of 1955
Reprinted from: *Medicina* 2020, 57, 12, doi:10.3390/medicina57010012 11

Derek F. H. Pheby, Diana Araja, Uldis Berkis, Elenka Brenna, John Cullinan, Jean-Dominique de Korwin, Lara Gitto, Dyfrig A. Hughes, Rachael M. Hunter, Dominic Trepel and Xia Wang-Steverding
A Literature Review of GP Knowledge and Understanding of ME/CFS: A Report from the Socioeconomic Working Group of the European Network on ME/CFS (EUROMENE)
Reprinted from: *Medicina* 2020, 57, 7, doi:10.3390/medicina57010007 21

John Cullinan, Derek F. H. Pheby, Diana Araja, Uldis Berkis, Elenka Brenna, Jean-Dominique de Korwin, Lara Gitto, Dyfrig A. Hughes, Rachael M. Hunter, Dominic Trepel and Xia Wang-Steverding
Perceptions of European ME/CFS Experts Concerning Knowledge and Understanding of ME/CFS among Primary Care Physicians in Europe: A Report from the European ME/CFS Research Network (EUROMENE)
Reprinted from: *Medicina* 2021, 57, 208, doi:10.3390/medicina57030208 39

Nina Muirhead, John Muirhead, Grace Lavery and Ben Marsh
Medical School Education on Myalgic Encephalomyelitis
Reprinted from: *Medicina* 2021, 57, 542, doi:10.3390/medicina57060542 51

Keng Ngee Hng, Keith Geraghty and Derek F. H. Pheby
An Audit of UK Hospital Doctors' Knowledge and Experience of Myalgic Encephalomyelitis
Reprinted from: *Medicina* 2021, 57, 885, doi:10.3390/medicina57090885 61

Timothy L. Wong and Danielle J. Weitzer
Long COVID and Myalgic Encephalomyelitis/Chronic Fatigue Syndrome (ME/CFS)—A Systemic Review and Comparison of Clinical Presentation and Symptomatology
Reprinted from: *Medicina* 2021, 57, 418, doi:10.3390/medicina57050418 81

Kenneth J. Friedman, Modra Murovska, Derek F. H. Pheby and Paweł Zalewski
Our Evolving Understanding of ME/CFS
Reprinted from: *Medicina* 2021, 57, 200, doi:10.3390/medicina57030200 95

Esme Brittain, Nina Muirhead, Andrew Y. Finlay and Jui Vyas
Myalgic Encephalomyelitis/Chronic Fatigue Syndrome (ME/CFS): Major Impact on Lives of Both Patients and Family Members
Reprinted from: *Medicina* 2021, 57, 43, doi:10.3390/medicina57010043 101

Elenka Brenna, Diana Araja and Derek F. H. Pheby
Comparative Survey of People with ME/CFS in Italy, Latvia, and the UK: A Report on Behalf of the Socioeconomics Working Group of the European ME/CFS Research Network (EUROMENE)
Reprinted from: *Medicina* **2021**, *57*, 300, doi:10.3390/medicina57030300 109

Laura Froehlich, Daniel B. R. Hattesohl, Leonard A. Jason, Carmen Scheibenbogen, Uta Behrends and Manuel Thoma
Medical Care Situation of People with Myalgic Encephalomyelitis/Chronic Fatigue Syndrome in Germany
Reprinted from: *Medicina* **2021**, *57*, 646, doi:10.3390/medicina57070646 121

Angelika Krumina, Katrine Vecvagare, Simons Svirskis, Sabine Gravelsina, Zaiga Nora-Krukle, Sandra Gintere and Modra Murovska
Clinical Profile and Aspects of Differential Diagnosis in Patients with ME/CFS from Latvia
Reprinted from: *Medicina* **2021**, *57*, 958, doi:10.3390/medicina57090958 135

Luis Nacul, François Jérôme Authier, Carmen Scheibenbogen, Lorenzo Lorusso, Ingrid Bergliot Helland, Jose Alegre Martin, Carmen Adella Sirbu, Anne Marit Mengshoel, Olli Polo, Uta Behrends, Henrik Nielsen, Patricia Grabowski, Slobodan Sekulic, Nuno Sepulveda, Fernando Estévez-López, Pawel Zalewski, Derek F. H. Pheby, Jesus Castro-Marrero, Giorgos K. Sakkas, Enrica Capelli, Ivan Brundsdlund, John Cullinan, Angelika Krumina, Jonas Bergquist, Modra Murovska, Ruud C. W. Vermuelen and Eliana M. Lacerda
European Network on Myalgic Encephalomyelitis/Chronic Fatigue Syndrome (EUROMENE): Expert Consensus on the Diagnosis, Service Provision, and Care of People with ME/CFS in Europe
Reprinted from: *Medicina* **2021**, *57*, 510, doi:10.3390/medicina57050510 149

Samaneh Khanpour Ardestani, Mohammad Karkhaneh, Eleanor Stein, Salima Punja, Daniela R. Junqueira, Tatiana Kuzmyn, Michelle Pearson, Laurie Smith, Karin Olson and Sunita Vohra
Systematic Review of Mind-Body Interventions to Treat Myalgic Encephalomyelitis/Chronic Fatigue Syndrome
Reprinted from: *Medicina* **2021**, *57*, 652, doi:10.3390/medicina57070652 175

Derek F. H. Pheby, Diana Araja, Uldis Berkis, Elenka Brenna, John Cullinan, Jean-Dominique de Korwin, Lara Gitto, Dyfrig A. Hughes, Rachael M. Hunter, Dominic Trepel and Xia Wang-Steverding
The Role of Prevention in Reducing the Economic Impact of ME/CFS in Europe: A Report from the Socioeconomics Working Group of the European Network on ME/CFS (EUROMENE)
Reprinted from: *Medicina* **2021**, *57*, 388, doi:10.3390/medicina57040388 219

About the Editors

Derek F. H. Pheby is recently retired. His most recent appointment was as Visiting Professor of Epidemiology at Buckinghamshire New University, UK. He was formerly a cancer epidemiologist, and was the UK permanent representative on the Steering Committee of the European Network of Cancer Registries and chairman of its Data Definitions Group. He was the founder and first chairman of the UK Association of Cancer Registries. More recently, he developed an interest in ME/CFS following the serious illness of a close family member. He was responsible for establishing the EUROMENE (European ME/CFS Network) research collaboration, and chaired its Socioeconomics Working Group. He was a trustee of the UK organisation Action for ME, and is a patron of the ME Association. He was awarded a Haldane Prize by the Royal Institute of Public Administration in 1983, and the Silver Medal of the European Society for Person-Centred Healthcare in 2018.

Kenneth J. Friedman, Ph.D. is an adjunct Associate Professor of Medicine at the School of Osteopathic Medicine, Rowan University, Stratford, NJ, USA. A neurophysiologist and pharmacologist by training, he taught medical, dental and graduate students at the New Jersey Medical School for 34 years while pursuing basic research in the area of membrane physiology. When medical science failed to diagnose, treat or cure his daughter's Chronic Fatigue Syndrome in the mid-1990s he began his research and pursuit of the science that underlies ME/CFS and similar chronic illnesses. Currently, he produces and disseminates educational materials for healthcare providers which assist them in providing care for patients suffering from Post Active Phase Infectious Syndromes (PAPIS).

Modra Murovska, MD, PhD, Associate Professor, Lead Researcher, Director of the Institute of Microbiology and Virology, Rīga Stradiņš University, Full Member of the Latvian Academy of Sciences. Her general interest is virology.

The ongoing projects under her guidance are "Reducing networking gaps between Rīga Stradiņš University (RSU) and internationally - leading counterparts in viral infection-induced autoimmunity research (VirA)" (H2020-WIDESPREAD-2018-2020); "Selection of biomarkers in ME/CFS for patient stratification and treatment surveillance/optimisation" (Project of the Latvian Council of Science). Her scientific interests are blood-borne viruses, persistent viral infections and their association with human pathologies, the implication of viral infections in the pathogenesis of chronic inflammatory and autoimmune diseases (including neural diseases), and the role of viral infections in cancer development. In 2000, M. Murovska received the American Society for Microbiology Morrison Rogosa Award.

Pawel Zalewski completed his postdoctoral training at Nicolaus Copernicus University in Torun (2011-2015), where his research work and interests focus on physiotherapy and the related areas of physical medicine, and applied and clinical physiology. He currently works in the Department of Exercise Physiology and Functional Anatomy, Faculty of Health Sciences, Nicolaus Copernicus University. His scientific achievements largely concern the influence of environmental and disease factors on physiological adaptation of the autonomic nervous system, as well as on biological mechanisms underlying the development of dysautonomia and related chronic fatigue. A major recent focus of research by his research group is on pathological mechanisms, biomarkers, diagnosis and therapy of chronic fatigue syndrome (ME/CFS), which is being undertaken in collaboration with international colleagues at the Universities of Newcastle and Oxford in the UK, Griffith University in Australia, and many others. He also actively promotes public understanding of science in these areas of interest, and in the effectiveness of the therapeutic influence of physical training in various clinical conditions.

Preface to "ME/CFS: Causes, Clinical Features and Diagnosis"

This volume aims to focus on the early stages of ME/CFS and the underlying factors predisposing to it, by addressing the causes of the illness, its clinical features, and diagnosis. We were motivated both by the plight of the individual patient, and also by the impact of the illness on society as a whole. We have reason to believe that patients and their families and carers frequently experience difficulties accessing care, and are subject to discriminatory attitudes on the parts of care providers and others. We also wish to create awareness of the impact of ME/CFS on society as a whole, which is considerable, in terms of both costs and social disruption. We also explore ways to reduce the public health burden of ME/CFS, and to mitigate the damaging effects of the illness on individual patients and their families.

Our aim is to provide content in this volume that will be of interest both to those undertaking scientific research and to those providing clinical care for ME/CFS patients. There is also plenty to interest, and provide food for thought, for social policy analysts, policy makers and governments, and those with an interest in social research and medical education. These considerations are of particular importance at the present time, when Long Covid-19 has moved post-viral syndromes to the forefront of the political agenda, and confronted society with new challenges in this area on a hitherto unprecedented scale.

Our themed issue is a truly international effort, with sixty-nine authors contributing from seventeen European countries, Canada, and the USA. We are very grateful to everyone who has contributed their high quality research. I am particularly grateful to my co-editors, Professor Modra Murovska, Professor Ken Friedman and Professor Pawel Zalewski, and also to our production editor at MDPI, Svetlana Miljanovic. Without their help and support, none of this would have been possible.

Cover picture

"The Heart Still Beats; the challenge and enigma of ME/CFS" The cover picture, "The Heart Still Beats", is original artwork of Christina Baltais, an ME/CFS patient and artist who resides in Toronto, Ontario, Canada. She uses art as a creative form of advocacy, to help raise ME/CFS awareness. Her work is directly inspired by living with ME/CFS for over fifteen years.

Derek F. H. Pheby, Kenneth J. Friedman, Modra Murovska, Pawel Zalewski
Editors

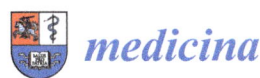

Editorial

Turning a Corner in ME/CFS Research

Derek F. H. Pheby [1,*,†], Kenneth J. Friedman [2], Modra Murovska [3] and Pawel Zalewski [4]

1. Society and Health, Buckinghamshire New University, High Wycombe HP11 2JZ, UK
2. School of Osteopathic Medicine, Rowan University, Stratford, NJ 08080, USA; kenneth.j.friedman@gmail.com
3. Institute of Microbiology and Virology, Riga Stradiņš University, LV-1067 Riga, Latvia; Modra.Murovska@rsu.lv
4. Department of Exercise Physiology and Functional Anatomy, Ludwik Rydygier Collegium Medicum in Bydgoszcz, Nicolaus Copernicus University in Torun, Swietojanska 20, 85-077 Bydgoszcz, Poland; p.zalewski@cm.umk.pl
* Correspondence: derekpheby@btinternet.com
† Retired.

Abstract: This collection of research papers addresses fundamental questions concerning the nature of myalgic encephalomyelitis/ chronic fatigue syndrome (ME/CFS), the problem of disbelief and lack of knowledge and understanding of the condition among many doctors and the origins of this problem, and its impact on patients and their families. We report briefly the growing knowledge of the underlying pathological processes in ME/CFS, and the development of new organizations, including Doctors with ME, the US ME/CFS Clinical Coalition and EUROMENE, to address aspects of the challenges posed by the illness. We discuss the implications of COVID-19, which has much in common with ME/CFS, with much overlap of symptoms, and propose a new taxonomic category, which we are terming post-active phase of infection syndromes (PAPIS) to include both. This collection of papers includes a number of papers reporting similar serious impacts on the quality of life of patients and their families in various European countries. The advice of EUROMENE experts on diagnosis and management is included in the collection. We report this in light of guidance from other parts of the world, including the USA and Australia, and in the context of current difficulties in the UK over the promulgation of a revised guideline from the National Institute for Health and Care Excellence (NICE). We also consider evidence on the cost-effectiveness of interventions for ME/CFS, and on the difficulties of determining the costs of care when a high proportion of people with ME/CFS are never diagnosed as such. The Special Issue includes a paper which is a reminder of the importance of a person-centred approach to care by reviewing mind–body interventions. Finally, another paper reviews the scope for prevention in minimizing the population burden of ME/CFS, and concludes that secondary prevention, through early detection and diagnosis, could be of value.

Keywords: ME/CFS; myalgic encephalomyelitis; chronic fatigue syndrome; knowledge and understanding; quality of life; guideline; clinical care

Myalgic encephalomyelitis/chronic fatigue syndrome (ME/CFS) is a relatively common and often misunderstood illness, which causes considerable distress to patients and their families, not least because of frequently encountered unhelpful and judgmental attitudes on the part of healthcare professionals. It also has considerable economic implications, and a focus group based in Ireland found that ME/CFS patients incurred wide-ranging costs, as well as wider societal costs including health care costs, lost productivity, and impacts on informal carers [1].

This collection of research papers concerning ME/CFS addresses some important issues. One such issue goes to the very heart of the debate within the medical profession about the very nature of the disease. Many doctors refuse to accept that ME/CFS is a genuine clinical entity, and ascribe it instead to a variety of psychiatric diagnoses. A major cause of doctors' disbelief in ME/CFS is the 1970 paper by McEvedy and Beard in the

BMJ, which determined that the 1958 Royal Free epidemic of ME/CFS was 'epidemic hysteria' [2]. However, the report in this collection by Underhill and Baillod [3], based on a focus group and interviews with survivors of the 1958 Royal Free epidemic, corroborates a paper published last year which invalidated the McEvedy/Beard paper on the basis of their having identified mathematical errors in the original publication [4]. The weaknesses in the McEvedy/Beard paper spotlighted by this triangulation of a mathematical and an historical approach should be sufficient to consign the hysteria hypothesis to the dustbin of history, where it belongs.

That ME/CFS is a clinical entity is underlined by an increasing corpus of knowledge of the pathological processes underlying ME/CFS. ME/CFS is a multi-system disorder, with dysregulation of the HPA axis and of metabolism of the central nervous system and of body systems generally. The range of abnormal responses includes alteration of autonomic nervous system function, in particular sensitization of the sympathetic nervous system, with lasting adaptations in energy metabolism and the immune response, orthostatic intolerance with reduction in cerebral blood flow on tilt testing, variations in cortisol levels associated with increased fatigue, disorganized circadian rhythms, increased immune system activation, as shown for example by increased pro-inflammatory cytokines and prolonged inflammatory responses, alterations in muscle anaerobic threshold, abnormal recovery after activity with post-exertional malaise, central sensitization, and changes in grey and white matter in the brain [5]. ME/CFS is neither a rare nor an orphan disease, with perhaps as many as 2.5 million people suffering from it in the USA, and there is now new evidence of underlying anatomical, physiological and electrical abnormalities in the brain, of chronic activation of the immune system, including autoantibodies directed at the central and autonomic nervous systems, of impaired energy metabolism with associated oxidative stress, of dysregulation of the autonomic nervous system, and of abnormalities of the gut microbiome [6]. Some blood test results differed in ME/CFS patients from those of healthy controls. In particular, creatine kinase and creatinine were reduced in ME/CFS patients [7]. Metabolic dysfunction, resulting from abnormal immune responses, has been identified as possibly underlying the major symptoms of ME/CFS [8]. Evidence for an infection-triggered autoimmune process involving dysfunctional ß2-adrenoreceptor antibodies has been published, which may indicate a therapeutic role for immunoadsorption therapy. The latter has shown promising results in a pilot study [9].

The persistence of dismissive attitudes among doctors is a consequence of inadequate teaching about ME/CFS, both in medical schools to undergraduates and at the postgraduate level to physicians in practice. Four of the papers in this collection consider aspects of knowledge of ME/CFS among doctors. A literature review of GP knowledge and understanding of ME/CFS included in this collection of papers concluded that between a one-third and a half of GPs did not accept ME/CFS as a genuine clinical entity, and that a similar proportion of patients were dissatisfied with the primary medical care they had received [10]. These proportions applied geographically irrespective of location, and had changed little in recent decades. Furthermore, the study of perceptions of ME/CFS experts across Europe indicated that this situation was current throughout Europe [11]. An exploratory survey of UK medical schools by Muirhead et al. indicated that undergraduate teaching about ME/CFS was generally inadequate [12], while, at the postgraduate level, evidence is evinced here of considerable misconceptions about the nature of ME/CFS, its diagnosis and management among UK junior hospital doctors [13]. It should be appreciated that this failure to recognize ME/CFS as a genuine clinical entity is not merely an interesting academic dispute. For patients deprived of medical care as a result, and, worse, labelled at best as being malingerers and at worst of being seriously psychiatrically disturbed, it is nothing short of disastrous.

The literature review referred to above [10] found that ignorance and denial among doctors were paralleled by widespread dissatisfaction with their medical care among patients. Where doctors (or their family members) are themselves patients, they experience a double problem: not only are they as subject to diagnostic error as any other patient, but they are uniquely qualified to know when they are subject to such errors. In addition, they may find themselves experiencing unsympathetic responses from colleagues who have little understanding of the condition. For these reasons, the establishment of Doctors with ME is to be welcomed. Not only does this constitute a source of support for doctors facing the social, medical and practical problems associated with ME/CFS, but it also creates a group of professionals who are uniquely qualified to comment on the experience of having this illness, especially on the experience of misdiagnosis and lack of understanding on the part of colleagues [14].

This is just one of many recent initiatives which are contributing to advancing the frontiers of knowledge in this area. Others elsewhere in the world include the establishment of the ME/CFS Clinical Coalition in the USA, and in Europe of the EUROMENE (European ME/CFS Research Network) collaboration, which involves more than thirty institutions in twenty-one European countries plus one COST near neighbor country, and means that at last there is in Europe a research infrastructure enabling us to complement the excellent research work being undertaken by our colleagues in North America and elsewhere in the world [15]. As a result, great progress is being made in unravelling underlying pathology, identifying biomarkers, developing better treatments, and discrediting damaging practices. In the UK, the Medical Research Council is at last allocating serious resources to ME/CFS research.

These reports come at a very opportune time. For decades, the study of ME/CFS has been very much a Cinderella specialization within the medical and scientific research community. However, interest has suddenly grown as a result of the increasing phenomenon of Long COVID-19, which has many similarities to ME/CFS. If the current COVID-19 catastrophe has any sort of silver lining, it is that sanity and common sense are beginning to come to the surface of the ME/CFS debate. No one is seriously suggesting that Long COVID-19 is a form of hysteria. Not only is it like ME/CFS, but in many ways it is ME/CFS. Indeed, if there is a silver lining to the current COVID-19 pandemic, it is that the message is finally being understood that long-term neurological and other sequelae following viral infections are genuine clinical entities.

One study found that 89.1% of participants with Long COVID-19 experienced post-exertional malaise, which is generally considered the defining symptom of ME/CFS [16], while a German study found that approximately half of all Long COVID-19 patients fulfilled the diagnostic criteria for ME/CFS [17]. A systemic review by Wong and Weitzer in this issue considered twenty-one studies, and reported much overlap of symptoms between Long COVID-19 and ME/CFS, including fatigue, reduced daily activity, and post-exertional malaise, and some common features in terms of pathophysiology [18]. ME/CFS and Long COVID-19 syndrome have similar symptoms, probably reflecting similar underlying pathological processes involving the central and autonomic nervous system, and a dysregulated immune system. Consequently, a likely consequence of the COVID-19 pandemic will be a considerable increase in the number of people with ME/CFS [19]. Biological abnormalities which appear common to both Long COVID-19 and ME/CFS include redox imbalance, systemic inflammation and neuroinflammation, an impaired ability to generate adenosine triphosphate, and a general hypometabolic state [20]. Such evidence has prompted the proposal of a new taxonomic classification, comprising both Long COVID and ME/CFS within a category entitled post-active phase of infection syndromes, or PAPIS [21].

With regard to the impact of ME/CFS on the quality of life of patients and their families, Brittain et al. [22] conducted a quantitative research study using postal questionnaires. Twenty-four adult volunteers responded, indicating that ME/CFS negatively affects the quality of life of the patient. Additionally, there was a significant correlation between the patient's reported quality-of-life scores and those of family members. The greatest reduction in the quality of life of ME/CFS patients was in terms of physical health, while that of family members was in terms of worry, family activities, frustration and sadness. Brenna et al. [23] demonstrated that the impact of the illness on net household incomes and quality of life was similar in three different European countries, Italy, Latvia, and the

UK. Respondents in all three countries reported similar difficulties in talking to doctors, though differences emerged in patterns and availability of medical and social care, and in societal attitudes. Similar impacts on quality of life have been reported in other contexts, including for example among university students, where stigmatization had a substantial negative impact on subjective self-esteem [24].

There are, not surprisingly, few first-hand accounts by patients with ME/CFS of their illness experiences. However, one seriously affected patient, who fell ill at the age of 21, has recently put his experiences on record. After a year, he was obliged to abandon his wedding photography business because of prolonged post-exertional malaise. He describes his experience of very severe ME/CFS, and reports that he is now bedridden most of the time, and has been unable to leave his room for seven years, except to go to hospital. He has been unable to speak, eat or drink, and has been tube fed. He cannot shower, cut his toe nails, clean his teeth or go to the lavatory, and has had no physical contact with another human being in all that time. It took eight years though, and numerous medical consultations, before he received a diagnosis, but nevertheless he still found himself stigmatized because of lack of knowledge or understanding of the condition. He reports a patient with severe ME/CFS who was forcibly incarcerated in a psychiatric ward and who while there was thrown into a swimming pool to get her to "snap her out of it" and who nearly drowned as a result [25].

Three papers in this Special Issue report on the status of ME/CFS patients in different European countries. In Germany, there may be over 300,000 patients, and Froehlich et al. concluded, on the basis of an online survey completed by 499 respondents who fulfilled the Canadian Consensus Criteria and reported post-exertional malaise, that they were medically underserved. Reported levels of satisfaction with medical care were low, and there were geographical and financial factors limiting the accessibility of medical services [26]. Krumina et al. studied 65 outpatients with fatigue, 55 of whom were diagnosed with ME/CFS. They concluded that patients with more severe ME/CFS were more likely also to have comorbidities, of which fibromyalgia, chronic hepatitis and Lyme disease were of the most frequent occurrences. Fatigue, myalgia, arthralgia and sleep disturbances were more frequently encountered among the ME/CFS patients than among those not diagnosed as having ME/CFS. All the ME/CFS patients reported fatigue and post-exertional malaise. Other symptoms most frequently reported were myalgia, headache, arthralgia and difficulty concentrating. The number of symptoms reported was associated with increased age and longer duration of fatigue. Many of the ME/CFS patients identified physical or mental stress and other chronic diseases as contributing to the development of their illness. Self-help strategies adopted by ME/CFS patients involved physical activities, sleep hygiene, physiotherapy and walking. A total of 90% had taken non-steroidal anti-inflammatory drugs [27]. A comparative survey of ME/CFS patients in Latvia, Italy and the UK found that demographic details were similar in the three countries, as was the impact of the illness on household incomes and quality of life. However, there are differences in illness progression and management, which may be associated with variations in health care patterns and attitudes in society [23].

On the management of ME/CFS in England, the National Institute for Health and Care Excellence (NICE) produced guidance on ME/CFS in 2007 [28]. This proved very unpopular with patients and many professionals, largely because of its espousal of graded exercise therapy (GET) for people with mild or moderate disease [28]. A draft of revised guidance was published in November 2020 which reversed this previous advice, stating 'Do not offer people with ME/CFS ... any therapy based on physical activity or exercise as a treatment or cure for ME/CFS' [29]. This document was due to be promulgated in its final, definitive form on 18 August 2021, but was withdrawn on the eve of publication because certain elements in the UK medical establishment objected to this change of position [30]. Such a withdrawal of guidance on the eve of publication is unprecedented. There is no provision in the NICE working procedures for this to happen, and it calls into question the much vaunted independence of NICE. GET is simply the immediate casus belli; what is really the issue here is a clash between two opposed points of view as to the nature of ME/CFS, which may be identified as the biomedical and psychosocial paradigms, respectively. NICE has now indicated that a round table meeting, with an independent chairman, will be convened during September 2021, with the intention of bringing the two schools of thought together in order to negotiate an acceptable compromise. However, the chances of success appear slight, as there is absolutely no common ground between the two viewpoints, and in the meantime a letter signed by one hundred and twenty-five of the world's leading scientific and clinical experts on ME/CFS, including many contributors to this current collection of research papers, has been sent to the Chief Executive of NICE calling for the immediate reinstatement of the withdrawn guidance [31].

If NICE accepts the position of those lobbying for changes to the new guideline on ME/CFS, it will be putting itself at variance with expert opinion in much of the rest of the world. The clinical working group of the European Network on ME/CFS (EUROMENE) has produced guidelines on diagnosis, management and service provision for ME/CFS, and these are published in this Special Issue [32]. They outline impediments to effective clinical care, including unavailability or inaccessibility of services, and unsympathetic attitudes or disbelief on the part of medical practitioners. On diagnosis, EUROMENE recommends use of the Canadian Consensus Criteria [33]. It states that the CDC-1994 (Fukuda) case definition [34] can be used for screening purposes, with the addition of post-exertional malaise as an essential symptom. It goes into considerable detail about the conduct of the consultation and the treatment options available, with the notable omission of graded exercise therapy (GET). In this, the EUROMENE expert consensus is consistent with recent guidance from the US ME/CFS Clinical Coalition, which goes further in stating that GET can worsen the patient's condition, and that it represents 'an outdated standard of care' [35]. It should be noted that, in the paper by Brenna et al. comparing the position of ME/CFS patients in three European countries, only in the UK had respondents received GET, and, of seventy people who had experienced it, only one reported any positive benefit from it [23].

This increasing concern about the use of GET is mirrored in other parts of the world. The Royal Australasian College of Physicians published guidance in 2002 [36]. However, the Australian ME/CFS Advisory Committee reported in 2019 that this guidance has more recently been a cause for concern, partly because of its espousal of graded exercise therapy, and commented: " . . . the historical context of this guideline must be noted, as they were developed at a time when not much was known about ME/CFS" [37], and stated that, for patients with a significant disability wishing to access care through the National Disability Insurance Scheme, or in receipt of a Disability Support Pension, graded exercise therapy may be inappropriate [38].

A systematic review on the cost-effectiveness of ME/CFS interventions considered ten economic evaluations based in randomized controlled trials, with varying results. It appeared from three studies that cognitive behavior therapy (CBT) may be cost-effective, but this may depend on context, and there was some suggestion from two trials that GET may be cost-effective [39]. However, such equivocal evidence of cost-effectiveness is far from indicating that such treatments may be curative, as their proponents have argued. The socioeconomics working group of EUROMENE drew attention to the costs incurred by those large numbers of patients with ME/CFS whose condition is never diagnosed, often because of the refusal of many doctors to recognize it as a genuine clinical entity [40]. In Latvia, it is thought that the number of undiagnosed patients may be five times greater than those who are diagnosed. It is estimated that the direct medical costs alone for these undiagnosed patients may have been more than €15 million p.a. before the start of the COVID-19 pandemic, and may now be in the region of €17 million [41].

There is general agreement that management of ME/CFS needs to be very much patient centred, and that it is essential for patients to be at the centre of, and very much involved in, clinical decision making in respect of their treatment. In this context, the paper by Ardestani et al., in this collection, is a valuable reminder of the importance of such a person-centred, holistic approach. Their review is of twelve studies of mind–body interventions, including seven randomized controlled trials. The outcomes which they observed were mostly severity of fatigue, anxiety/depression, quality of life, and physical and mental functioning. They found general improvements in these outcome parameters. However, these findings must be regarded as provisional, due to small sample sizes, heterogeneous diagnostic criteria, and the possibility of various biases [42].

To complete the contribution of this Special Issue to the management of patients with ME/CFS, Pheby et al., on behalf of EUROMENE, considered the possible role of preventive programs in minimizing the impact of ME/CFS. They considered in detail the economic case for prevention, as well as the possible health benefits. They concluded that primary prevention would be of little benefit, as not enough is known about modifiable risk factors which could be the subject of such programs. The only exception was in the use of agricultural chemicals, in particular organophosphates. However, secondary prevention is a different matter altogether, and programs to minimize diagnostic delays would have a beneficial effect on both health and the costs of care, by reducing the incidence of prolonged and severe disease [43]. An important element in implementing such a secondary prevention strategy must be measures to address the problems of disbelief and lack of knowledge and understanding among doctors referred to above [10–13].

In conclusion, the reconsideration in this Special Issue of the 1950s epidemic outbreak of ME/CFS known as Royal Free disease, and effective invalidation of the 'epidemic hysteria' hypothesis attached to it, comes at a very opportune time when knowledge of the underlying pathology of the disease is increasing rapidly. Four papers considered the problem of disbelief among many doctors, much of it undoubtedly fuelled by the 'epidemic hysteria' hypothesis, and lack of knowledge and understanding of ME/CFS among doctors, with consequent widespread dissatisfaction among patients. In this context, the formation of new organizations specifically concerned with particular aspects of ME/CFS is helpful. Doctors with ME addresses the problems faced by doctors themselves who have the misfortune to have the illness, and who as a result have not only the symptoms of the disease to contend with, but also the opprobrium of colleagues. EUROMENE, the European ME/CFS Research Network, was established to facilitate collaborative working between scientific and clinical colleagues across Europe, and to bring a more strategic approach to the research endeavor. The COVID-19 pandemic has brought with it an upsurge in the number of people experiencing a post-viral syndrome which in many cases is indistinguishable from ME/CFS. This is underlined by an important paper in this collection, and led us to propose a new taxonomic classification category which we are calling post-active phase of infection syndromes, or PAPIS. This Special Issue has also considered in detail the impact of ME/CFS on the lives of patients. One paper considered the quality of life of patients and their families in the UK, while another compared quality of life and other aspects of the illness in three European countries and found many similarities. Other papers reviewed the position of people with ME/CFS in Germany and Latvia, respectively. On management of ME/CFS, the EUROMENE expert consensus document comes at a very opportune moment, when in the UK a last-ditch attempt is being made to subvert and derail the NICE process of guideline development, and to undermine the intention of the draft guideline to abandon NICE's previous espousal of graded exercise therapy, which has proved very damaging to many patients in the past. This is very unfortunate. The hope is that this attempt will come to naught, as the draft guideline was in line with the growing body of expert opinion throughout the world, including not only the EUROMENE consensus document but also that of the US ME/CFS Clinical Coalition. There is general recognition that the treatment of ME/CFS needs to be very much patient-centred, and this is supported by the paper in this collection on mind–body interventions. Finally, the review of the scope for prevention in ME/CFS underlines once again the need for early detection in order to achieve secondary prevention and minimize the incidence of severe, prolonged disease. The impact of the errors of the past on patients and their families has been immense, particularly on those families of professionals working within the health care system. These are not victimless errors. The consequences can be observed in destroyed reputations, shattered families and family finances, wrecked careers, and blighted lives. However, at long last, there is the prospect of real progress being made through research to unravel the enigma of this very damaging disease. Many of us who have been working in this field for many years have ploughed a difficult furrow, but at last, though the challenges remain immense, the future is looking bright.

Author Contributions: Initial conceptualization, and original draft preparation, D.F.H.P.; additional writing contributions, review and editing, M.M., K.J.F., D.F.H.P. and P.Z. All authors have read and agreed to the published version of the manuscript.

Funding: This research received no external funding.

Data Availability Statement: Not applicable.

Conflicts of Interest: The authors declare no conflict of interest.

References

1. Cullinan, J.; Chomhraí, O.N.; Kindlon, T.; Black, L.; Casey, B. Understanding the economic impact of myalgic encephalomyelitis/chronic fatigue syndrome in Ireland: A qualitative study. *HRB Open Res.* **2020**, *3*. [CrossRef] [PubMed]
2. McEvedy, C.P.; Beard, A.W. Royal Free Epidemic of 1955: A Reconsideration. *BMJ* **1970**, *5687*, 7–11. [CrossRef] [PubMed]
3. Underhill, R.; Baillod, R. Myalgic Encephalomyelitis/Chronic Fatigue Syndrome: Organic Disease or Psychosomatic Illness? A Re-Examination of the Royal Free Epidemic of 1955. *Medicina* **2021**, *57*, 12. [CrossRef]
4. Waters, F.G.; McDonald, G.J.; Banks, S.; Waters, R.A. Myalgic Encephalomyelitis (ME) outbreaks can be modelled as an infectious disease: A mathematical reconsideration of the Royal Free Epidemic of 1955. *Fatigue: Biomed. Health Behav.* **2020**, *8*, 70–83. [CrossRef]
5. BACME (British Association for CFS/ME). An Introduction to Dysregulation in ME/CFS. August 2021. Available online: https://www.bacme.info/sites/bacme.info/files/BACME20An%20Introduction%20to%20Dysregulation%20in%20MECFS.pdf (accessed on 2 September 2021).
6. Komaroff, A.L. Myalgic Encephalomyelitis/Chronic Fatigue Syndrome: When suffering is multiplied. *Healthcare* **2021**, *9*, 919. [CrossRef]
7. Baklund, I.H.; Dammen, T.; Moum, T.Å.; Kristiansen, W.; Castro-Marrero, J.; Helland, I.B.; Strand, E.B. Evaluating routine blood tests according to clinical symptoms and diagnostic criteria in individuals with Myalgic Encephalomyelitis/Chronic Fatigue Syndrome (CFS/ME). *J. Clin. Med.* **2021**, *10*, 3105. [CrossRef]
8. Hoel, F.; Hoel, A.; Pettersen, I.K.N.; Rekeland, I.G.; Risa, K.; Alme, K.; Sørland, K.; Fosså, A.; Lien, K.; Herder, I.; et al. A map of metabolic phenotypes in patients with myalgic encephalomyelitis/chronic fatigue syndrome. *CI Insight* **2021**, *6*, e149217. [CrossRef]
9. Tölle, M.; Freitag, H.; Antelmann, M.; Hartwig, J.; Schuchardt, M.; van der Giet, M.; Eckardt, K.-U.; Grabowski, P.; Scheibenbogen, C. Myalgic Encephalomyelitis/Chronic Fatigue Syndrome: Efficacy of repeat immunoadsorption. *J. Clin. Med.* **2020**, *9*, 2443. [CrossRef]
10. Pheby, D.F.H.; Araja, D.; Berkis, U.; Brenna, E.; Cullinan, J.; de Korwin, J.-D.; Gitto, L.; Hughes, D.A.; Hunter, R.M.; Trepel, D.; et al. A Literature Review of GP Knowledge and Understanding of ME/CFS: A Report from the Socioeconomic Working Group of the European Network on ME/CFS (EUROMENE). *Medicina* **2021**, *57*, 7. [CrossRef]
11. Cullinan, J.; Pheby, D.F.H.; Araja, D.; Berkis, U.; Brenna, E.; de Korwin, J.-D.; Gitto, L.; Hughes, D.A.; Hunter, R.M.; Trepel, D.; et al. A Perceptions of European ME/CFS Experts Concerning Knowledge and Understanding of ME/CFS among Primary Care Physicians in Europe: A Report from the European ME/CFS Research Network (EUROMENE). *Medicina* **2021**, *57*, 208. [CrossRef]
12. Muirhead, N.; Muirhead, J.; Lavery, G.; Marsh, B. Medical School Education on Myalgic Encephalomyelitis. *Medicina* **2021**, *57*, 542. [CrossRef] [PubMed]
13. Hng, K.N.; Geraghty, K.; Pheby, D.F.H. An Audit of UK Hospital Doctors' Knowledge and Experience of Myalgic Encephalomyelitis. *Medicina* **2021**, *57*, 885. [CrossRef]
14. Doctors with ME. Available online: https://doctorswith.me/home/about (accessed on 8 September 2021).
15. EUROMENE. Available online: www.euromene.eu (accessed on 31 August 2021).
16. Davis, H.E.; Assaf, G.S.; McCorkell, L.; Wei, H.; Low, R.J.; Re'em, Y.; Redfield, S.; Austin, J.P.; Akrami, A. Characterizing Long COVID in an international cohort: 7 months of symptoms and their impact. *EClinicalMedicine* **2021**, *38*, 101019. [CrossRef]
17. Kedor, C.; Freitag, H.; Meyer-Arndt, L. Chronic COVID-19 Syndrome and Chronic Fatigue Syndrome (ME/CFS) following the first pandemic wave in Germany—A first analysis of a prospective observational study. *medRxiv* **2021**. [CrossRef]
18. Wong, T.L.; Weitzer, D.J. Long COVID and Myalgic Encephalomyelitis/Chronic Fatigue Syndrome (ME/CFS)-A Systemic Review and Comparison of Clinical Presentation and Symptomatology. *Medicina* **2021**, *57*, 418. [CrossRef]

19. Komaroff, A.l.; Lipkin, I. Insights from myalgic encephalomyelitis/chronic fatigue syndrome may help unravel the pathogenesis of postacute COVID-19 syndrome. *Trends Mol. Med.* **2021**, *27*, 895–906. [CrossRef]
20. Paul, B.D.; Lemle, M.D.; Komaroff, A.L.; Snyder, S.H. Redox imbalance links COVID-19 and myalgic encephalomyelitis/chronic fatigue syndrome. *Proc. Natl. Acad. Sci. USA* **2021**, *118*, e2024358118. [CrossRef] [PubMed]
21. Friedman, K.J.; Murovska, M.; Pheby, D.F.H.; Zalewski, P. Our Evolving Understanding of ME/CFS. *Medicina* **2021**, *57*, 200. [CrossRef] [PubMed]
22. Brittain, E.; Muirhead, N.; Finlay, A.Y.; Vyas, J. Myalgic Encephalomyelitis/Chronic Fatigue Syndrome (ME/CFS): Major Impact on Lives of Both Patients and Family Members. *Medicina* **2021**, *57*, 43. [CrossRef]
23. Brenna, E.; Araja, D.; Pheby, D.F.H. Comparative Survey of People with ME/CFS in Italy, Latvia, and the UK: A Report on Behalf of the Socioeconomics Working Group of the European ME/CFS Research Network (EUROMENE). *Medicina* **2021**, *57*, 300. [CrossRef]
24. Waite, F.; Elliot, D.L. Feeling like 'a damaged battery': Exploring the lived experiences of UK university students with ME/CFS. *Fatigue Biomed. Health Behav.* **2021**, *9*, 159–174. [CrossRef]
25. Dafoe, W. Extremely Severe ME/CFS—A Personal Account. *Healthcare* **2021**, *9*, 504. [CrossRef]
26. Froehlich, L.; Hattesohl, D.B.R.; Jason, L.A.; Scheibenbogen, C.; Behrends, U.; Thoma, M. Medical Care Situation of People with Myalgic Encephalomyelitis/Chronic Fatigue Syndrome in Germany. *Medicina* **2021**, *57*, 646. [CrossRef] [PubMed]
27. Krumina, A.; Vecvagare, K.; Svirskis, S.; Gravelsina, S.; Nora-KruklE, Z.; Gintere, S.; Murovska, M. Clinical profile and aspects of differential diagnosis in patients with ME/CFS from Latvia. *Medicina* **2021**, *57*, 958. [CrossRef]
28. National Institute for Health and Care Excellence (NICE). Chronic Fatigue Syndrome/Myalgic Encephalomyelitis (or Encephalopathy): Diagnosis and Management. London, NICE, 2007. Para. 1.6.2.4. Available online: https://www.nice.org.uk/Guidance/CG53 (accessed on 6 September 2021).
29. National Institute for Health and Care Excellence. Guideline: Myalgic Encephalomyelitis (or Encephalopathy)/Chronic Fatigue Syndrome: Diagnosis and Management. Draft for Consultation, November 2020, Para. 1.11.16. Available online: https://www.nice.org.uk (accessed on 14 November 2020).
30. Grover, N. Withdrawal of Planned Guidance on ME Upsets Patients. *Guardian*, 30 August 2021. Available online: https://www.theguardian.com/society/2021/aug/30/withdrawal-planned-guidance-me-leaves-patients-distraught (accessed on 6 September 2021).
31. Tuller, D.; Ablashi, D.V.; Adler, J.R.; Akam, N.; Allen, M.; Amitay, O.; Armstrong, A.; Atherton, P.; Barcellos, L.F.; Barham, A.; et al. Trial by Error: A Letter Urging NICE to publish ME/CFS Guideline Without Delay. 1 September 2021. Available online: https://www.virology.ws/2021/09/01/trial-by-error-a-letter-urging-nice-to-publish-me-cfs-guideline-without-delay/ (accessed on 6 September 2021).
32. Nacul, L.; Authier, F.J.; Scheibenbogen, C.; Lorusso, L.; Helland, I.B.; Martin, J.A.; Sirbu, C.A.; Mengshoel, A.M.; Polo, O.; Behrends, U.; et al. European Network on Myalgic Encephalomyelitis/ Chronic Fatigue Syndrome (EUROMENE): Expert Consensus on the Diagnosis, Service Provision, and Care of People with ME/CFS in Europe. *Medicina* **2021**, *57*, 510. [CrossRef] [PubMed]
33. Carruthers, B.; Jain, A.K.; de Meirleir, K.L.; Peterson, D.L.; Klimas, N.G.; Lerner, A.M.; Bested, A.C.; Flor-Henry, P.; Joshi, P.; Powles, A.P.; et al. Myalgic encephalomyelitis/chronic fatigue syndrome: Clinical working case definition, diagnostic and treatment protocols. *J. Chronic Fatigue Syndr.* **2003**, *11*, 7–115. [CrossRef]
34. Fukuda, K.; Straus, S.E.; Hickie, I.; Sharpe, M.C.; Dobbins, J.G.; Komaroff, A. The chronic fatigue syndrome: A comprehensive approach to its definition and study. International Chronic Fatigue Syndrome Study Group. *Ann. Intern. Med.* **1994**, *121*, 953–959. [CrossRef]
35. Lucinda Bateman, L.; Bested, A.C.; Bonilla, H.F.; Chheda, B.V.; Chu, L.; Curtin, J.M.; Dempsey, T.T.; Dimmock, M.E.; Dowell, T.G.; Felsenstein, D.; et al. Myalgic Encephalomyelitis/Chronic Fatigue Syndrome: Essentials of diagnosis and management. *Mayo Clin. Proc.* **2021**, 1–18, in press. [CrossRef]
36. Royal Australasian College of Physicians. Chronic fatigue Syndrome: Clinical practice guidelines 2002 Sydney, RACP, 2002. *MJA* **2002**, *176*, S17–S58.
37. Myalgic Encephalomyelitis. Chronic Fatigue Syndrome Advisory Committee. Report to the NHMRC Chief Executive Officer (April 2019), Para. 3.2.1. Available online: https://www.nhmrc.gov.au/about-us/publications/mecfs-advisory-committee-report-nhmrc-chief-executive-officer (accessed on 13 September 2021).
38. Myalgic Encephalomyelitis. Chronic Fatigue Syndrome Advisory Committee. Report to the NHMRC Chief Executive Officer (April 2019), Para. 4.5.3. Available online: https://www.nhmrc.gov.au/about-us/publications/mecfs-advisory-committee-report-nhmrc-chief-executive-officer (accessed on 13 September 2021).
39. Cochrane, M.; Mitchell, E.; Hollingworth, W.; Crawley, E.; Trépel, D. Cost-effectiveness of Interventions for Chronic Fatigue Syndrome or Myalgic Encephalomyelitis: A Systematic Review of Economic Evaluations. *Appl. Health Econ. Health Policy* **2021**, *19*, 473–486. [CrossRef]
40. Pheby, D.F.H.; Araja, D.; Berkis, U.; Brenna, E.; Cullinan, J.; de Korwin, J.-D.; Gitto, L.; Hughes, D.A.; Hunter, R.M.; Trepel, D.; et al. The Development of a Consistent Europe-Wide Approach to Investigating the Economic Impact of Myalgic Encephalomyelitis (ME/CFS): A Report from the European Network on ME/CFS (EUROMENE). *Healthcare* **2020**, *8*, 88. [CrossRef]

41. Araja, D.; Berkis, U.; Lunga, A.; Murovska, M. Shadow Burden of Undiagnosed Myalgic Encephalomyelitis/Chronic Fatigue Syndrome (ME/CFS) on Society: Retrospective and Prospective—In Light of COVID-19. *J. Clin. Med.* **2021**, *10*, 3017. [CrossRef] [PubMed]
42. Ardestani, S.K.; Karkhaneh, M.; Stein, E.; Punja, S.; Junqueira, D.R.; Kuzmyn, T.; Pearson, M.; Smith, L.; Olson, K.; Vohra, S. Systematic Review of Mind-Body Interventions to Treat Myalgic Encephalomyelitis/ Chronic Fatigue Syndrome. *Medicina* **2021**, *57*, 652. [CrossRef] [PubMed]
43. Pheby, D.F.H.; Araja, D.; Berkis, U.; Brenna, E.; Cullinan, J.; de Korwin, J.-D.; Gitto, L.; Hughes, D.A.; Hunter, R.M.; Trepel, D.; et al. The Role of Prevention in Reducing the Economic Impact of ME/CFS in Europe: A Report from the Socioeconomics Working Group of the European Network on ME/CFS (EUROMENE). *Medicina* **2021**, *57*, 388. [CrossRef] [PubMed]

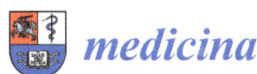

Article

Myalgic Encephalomyelitis/Chronic Fatigue Syndrome: Organic Disease or Psychosomatic Illness? A Re-Examination of the Royal Free Epidemic of 1955

Rosemary Underhill [1],* and Rosemarie Baillod [2]

1   Independent Researcher, 7 Avenue De La Mer #506, Palm Coast, FL 32137, USA
2   Independent Researcher, 2, Wold Rd. Hull, Yorkshire HU5 5UN, UK; rabaillod@aol.com
*   Correspondence: petro8888@aol.com

Abstract: *Background and Objectives:* Controversy exists over whether myalgic encephalomyelitis/chronic fatigue syndrome (ME/CFS) is an organic disease or a psychosomatic illness. ME/CFS usually occurs as sporadic cases, but epidemics (outbreaks) have occurred worldwide. Myalgic encephalomyelitis was named to describe an outbreak affecting the lymphatic, muscular, and nervous systems that closed the Royal Free hospital for three months in 1955. Fifteen years later, two psychiatrists concluded that epidemic hysteria was the likely cause. ME/CFS research studies show multiple pathophysiological differences between patients and controls and a possible etiological role for infectious organisms, but the belief that ME/CFS is psychosomatic is widespread and has been specifically supported by the epidemic hysteria hypothesis for the Royal Free outbreak. Our objective was to obtain accounts from ex-Royal Free hospital staff who personally experienced the 1955 outbreak and evaluate evidence for it being an infectious illness versus epidemic hysteria. *Materials and Methods:* Statements in the newsletters of two organizations for staff who had worked at the Royal Free hospital invited anyone who had experienced the 1955 Royal Free outbreak to contact the authors. Accounts of the outbreak from telephone interviews and letters were evaluated against the "epidemic hysteria hypothesis" paper and original medical staff reports. *Results:* Twenty-seven ex-Royal Free hospital staff, including six who had developed ME, provided descriptions typical of an infectious illness affecting the lymphatic, muscular, and nervous systems, and were not consistent with epidemic hysteria. *Conclusions:* The 1955 Royal Free hospital epidemic of myalgic encephalomyelitis was an organic infectious disease, not psychogenic epidemic hysteria.

Keywords: Chronic fatigue syndrome; epidemic hysteria; mass hysteria; myalgic encephalomyelitis; psychosomatic illness; Royal Free epidemic

Citation: Underhill, R.; Baillod, R. Myalgic Encephalomyelitis/Chronic Fatigue Syndrome: Organic Disease or Psychosomatic Illness? A Re-Examination of the Royal Free Epidemic of 1955. *Medicina* **2020**, *57*, 12. https://dx.doi.org/10.3390/medicina57010012

Received: 20 November 2020
Accepted: 22 December 2020
Published: 26 December 2020

Publisher's Note: MDPI stays neutral with regard to jurisdictional claims in published maps and institutional affiliations.

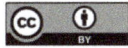

Copyright: © 2020 by the authors. Licensee MDPI, Basel, Switzerland. This article is an open access article distributed under the terms and conditions of the Creative Commons Attribution (CC BY) license (https://creativecommons.org/licenses/by/4.0/).

1. Introduction

Controversy exists over whether myalgic encephalomyelitis (ME), also known as chronic fatigue syndrome (CFS) and as ME/CFS, is an organic disease, a psychosomatic illness, or even exists as a disease entity. ME/CFS usually occurs as sporadic cases, but epidemics (outbreaks) have occurred worldwide [1,2]. In the summer of 1955, an illness, that had not been described in existing medical textbooks, affected more than 300 members of the medical, nursing, and ancillary staff at the Royal Free Group of hospitals in London [2–4]. The hospital medical staff reported that "this was an outbreak of an obscure, highly infectious illness with evidence of involvement of lymphoreticular structures and the central and peripheral nervous systems" and called it an encephalomyelitis [3,4]. The outbreak lasted from July to November and resulted in the main hospital being closed for three months. In spite of intensive investigation, no causal pathogen was identified [2–4]. No evidence was found that contaminated water, milk, or food was the source of infection and no toxins were found [3,4]. The illness was initially named Royal Free disease but the following year the name benign myalgic encephalomyelitis was coined to describe this and several other similar outbreaks [5]. The name chronic fatigue syndrome (CFS) was introduced in 1988 to describe a comparable disease, in Nevada, USA [6].

Fifteen years after the Royal Free outbreak, two psychiatrists (McEvedy CP, and Beard AW) published a hypothesis stating: "From a re-analysis of the case notes of patients with Royal Free disease, it is concluded that there is little evidence of an organic disease affecting the central nervous system and that epidemic hysteria is a much more likely explanation. The data which support this hypothesis are the high attack rate in females compared with males; the intensity of the malaise compared with the slight pyrexia; the presence of subjective features similar to those seen in a previous epidemic of hysterical over-breathing; the glove-and-stocking distribution of the anesthesia; and the normal findings in special investigations. Finally, a deliberate attempt by one of the authors to produce an electromyographic record similar to that reported in Royal Free disease was successful" [7]. They based their hypothesis on a study of 198 case notes selected from 255 hospitalized patients [3,7]. McEvedy and Beard also reviewed 14 other outbreaks identified as ME and proposed that they were psychosocial phenomena caused by mass hysteria on the part of the patients or altered medical perception of the community [8]. The concept of hysteria as the cause of the Royal Free outbreak was strongly opposed by the Royal Free medical staff on the grounds that there were characteristic physical signs, the disease was endemic in North London at the time of the outbreak, the disease course was prolonged, and epidemics had occurred worldwide [9,10].

The publication of the McEvedy and Beard papers ignited controversy over whether ME was an organic disease or a psychosomatic illness [2]. The following factors have been employed to support a psychosomatic hypothesis. The etiology is uncertain. There is no biomarker. Diagnostic criteria are based on clinical symptoms and the exclusion of other fatiguing illnesses. There are no pathognomonic physical signs. Patients frequently do not look ill even when severely affected by the disease. There is no curative medication. The concept that ME/CFS is a psychosomatic illness is widespread [11–13] and has resulted in the stigmatization of patients and patient complaints of sensing hostility from their health care providers [14,15].

Research studies in patients with ME/CFS have shown multiple pathophysiological differences between patients and healthy controls in the immune system, the nervous system, and metabolic processes including energy metabolism [16–18]. Although no causal pathogen has been identified, studies have shown that patients harbor a variety of infectious agents and have pointed towards a possible aetiological role for infectious organisms [19,20]. The psychosomatic hypothesis does not explain these pathophysiological changes. Mathematical modeling of the Royal Free outbreak also validates an infectious disease aetiology and refutes the epidemic hysteria hypothesis [21].

The question of hysteria or psychoneurosis as a possible cause was raised in the Royal Free outbreak [2,3], the 1934 Los Angeles county general hospital outbreak [22], and in three other outbreaks classified as ME [23]. Manifestations of psychoneurosis were seen in a few cases in all these outbreaks, but the authors concluded that hysteria did not explain the observed clinical features. Psychogenic anxiety reactions, evidenced by non-specific symptoms have been described in people exposed to outbreaks of organic disease, or people present during a disaster [24–26] and have been labeled "reactive psychological disaster syndrome" [26]. Reactive psychological disaster syndrome might account for some patients showing hysterical manifestations in various outbreaks of ME.

Our objective was to obtain first-hand observational accounts of the 1955 outbreak of ME from ex-Royal Free hospital staff and patients who had experienced it and to review evidence for the underlying cause being an organic infectious illness versus psychogenic epidemic hysteria. No other follow-up studies have been published.

Etymology: ME/CFS has been labeled psychosomatic, psychosocial, somatoform, and a biopsychosocial illness. This paper uses the term psychosomatic.

2. Materials and Methods

Statements were placed in the 'Royal Free Association' newsletter and the 'Royal Free Nurses League' magazine. These organizations were established for doctors and nurses respectively who trained or worked at the Royal Free Group of hospitals. The statements invited anyone who had experienced the Royal Free disease outbreak of 1955 to contact the authors to provide information about their experiences. We asked for information from both those who became ill and those who remained healthy. Volunteers contacted us by email and letters. Those who supplied a telephone number were interviewed using a semi-structured interview. Telephone participants were asked for their age and occupation at the time of the outbreak and were asked what they remembered about the event. Participants were included in the study if they had personally experienced the outbreak. The authors of this study were medical students at the Royal Free medical school and as such, were not permitted to enter the hospital at the time of the outbreak. Therefore, we did not meet the inclusion criteria for the study group. To avoid individual identification, descriptions of the outbreak in this paper are a compilation of individual accounts. Evidence for the outbreak being an infectious encephalomyelitis versus epidemic hysteria was evaluated by comparing the study group's accounts and the original published medical staff reports [3,4] with data given for the epidemic hysteria hypothesis [7].

3. Results

3.1. Study Group

This study took place 58 years after the outbreak. Thirty people contacted the authors. Of these, 27 had personally experienced the outbreak and met inclusion criteria for the study group. Two responders provided information about friends who had developed Royal Free disease, and one told us about developing ME subsequent to the outbreak. Nineteen participants who provided a phone number were interviewed by phone. Participants' data are given in Table 1.

Table 1. Study Group Participants.

Participants	Number
Age: 75–85 years	27
Gender	26 females, 1 male
Occupation in 1955	9 doctors, 5 nurses, 12 medical students, 1 physiotherapist
Royal Free disease diagnosis	19 remained healthy, 6 were diagnosed with Royal Free disease, 2 had mild symptoms possibly, abortive Royal Free disease

3.2. Descriptions of the Outbreak

The study group confirmed that the outbreak started in July of 1955 and lasted several months. Importantly, staff in all five hospitals of the Royal Free Group were affected. People from the local community outside the hospital with symptoms of the disease were also seen in the casualty (Accident and Emergency) departments of the Royal Free and other London hospitals. The main Royal Free hospital in Gray's Inn Road was closed to new admissions for three months due to a lack of healthy staff. Affected hospital staff were isolated at the Liverpool Road branch of the hospital, or were sent home. The epidemic was covered widely in national newspapers. The disease affected men and women, and both young and older, junior and senior staff. Very few existing hospital inpatients were affected. Most of those affected were nurses. Two study participants described secondary cases following close contact with a patient. The incubation period was "4–5 days" in one and "a few days" in the other. No secondary cases were reported following immediate visual exposure to a patient.

3.3. Descriptions of the Illness

Six study group participants developed the disease. Their experiences are compiled in Table 2.

Table 2. Patients who developed Royal Free disease.

Features of the Disease	Patient Experiences
Initial prodromal symptoms	Severe pressure headache, malaise, exhaustion, feeling weak, feeling hot, dizziness, feeling drowsy, hypersomnia, and sore throat
Initial physical signs	Fever, pharyngitis, enlarged cervical glands
New symptoms and signs manifested a few days after onset	Severe weakness in one or both legs causing difficulty in walking, painful muscular twitching or spasms, hemiparesis, difficulty focusing eyes
Testing	Blood testing not done routinely. EMG done on one patient *
Severity	Mild or moderate
Hospitalization	Two to five weeks
Treatment/management	Complete bed rest while symptoms lasted, (except for walking to the toilet). Convalescence for the same length of time as illness duration
Length of illness	Two to three weeks to two to three months
Recovery and return to work	Return to work in one to six months. Recovery was often incomplete because easily tired. Some returned to work part-time
Relapse	Relapse after two months back at work
Long term effects	Unusual fatigue persisting for 2–3 years. A return of muscular twitching when under stress in later life. A muscle paralysis

* The electromyogram (EMG) showed changes that were associated with Royal Free disease.

The study group described a biphasic illness. Initially, there were prodromal symptoms and signs (see Table 2). Tender enlarged posterior cervical glands were a defining diagnostic feature. Initial symptoms persisted into the second phase of the illness. A few days after illness onset, diverse muscular and neurological manifestations developed in many patients. Muscular pain and tenderness occurred in the neck, back, and/or limbs. Reported neurological manifestations included ptosis, difficulty with focusing eyes, hemiparesis, mono-paresis, weakness of hand muscles, foot drop, various sensory losses, and hyperesthesia. Other reported symptoms included difficulty urinating, anorexia, nausea, and vomiting. Hyperventilation was not reported. Patients often delayed seeking medical care until several days after illness onset. Symptom severity ranged from mild to very severe. Myalgia was sometimes extreme, causing patients to cry with pain. A putative diagnosis of abortive Royal Free disease was proposed for patients with mild symptoms who lacked physical signs. The study group also reported that there were some patients lacking physical signs, who were thought to be neurotic or to have exaggerated their symptoms.

Many patients were diagnosed clinically without blood testing, but in patients who were tested, leukopenia, or lymphocytes typical of viral diseases were found. Leucocytes, characteristic of glandular fever (infectious mononucleosis) were not found. Paul Bunnell tests were negative except in a patient diagnosed with glandular fever. Cerebro-spinal fluid testing did not show changes typical of poliomyelitis. Electromyograms (EMGs) (carried out in some patients) showed unspecified findings regarded as characteristic of the disease. Possible causal pathogens were sought but none identified.

Treatment was symptomatic. Severe muscle pain sometimes required the strongest analgesics. Complete bed rest while symptoms lasted (except for walking to the toilet) was insisted on, followed by slow mobilization. Convalescence was advised for the same period of time as the duration of symptoms because an early return to work could precipitate a relapse. Patients were hospitalized for two weeks and upwards. A few very severely ill patients, some with paralyzses, were hospitalized for over six months and were widely investigated for many bizarre symptoms.

The time for recovery varied from a few days in those with the possible abortive disease to several weeks or months in others. Prolonged time to recovery also occurred in patients isolated at home. Some affected staff were only able to return to work part-time, and in several individuals, an unusual fatigue persisted for up to two to three years. Some patients appeared to recover but later relapsed. One patient committed suicide. Patients with persisting paralysis were transferred to a rehabilitation unit. A number of patients remained disabled and were unable to return to their previous occupations. We received a report of one patient in whom ME/CFS symptoms persisted long term.

Initially, a glandular fever (infectious mononucleosis)-like illness was diagnosed, but this was rejected because diverse neurological signs occurred and Paul Bunnell tests were negative. A poliomyelitis diagnosis was also rejected because muscle weakness clearly differed from the paralysis seen in poliomyelitis and lumbar puncture testing was inconclusive. The question of hysteria was raised as some patients were thought to be neurotic. However, since a large number of patients were seriously ill with significant physical signs, the study group indicated that most hospital staff believed that the outbreak was an infectious illness.

3.4. Long Term Health Effects Attributed to the Illness

We were told of five people who developed a persisting paralysis. They included one person each with ptosis, weakness of one hand, foot drop, wasting of hypothenar muscles of both hands, and severe weakness of one leg that required arthrodesis of the knee and ankle.

4. Discussion

Based on the recollections of all the 27 ex-Royal Free hospital staff and medical students who provided data for this study, hysteria as the underlying cause of the Royal Free outbreak seems inconceivable. Our study group's accounts are based on their first-hand personal experiences. McEvedy and Beard based their epidemic hysteria hypothesis on an analysis of some selected patient case notes [7]. They did not provide any evidence from the follow-ups of patients who had had the disease or from hospital staff. Epidemic hysteria is a diagnosis of exclusion, but McEvedy and Beard provided no data to exclude an infectious disease as a cause of the outbreak.

4.1. Evidence for Infectious Illness

Although no causal pathogen was found in the Royal Free outbreak, epidemiological and clinical features were consistent with an outbreak of an infectious illness. The disease was present in the wider community of north London as well as in all five hospitals of the Royal Free group. It affected male and female, young and older staff. Case to case infection clearly showed an incubation period of several days and no immediate visual transmission. Initially, prodromal constitutional symptoms and upper respiratory signs of low-grade fever, pharyngitis, and cervical lymphadenopathy were present. After a few days, diverse muscular and neurological symptoms and signs appeared in many patients. Lymphocytes typical of viral infection were seen in some patients. The duration of the illness ranged from a few days to many months. Its severity ranged from patients with the possible abortive disease to patients with severe disease. The authors of this paper consider that the closure of a large teaching hospital in London for three months might be necessary to control an outbreak of a persisting, highly infectious disease, that affected a large number of hospital staff and that might be transmitted to hospital patients. On the other hand, an outbreak of epidemic hysteria would not be a sufficient cause to close a hospital.

4.2. Arguments for Epidemic Hysteria

McEvedy and Beard asserted that there was little evidence of organic disease affecting the central nervous system [7]. Our study group contradicted this assertion and reported diverse neurological manifestations in many patients and permanent paralysis in a few. The original hospital medical staff report describes 148 patients with involvement of cranial nerves and/or motor or sensory defects in the limbs and trunk [3]. The undoubted neurological manifestations in this outbreak are not found in epidemic hysteria.

Our study group confirmed that the majority of those affected were female nurses. In McEvedy and Beard's cases selected for study, they found an attack rate of 0.8% in males and 11% in females and said this supported their epidemic hysteria hypothesis [7]. However, the original Royal Free hospital staff reports showed that females comprised 70% of the population at risk, and the attack rate was 10.4% for females and 2.8% for males [4]. These attack rates are comparable to those found in other outbreaks of ME, which ranged from 1.6% to 4% in males and 6.4% to 8.4% in females [23]. A high attack rate in females compared with males does not distinguish epidemic hysteria from ME.

McEvedy and Beard stated that the intensity of the malaise compared with the slight pyrexia supported their epidemic hysteria hypothesis [7]. Our study group confirmed malaise and mild pyrexia. Severe malaise that worsens with exertion is a cardinal feature of ME, but malaise and pyrexia are not features of mass hysteria [27,28]. Pyrexia is characteristic of infectious disease.

McEvedy and Beard noted the presence of subjective features similar to those seen in a previous epidemic (described by McEvedy [29]), of hysterical over-breathing in schoolgirls as evidence of epidemic hysteria. In this previous epidemic, many reported symptoms resembled the constitutional prodromal symptoms exhibited in the Royal Free outbreak. However, notably, hyperventilation was reported in 40% of the schoolgirls and tetany occurred in one-third of them [29]. Hyperventilation has been reported in 19%–32% of cases in outbreaks of mass hysteria [27,28]. McEvedy and Beard noted a raised respiratory rate only in four severely ill, Royal Free patients and speculated "this was a frightened and hysterical population whose over-breathing was intermittent and covert" [7]. Hyperventilation cannot be covert. Overt hyperventilation was not reported by our study group, nor reported in the original medical staff reports [3,4]. The notable absence of hyperventilation does not support the argument that the Royal Free outbreak resembled this outbreak of hysterical over-breathing in schoolgirls.

McEvedy and Beard noted "the glove-and-stocking distribution of the anesthesia" as evidence of epidemic hysteria and commented "It seems fair to say that the characteristic pattern of sensory loss is a classically hysterical one" [7]. They found a glove-and-stocking type of anesthesia recorded in the charts of 13 patients, 11 of whom were also severely ill [7]. Our study group did not report details of sensory losses, but the original medical staff reports stated that "objective sensory loss was usually maximal peripherally, and frequently coincided with motor weakness" [3]. Glove-and-stocking anesthesia may occur in patients with a hysterical conversion disorder, but it can also be due to peripheral neuropathy in many serious organic diseases. This type of conversion disorder has not been reported in any published outbreaks of mass hysteria [27,28] and its presence in patients who are also seriously ill is questionable. A glove-and-stocking type of anesthesia in a few seriously ill patients does not support a diagnosis of epidemic hysteria.

Our study group said that EMG recordings of muscles affected by Royal Free disease showed characteristic features. To support their epidemic hysteria hypothesis, McEvedy and Beard stated that "a deliberate attempt by one of the authors to produce an electromyographic record similar to that reported in Royal Free disease was successful" [7], with the implication that abnormal EMG tracings of patients with Royal Free disease might have been fabricated. They published an EMG tracing of the extensor digitorum of the arm from a healthy person while encouraging the outstretched arm to tremble and suggested a similarity between this tracing and the EMG tracing of a weak tibialis anterior muscle affected by Royal Free disease during maximal sustained volition, that had been published by the Royal Free medical staff [4,7]. They proposed that the EMGs in the Royal Free patients could have been produced by "maximum effort" [7]. Whether an EMG of a healthy arm muscle, while encouraging the arm to tremble should be equated with an EMG of a weak leg muscle under maximal sustained volition from a patient suffering from Royal Free disease is questionable, but this attempt to imply that the experienced Royal Free medical staff might have misinterpreted EMG data or that one Royal Free patient might have fabricated an abnormal EMG does not provide evidence that the Royal Free outbreak was epidemic hysteria.

Distinguishing epidemic hysteria from an organic illness can be difficult, but characteristic features can help with diagnosis. In epidemic hysteria outbreaks, person-to-person i.e., visual transmission usually occurs within minutes [27,28]. Contrary to this, our study group reported an incubation period of several days. In epidemic hysteria, symptoms usually quickly resolve in patients separated from other patients and from the environment where the outbreak began [27,28]. In the Royal Free outbreak, patients sent home did not recover quickly. The incubation period and the failure of symptoms to resolve in isolated patients is not consistent with epidemic hysteria.

4.3. Reactive Psychogenic Symptoms

Diagnostic difficulties occurred in a minority of patients who were thought to be neurotic or to have exaggerated their symptoms. We suggest that at least some patients might have developed "reactive psychological disaster syndrome" [26] as a result of knowing that they had been exposed to a serious, debilitating, infectious disease of an unknown cause. A minority of patients with possible reactive psychogenic symptoms does not invalidate an organic cause for the outbreak.

4.4. SARS CoV 2

Recent reports show that some patients infected with SARS CoV 2 have developed post-viral symptoms characteristic of ME/CFS [30]. Given the growing recognition of similarities between ME/CFS and post-viral SARS CoV 2 [30], we hope that these patients are not regarded as having a psychosomatic illness. We also hope that future studies investigating features of both diseases may lead to new treatments that could potentially be of benefit for both groups of chronically ill patients.

4.5. Strengths and Limitations

The study group all experienced the Royal Free outbreak of ME as hospital staff, medical students, and some as patients. The outbreak was dramatic and the participants provided clear first-hand eye-witness accounts. The authors of this study were medical students at the Royal Free medical school at the time of the outbreak. Our recollections are consistent with the findings of this study. The study participants were self-selected members of two organizations for staff who worked or trained at the Royal Free hospital and may not be representative of the hospital staff at the time of the outbreak. This study took place 58 years after the outbreak and the participants' recollected accounts are subject to recall bias, are dimmed by the passage of time, and lack specific details of clinical findings.

5. Conclusions

This study obtained new eye-witness accounts of the 1955 Royal Free outbreak of ME from ex-Royal Free hospital staff, medical students, and patients who had developed the disease. Clinical and epidemiological features described by them, are consistent with an outbreak of an infectious illness affecting the lymphatic, muscular, and nervous systems, with long-term neurological defects in a few cases. Their accounts did not describe the expected features of epidemic hysteria. McEvedy and Beard's hypothesis that epidemic hysteria was the cause of this outbreak was based solely on the examination of selected patient case notes. We show that data given by McEvedy and Beard to support their epidemic hysteria hypothesis are flawed. Specifically, some data was contradicted by the study group's first-hand accounts of the outbreak. Some data did not distinguish between epidemic hysteria and ME. Some data preferentially supported an organic etiology, and some data was of doubtful validity. This study confirms that ME/CFS is an organic disease and repudiates the hypothesis of it being a psychosomatic illness.

Author Contributions: Conceptualization, R.U. and R.B.; Data curation, R.U.; Formal analysis, R.U.; Investigation, R.U. and R.B.; Methodology, R.U. and R.B.; Project administration, R.B.; Writing— Original draft, R.U.; Writing—Review & editing, R.B. All authors have read and agreed to the published version of the manuscript.

Funding: This research did not receive any specific grant from funding agencies in the public, commercial, or not-for-profit sectors.

Institutional Review Board Statement: Not applicable as no experiments were done on humans or animals.

Informed Consent Statement: Not Applicable as all participants volunteered to provide recalled information on the outbreak

Data Availability Statement: Enough data is given in the paper to show exactly how the was done. There is no further data.

Acknowledgments: The authors thank the ex-staff of the Royal Free Hospital who experienced the 1955 outbreak of ME and who participated in this survey. The authors also thank Alan Gurwitt, MD, Yale Child Study Center and University of Connecticut School of Medicine, Harvard Medical School (retired) for reviewing psychiatric data in this paper.

Conflicts of Interest: The authors declare no conflict of interest.

References

1. Parish, G.; Hyde, B.M. A Bibliography of ME/CFS Epidemics. In *The Clinical and Scientific Basis of Myalgic Encephalomyelitis Chronic Fatigue Syndrome*; Hyde, B.M., Goldstein, J., Levine, P., Eds.; The Nightingale Research Foundation: Ottawa, ON, Canada, 1992; pp. 176–186.
2. Ramsey, A.M. Myalgic encephalomyelitis and postviral fatigue states. In *The Saga of Royal Free Disease*, 2nd ed.; Gower Medical Publishing: London, UK, 1988.
3. The Medical Staff of the Royal Free Hospital. An outbreak of encephalomyelitis in the Royal Free Hospital Group, London, in 1955. *Br. Med. J.* **1957**, *2*, 895–904. [CrossRef]
4. Crowley, N.; Nelson, M.; Stovin, S. Epidemiological aspects of an outbreak of encephalomyelitis at the Royal Free Hospital, London, in the summer of 1955. *J. Hyg. (Lond.)* **1957**, *55*, 102–122. [CrossRef] [PubMed]
5. Sigurdsson, B. A new clinical entity? Editorial. *Lancet* **1956**, *270*, 789–790.
6. Holmes, G.P.; Kaplan, J.E.; Gantz, N.M.; Komaroff, A.L.; Schonberger, L.B.; Straus, S.E.; Jones, J.F.; Dubois, R.E.; Cunningham-Rundles, C.; Pahwa, S.; et al. Chronic fatigue syndrome: A working case definition. *Ann. Intern. Med.* **1988**, *108*, 387–389. [CrossRef]
7. McEvedy, C.P.; Beard, A.W. Royal Free epidemic of 1955: A reconsideration. *Br. Med. J.* **1970**, *1*, 7–11. [CrossRef]
8. McEvedy, C.P.; Beard, A.W. Concept of Benign Myalgic Encephalomyelitis. *Br. Med. J.* **1970**, *1*, 11. [CrossRef]
9. Ramsey, A.M. Hysteria and "Royal Free Disease". *Br. Med. J.* **1965**, *2*, 1062. [CrossRef]
10. Compston, N.D.; Dimsdale, H.E.; Ramsay, A.M.; Richardson, A.T. Epidemic Malaise. *Br. Med. J.* **1970**, *1*, 362–363. [CrossRef]
11. Wojcik, W.; Armstrong, D.; Kanaan, R. Is chronic fatigue syndrome a neurological condition? A survey of UK neurologists. *J. Psychosom. Res.* **2011**, *70*, 573–574. [CrossRef]
12. Van Houdenhove, B.; Kempke, S.; Luyten, P. Psychiatric aspects of chronic fatigue syndrome and fibromyalgia. *Curr. Psychiatry Rep.* **2010**, *12*, 208–214. [CrossRef]
13. Wessely, S. Old wine in new bottles: Neurasthenia and 'ME'. *Psychol. Med.* **1990**, *20*, 35–53. [CrossRef] [PubMed]
14. Geraghty, K.J.; Esmail, A. Chronic fatigue syndrome: Is the biopsychosocial model responsible for patient dissatisfaction and harm? *Br. J. Gen. Pract.* **2016**, *66*, 437–438. [CrossRef] [PubMed]
15. Dickson, A.; Knussen, C.; Flowers, P. Stigma and the delegitimation experience: An interpretative phenomenological analysis of people living with chronic fatigue syndrome. *Psychol. Health* **2007**, *22*, 851–867. [CrossRef]
16. Committee on the Diagnostic Criteria for Myalgic Encephalomyelitis/Chronic Fatigue Syndrome; Board on the Health of Select Populations; Institute of Medicine. *Beyond Myalgic Encephalomyelitis/Chronic Fatigue Syndrome: Redefining an Illness*; National Academies Press (US): Washington, DC, USA, 2015.

17. Nagy-Szakal, D.; Barupal, D.K.; Lee, B.; Che, X.; Williams, B.L.; Kahn, E.J.R.; Ukaigwe, J.E.; Bateman, L.; Klimas, N.G.; Komaroff, A.L.; et al. Insights into myalgic encephalomyelitis/chronic fatigue syndrome phenotypes through comprehensive metabolomics. *Sci. Rep.* **2018**, *8*, 10056. [CrossRef]
18. Tomas, C.; Newton, J. Metabolic abnormalities in chronic fatigue syndrome/myalgic encephalomyelitis: A mini-review. *Biochem. Soc. Trans.* **2018**, *46*, 547–553. [CrossRef]
19. Rasa, S.; Nora-Krukle, Z.; Henning, N.; Eliassen, E.; Shikova, E.; Harrer, T.; Scheibenbogen, C.; Murovska, M.; Prusty, B.K. Chronic viral infections in myalgic encephalomyelitis/chronic fatigue syndrome (ME/CFS). *J. Transl. Med.* **2018**, *16*, 268. [CrossRef]
20. Underhill, R.A. Myalgic encephalomyelitis, chronic fatigue syndrome: An infectious disease. *Med. Hypotheses* **2015**, *85*, 765–773. [CrossRef]
21. Waters, F.G.; McDonald, G.J.; Banks, S.; Waters, R.A. Myalgic Encephalomyelitis (ME) outbreaks can be modelled as an infectious disease: A mathematical reconsideration of the Royal Free Epidemic of 1955. *Fatigue Biomed. Health Behav.* **2020**, *8*, 70–83. [CrossRef]
22. Gilliam, A.G. *Epidemiological Study of an Epidemic Diagnosed as Poliomyelitis Occurring Among the Personnel of the Los Angeles County General Hospital during the Summer of 1934*; Public Health Bulletin U.S. Treasury Dept. No. 240: Washington, DC, USA, 1938.
23. Acheson, E.D. The clinical syndrome variously called benign myalgic encephalomyelitis, Iceland disease and epidemic neuromyasthenia. *Am. J. Med.* **1959**, *26*, 569–595. [CrossRef]
24. Brooks, S.K.; Dunn, R.; Amlôt, R.; Greenberg, N.; Rubin, G.J. Social and occupational factors associated with psychological distress and disorder among disaster responders: A systematic review. *BMC Psychol.* **2016**, *4*, 18. [CrossRef]
25. Makwana, N. Disaster and its impact on mental health: A narrative review. *J. Fam. Med. Prim. Care* **2019**, *8*, 3090–3095. [CrossRef] [PubMed]
26. López-Ibor, J.J., Jr.; Soria, J.; Cañas, F.; Rodriguez-Gamazo, M. Psychopathological aspects of the toxic oil syndrome catastrophe. *Br. J. Psychiatry.* **1985**, *147*, 352–365. [CrossRef] [PubMed]
27. Jones, T.F. Mass psychogenic illness: Role of the individual physician. *Am. Fam. Physician* **2000**, *62*, 2649–2653. [PubMed]
28. Boss, L.P. Epidemic hysteria: A review of the published literature. *Epidemiol. Rev.* **1997**, *19*, 233–243. [CrossRef]
29. Moss, P.D.; McEvedy, C.P. An epidemic of over breathing among school girls. *Br. Med. J.* **1966**, *2*, 1295. [CrossRef]
30. Mardani, M. Post COVID Syndrome. *Arch. Clin. Infect. Dis.* **2020**, *15*, e108819. [CrossRef]

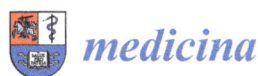

Review

A Literature Review of GP Knowledge and Understanding of ME/CFS: A Report from the Socioeconomic Working Group of the European Network on ME/CFS (EUROMENE)

Derek F. H. Pheby [1,*], Diana Araja [2], Uldis Berkis [3], Elenka Brenna [4], John Cullinan [5], Jean-Dominique de Korwin [6,7], Lara Gitto [8], Dyfrig A. Hughes [9], Rachael M. Hunter [10], Dominic Trepel [11,12] and Xia Wang-Steverding [13]

1. Society and Health, Buckinghamshire New University, High Wycombe HP11 2JZ, UK
2. Department of Dosage Form Technology, Faculty of Pharmacy, Riga Stradins University, Dzirciema Street 16, LV-1007 Riga, Latvia; diana.araja@rsu.lv
3. Institute of Microbiology and Virology, Riga Stradins University, Dzirciema Street 16, LV-1007 Riga, Latvia; Uldis.Berkis@rsu.lv
4. Department of Economics and Finance, Università Cattolica del Sacro Cuore, Largo Agostino Gemelli 1, 20123 Milan, Italy; elenka.brenna@unicatt.it
5. School of Business & Economics, National University of Ireland Galway, University Road, H91 TK33 Galway, Ireland; john.cullinan@nuigalway.ie
6. Internal Medicine Department, University of Lorraine, 34, cours Léopold, CS 25233, CEDEX F−54052 Nancy, France; jean-dominique.dekorwin@univ-lorraine.fr
7. University Hospital of Nancy, Rue du Morvan, 54511 Vandœuvre-Lès-Nancy, France
8. Department of Economics, University of Messina, Piazza Pugliatti 1, 98122 Messina, Italy; lara.gitto@unime.it
9. Centre for Health Economics & Medicines Evaluation, Bangor University, Bangor LL57 2PZ, UK; d.a.hughes@bangor.ac.uk
10. Institute of Epidemiology & Health, Royal Free Medical School, University College London, London NW3 2PF, UK; r.hunter@ucl.ac.uk
11. School of Medicine, Trinity College Dublin, College Green, D02 PN40 Dublin 2, Ireland; trepeld@tcd.ie
12. Global Brain Health Institute, School of Medicine, Trinity College Dublin, College Green, D02 PN40 Dublin 2, Ireland
13. Warwick Medical School, University of Warwick, Coventry CV4 7AL, UK; xiasteverding@gmail.com
* Correspondence: derekpheby@btinternet.com

Abstract: *Background and Objectives:* The socioeconomic working group of the European myalgic encephalomyelitis/chronic fatigue syndrome (ME/CFS) Research Network (EUROMENE) has conducted a review of the literature pertaining to GPs' knowledge and understanding of ME/CFS; *Materials and Methods:* A MEDLINE search was carried out. The papers identified were reviewed following the synthesis without meta-analysis (SWiM) methodology, and were classified according to the focus of the enquiry (patients, GPs, database and medical record studies, evaluation of a training programme, and overview papers), and whether they were quantitative or qualitative in nature; *Results:* Thirty-three papers were identified in the MEDLINE search. The quantitative surveys of GPs demonstrated that a third to a half of all GPs did not accept ME/CFS as a genuine clinical entity and, even when they did, they lacked confidence in diagnosing or managing it. It should be noted, though, that these papers were mostly from the United Kingdom. Patient surveys indicated that a similar proportion of patients was dissatisfied with the primary medical care they had received. These findings were consistent with the findings of the qualitative studies that were examined, and have changed little over several decades; *Conclusions:* Disbelief and lack of knowledge and understanding of ME/CFS among GPs is widespread, and the resultant diagnostic delays constitute a risk factor for severe and prolonged disease. Failure to diagnose ME/CFS renders problematic attempts to determine its prevalence, and hence its economic impact.

Keywords: ME/CFS; myalgic encephalomyelitis; chronic fatigue syndrome; primary care; GP knowledge and understanding

1. Introduction

Myalgic encephalomyelitis/chronic fatigue syndrome (ME/CFS) is a poorly understood, serious, complex, multi-system disorder, characterized by symptoms lasting at least six months, with severe incapacitating fatigue not alleviated by rest, and other symptoms, many autonomic or cognitive in nature, including cognitive dysfunction, sleep disturbances, muscle pain, and post-exertional malaise, which lead to marked reductions in functional activity and quality of life [1–3]. Symptomatology, severity and disease progression are all very variable. ME/CFS is most common between the ages of 20 to 50 years, but it can affect all age groups. Around three quarters of patients are female [4–6]. There are no Europe-wide prevalence data, but there is a commonly held belief that there are some 250,000 sufferers in the U.K. [7]. If this is correct, there may be some two million patients in Europe as a whole.

The European ME/CFS Research Network (EUROMENE) was established to promote collaborative research on the condition across Europe. It is currently in receipt of EU funding from the Collaboration on Science and Technology Association (COST, https://www.cost.eu) to support network activities. It seeks to review the current state of the art and to identify gaps in knowledge of ME/CFS. EUROMENE also aims to shed light on the overall burden of disease, and also to investigate possible biomarkers, diagnosis and treatment [8].

Previous work by the socioeconomic working group of EUROMENE identified widespread failure by GPs to diagnose ME/CFS as an important factor contributing to underestimation of the incidence and prevalence of the illness, and hence of its economic impact [9]. The group conducted a pilot survey among EUROMENE participants to assess the position regarding GP diagnoses of ME/CFS [10]. The survey findings suggested that under-diagnosis in primary care was a Europe-wide problem, and that estimates of the public health burden of the illness, even where these exist, are therefore likely to underestimate substantially its true prevalence.

A systematic review of qualitative studies published in 2013 and concerned with barriers to the diagnosis and management of CFS/ME in primary care identified 21 studies. This review demonstrated a limited understanding of ME/CFS by GPs [11]. We conducted a comprehensive literature review with the aim of assessing whether primary care doctors' awareness, understanding and acceptance of ME/CFS as a disease has changed in the intervening years.

2. Materials and Methods

A MEDLINE search was carried out, covering the period from 1946 until 20 August 2020. The inclusion criteria were focuses on general practice, family practice, primary care or primary health care, and myalgic encephalomyelitis or chronic fatigue syndrome (including ME/CFS, CFS/ME, and post-viral fatigue syndrome). Exclusions were papers not addressing GP attitudes, knowledge or understanding of ME/CFS or any of its synonyms.

The papers were sorted into categories following the synthesis without meta-analysis (SWiM) methodology. Categories were defined on the basis of the focus of the enquiry (patients, GPs, database and medical record studies, evaluation of a training programme, and overview papers), and whether the studies were quantitative or qualitative in nature. These are summarised in Table 1 below. One of the papers was the review referred to above [11].

Table 1. Search Strategy.

Step	Description	No. Records
1	General Practice or family practice	75,004
2	limit 1 to abstracts	35,740
3	Primary care, or primary health care	133,124
4	limit 3 to abstracts	104,892
5	2 or 4	129,775

Table 1. Cont.

Step	Description	No. Records
6	Myalgic encephalomyelitis, or fatigue syndrome, chronic	5606
7	limit 6 to abstracts	3936
8	5 and 7	176
9	After exclusions (because not conforming to inclusion criteria)	33
10	After exclusions (because of unavailability of full texts)	30

3. Results
3.1. Search Strategy
3.1.1. Implementation

The search strategy and its outcomes are summarised in Table 1 and Figure 1 below:

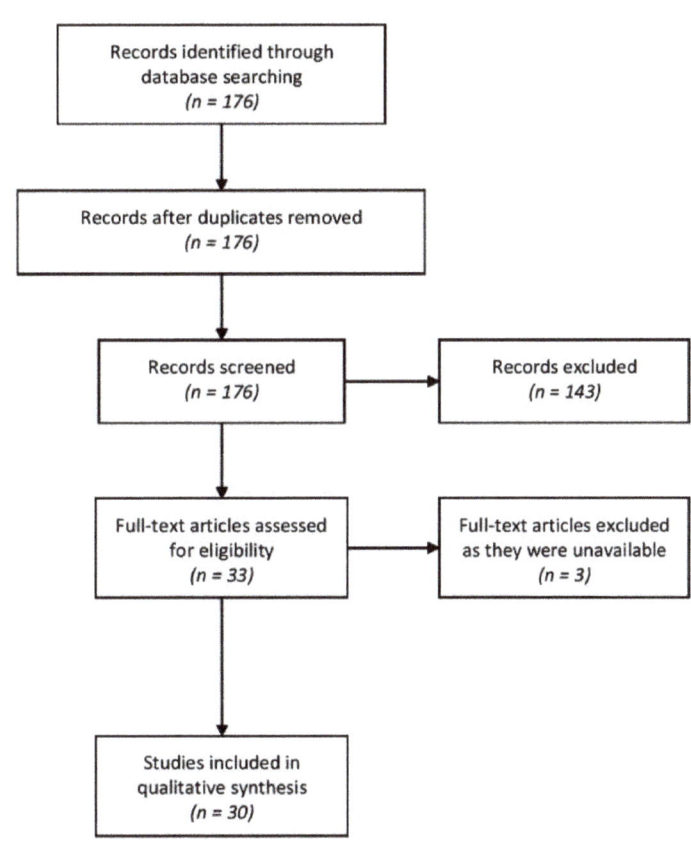

Figure 1. PRISMA Diagram.

At step 9, 143 papers were excluded, either because the focus was not primary care, or because they were not about ME/CFS, or because, although they did concern ME/CFS in primary care, they did not address knowledge or understanding of the condition. The papers identified were extremely heterogeneous with respect to the populations studied, research questions addressed, and methodologies followed, as to preclude any form of meta- synthesis or meta-analysis. Consequently, the synthesis without meta-analysis (SWiM) methodology, which was developed specifically to ensure an adequate standard of review in such circumstances, was utilised [12].

3.1.2. Papers Identified

The papers identified in the MEDLINE search were considered in detail within the categories identified in Table 2.

Table 2. Summary of papers identified.

Type of Study	No. Papers Identified *
Reviews	1
GP surveys—quantitative	7
Patient surveys—quantitative	7
Database studies—quantitative	2
Medical record review—quantitative	1
Evaluation of training programme—quantitative	1
GP studies—qualitative	6
Patient studies—qualitative	9
Overview papers on myalgic encephalomyelitis/chronic fatigue syndrome (ME/CFS)	4

* Note that the total is greater than the number identified in the MEDLINE search, because some qualitative papers are included in more than one category.

3.2. Quantitative Studies

3.2.1. Surveys of GPs

Seven papers were identified. Saidi and Haines (2006) distributed a postal questionnaire to GPs throughout the U.K., to assess the proportion of practices with children diagnosed with ME/CFS [13]. Of the 112 practices contacted, 62 (55%) had diagnosed children or adolescents with chronic fatigue.

For each of the other six studies, the outcome metric was the proportion of GP respondents to questionnaires who recognised ME/CFS as a genuine clinical entity, and these are summarised in Table 3. Three of these studied GPs were in different parts of the U.K., namely, South Wales [14], Scotland [15] and south-west England [16], while the other papers were from Australia [17], the Netherlands [18] and Ireland [19]. The Australian study reported that 31% of GPs surveyed did not accept ME/CFS as a distinct syndrome [17], but we lacked a full text of this paper.

Table 3. Acceptance in general practice of ME/CFS as a genuine clinical entity.

Authors	Year of Publication	Location	Sample Size	Principal Finding: % Respondents Accepting Existence of ME/CFS as a Genuine Clinical Entity	Definition of Outcome
Ho-Yen DO, McNamara I. [15]	1991	Scotland	178	71	Response to question as to whether respondent accepted the existence of chronic fatigue syndrome, requiring 'yes', 'no' or 'undecided' response.
Fitzgibbon EJ, Murphy D, O'Shea K et al. [19]	1997	Ireland	118	58	Response to question: 'Do you accept CFS as a distinct clinical entity?', requiring 'accept', 'do not accept' or 'undecided' response.
Bazelmans E, Vercoulen JH, Swanink CM et al. [18]	1999	Netherlands	3881	99	Inferred from number of invitees who cited disbelief in the syndrome as their reason for non-response
Thomas MA, Smith AP. [14]	2005	South Wales	45	56	Proportion of respondents agreeing that the syndrome actually exists (specific question not reported)
Bowen J, Pheby D, Charlett A, McNulty C. [16]	2005	South-west England	811	72	Responses agreeing or strongly agreeing to proposition via a 5-point Likert scale

In the Dutch study [18] respondents were not specifically asked whether they accepted the existence of ME/CFS as a genuine clinical entity, and the proportion of GPs who reported that they did not accept ME/CFS as a genuine clinical entity was inferred from the number of those contacted who indicated, via a free text response, that this was their opinion. However, 73% of respondents reported that they had at least one patient with chronic fatigue syndrome, and 83% that they had at least one patient with post-viral fatigue syndrome.

The heterogeneous nature of populations studied, and the research methodologies utilised precluded a formal meta-analysis, but for comparison purposes we have calculated 95% confidence intervals for the British and Irish studies which specifically enquired about the acceptance of ME/CFS as a genuine diagnosis. The higher levels of acceptance of ME/CFS in Scotland and south-west England may demonstrate the impact of secondary referral facilities and active programmes of GP education in those areas. The results are itemised in Table 4.

There were additional findings of relevance in the studies examined. Bowen et al. [16] found that only 52% of respondents expressed confidence in their ability to diagnose the condition, and 59% in their ability to manage it. Sixty-eight percent of respondents to the study in South Wales had diagnosed the condition [14]. In the Irish study, 78% of respondents had patients with chronic debilitating fatigue in their practices [19].

These studies were published over a fourteen-year period, and are consistent in demonstrating that a substantial proportion of GPs, which changed little over that time, did not accept ME/CFS as a genuine clinical entity.

Table 4. Acceptance by GPs of ME/CFS—summary statistics.

Reference	Respondents Accepting ME/CFS as Genuine Diagnosis		95% Confidence Interval
	No./Sample Size	%	
Ho-Yen and McNamara [15]	127/178	71.0	33.0–47.2
Fitzgibbon et al. [19]	68/118	58.0	48.6–66.2
Thomas and Smith [14]	25/45	56.0	41.1–69.1
Bowen et al. [16]	584/811	72.0	68.8–75.0
TOTAL	804/1152	69.8	67.1–72.4

3.2.2. Surveys of ME/CFS Patients

Seven papers were identified in this section, but three could not be included in the overall comparative analysis, one for the lack of a full text, and the others for absence of relevant numerical information. The first of these, a Belgian study of 177 patients with different GPs, attending a tertiary clinic, found that only 35% of respondents thought that their GPs had experience of the condition, and only 23% felt their GP had sufficient knowledge to treat it [20]. Another Belgian study of 155 patients with ME/CFS recruited via primary care practitioners reported that 43% of subjects self-assessed as having interpersonal problems with their GPs. A disparity with physician assessments was asserted, and the authors concluded that this disparity had to be seen in the context of previous research, demonstrating that patients with ME/CFS tended to feel misunderstood and disrespected. However, this disparity was not reported numerically [21]. Finally, a French report on 231 participants in a clinical trial undertaken in general practice found a tendency in primary care to attribute fatigue to somatic causes in cases with more reported symptoms. They attributed this to a predilection not to entertain somatic explanations of mild or moderate fatigue, but this could not be quantified from the information presented [22].

The remaining four papers are summarised in Table 5. Three of them, from Norway, are interrelated [23–25], and it can be noted that, although the outcome measures in these studies were not precisely the same as that in an American study by Jason et al. [26], and the populations studied and the modes of selection of participants were different, the proportions of respondents expressing reservations about aspects of the quality of primary care were similar in magnitude.

Table 5. Patients' opinions about GP care of people with ME/CFS.

Authors	Year of Publication	Location	Sample Size	Source of Recruitment	Principal Relevant Outcome Measure	
					Description	Numerical Value
Jason LA; Ferrari JR; Taylor RR; Slavich SP; Stenzel CL [26]	1996	U.S.A.	1073	Self-selected respondents to a survey published in the CFIDS Chronicle.	% respondents reporting a need for better education of health care professionals (including in primary care) about ME/CFS	65
Hansen AH; Lian OS [23]	2016	Norway	488	Norwegian ME Association (cross-sectional survey)	% respondents reporting poor continuity of GP care: - Informational - Management - Relational	35 35 33

Table 5. Cont.

Authors	Year of Publication	Location	Sample Size	Source of Recruitment	Principal Relevant Outcome Measure	
					Description	Numerical Value
Hansen AH; Lian OS [24].	2016	Norway	431	Norwegian ME Association (cross-sectional survey)	% assessing overall quality of primary care to be poor or very poor	61
Lian OS; Hansen AH [25].	2016	Norway	431	Norwegian ME Association (cross-sectional survey)	% reporting satisfaction (to a large extent or to some extent) with GP support during initial phase of illness	46

3.2.3. Other Quantitative Studies

Other quantitative studies identified included two database studies [27,28] a review of medical records [29], and an evaluation of a training programme [30].

Gallagher et al., [27] in an analysis of data from the U.K. General Practice Research Database (now the Clinical Practice Research Datalink), found that, between 1990 and 2001, there was a marked decline in diagnoses of post-viral fatigue syndrome, paralleled by increases in diagnoses of ME/CFS and fibromyalgia, suggesting that diagnostic fashion has a significant part to play in the allocation of diagnostic labels by GPs. A study based on the Norwegian Patient Register found that there were substantial delays in the primary care diagnosis of ME/CFS in children and adolescents. Three-quarters of those patients identified were initially diagnosed with weakness/general tiredness, and for nearly half of them the interval between this initial diagnosis and the definitive diagnosis of ME/CFS was over a year. A comparison with diagnoses of type 1 diabetes mellitus found that only 3.5% of patients were initially diagnosed with weakness/general tiredness, and there was no comparable diagnostic delay [28].

A comparative study of the primary care prevalence of ME/CFS in Sao Paolo and London was carried out by means of a review of medical records [29]. The overall prevalence of chronic fatigue syndrome plus unexplained chronic fatigue was similar in both countries. However, a slightly higher prevalence of chronic fatigue syndrome was apparent among the U.K. patients. The authors attributed this to a cultural factor, namely, a relative lack of recognition of chronic fatigue syndrome among Brazilian doctors, but in fact the difference in prevalence of CFS between the Brazilian and English samples was not statistically significant (prevalence: Brazil 1.6%; U.K. 2.1%. $p = 0.09$).

An American study evaluated a series of five two-day "Train-the-Trainer" workshop training programmes directed towards increasing ME/CFS understanding in primary care [30]. There were marked improvements in both knowledge and self-efficacy, leading to increased confidence in making the diagnosis, but the point was made that the participants were self-selected.

3.3. Qualitative Studies

3.3.1. Studies of GPs

We identified six papers reporting qualitative studies involving GPs dating from 1993 to 2016. The earliest was from New Zealand [31], and the others were all from the U.K., the most recent four coming from the same team based in north-west England [32–36]. The papers are summarised in Table 6:

All the papers reviewed were consistent in concluding that there were substantial gaps in levels of knowledge and understanding of ME/CFS.

3.3.2. Studies of Patients

Nine papers were identified in this category. Our detailed analysis is summarised in Table 7.

It will be noted that the methodologies followed were extremely heterogeneous, precluding any sort of meta-synthesis, but the overall conclusions in all cases were very similar. Concern was expressed in most cases about the lack of legitimation of the condition, and many GPs were seen as being unsympathetic and lacking in knowledge of the condition, and therefore not a good source of advice. By contrast, a good rapport with the doctor was seen to be very positive, though frequently missing.

3.4. Overview Papers

The final category identified in this analysis was of a small number of publications which made reference to problems of GP knowledge and understanding of the condition, but presented no empirical research. Bansal wrote a wide-ranging paper centred on the use of a simplified scoring system for the diagnosis of ME/CFS in general practice, in which he described ME/CFS as poorly understood, and refers to disagreements concerning investigation and management [37]. Wearden and Chew-Graham reviewed the evidence on the primary care treatment of ME/CFS. They acknowledged that some primary care physicians find ME/CFS hard to diagnose, but argued that early diagnosis and coherent explanation of symptoms would be of benefit [38]. Murdoch produced a straightforward, easy-to-follow guide to the diagnosis and care of patients with ME/CFS, via an illustrative clinical scenario, and asserted that ME/CFS is best managed by the patient's GP in a primary care setting [39]. Campion, in a letter to the British Journal of General Practice, stated that the biopsychosocial model of ME/CFS had caused disagreement between doctors and patients, and that doctors should respect patients, and, given our ignorance of the precise causes of the condition, show humility [40].

Table 6. Papers reporting qualitative studies of GPs' knowledge and understanding of ME/CFS.

Authors	Year of Publication	Location	Methodology	GP Sample Size	Relevant Outcome Measures	Findings
Denz-Penhey H, Murdoch JC [31]	1993	New Zealand	Action research in a general practice	10	Identification of GP tasks (illness acknowledgement, symptom control, recommendation of health behaviours, relapse prevention), and service and delivery mechanisms	The authors concluded that medical models of illness were unhelpful, and patients suffered as failure to legitimate their conditions led to denial of access to medical care. They wrote: "Doctors ... have a weighty bias towards the biomedical model even when it has manifestly failed to meet the needs of our patients."
Raine R; Carter S; Sensky T [32]	2004	England	Focus group discussions of clinical scenarios	46	Thematic analysis of focus group transcripts, examined against field notes.	Findings support research indicating that outcomes are poorer where doctors and patients disagree. Doctors' beliefs could result in negative stereotyping of patients with CFS, which constituted a barrier to effective clinical management.
Chew-Graham C; Dowrick C; Wearden A; Richardson V; Peters S [33]	2010	NW England	Semi-structured interviews with patients participating in a primary care-based randomised controlled trial (the FINE Trial)	22	Five themes were identified: defining CFS/ME, excluding physical causes, potential harm from the label, the role of referral and moving on from making the diagnosis.	There was lack of confidence among GPs about making the diagnosis and uncertainty about CFS/ME as a medical condition. Hence, GPs were reluctant to make the diagnosis of CFS/ME, with resultant diagnostic delays and lack of appropriate primary care.
Hannon K, Peters S, Fisher L, Riste L, Wearden A, Lovell K, Turner P, Leech Y, Chew-Graham C [34]	2012	NW England	Semi-structured interviews with patients, carers, practice nurses, ME/CFS specialists and GPs	9	Acquisition of information with the intention of developing a training resource on ME/CFS for primary care.	The GPs had varying degrees of understanding of ME/CFS; some questioned whether ME/CFS was a legitimate illness, and were unaware of the evidence base. There was concern about difficulties of referral to secondary care due to fragmented services and lack of collaboration.

Table 6. Cont.

Authors	Year of Publication	Location	Methodology	GP Sample Size	Relevant Outcome Measures	Findings
Bayliss K; Riste L; Fisher L; Wearden A; Peters S; Lovell K; Chew-Graham C [35]	2014	NW England	Semi-structured interviews with key stakeholders (11 BME patients, 2 carers, 9 GPs, 5 practice nurses, 4 ME/CFS specialists, 5 BME community leaders)	9	Key themes identified were: models of illness, access to care, language and understanding, family and community, religion and culture, stereotypes and racism.	Patients tended to be unwilling to consult GPs for fatigue, and also encountered impediments to accessing primary care. The high turnover of inner-city GPs may constitute a barrier to accessing care.
Bayliss K, Riste L, Band R, Peters S, Wearden A, Lovell K, Fisher L, Chew-Graham CA [36]	2016	NW England	Semi-structured interviews with GPs taking part in an ME/CFS training programme	28	GPs' experience of managing people with CFS/ME before participating in the study, and their opinions on the training programme.	There was difficulty recruiting GP practices, for reasons including scepticism about ME/CFS, the complexity of managing the condition, lack of time in a 10 min consultation, and limited specialist referral options.

Table 7. Qualitative studies of patients' views of GPs' knowledge and understanding of ME/CFS.

Authors	Year of Publication	Location	Methodology	Patient Sample Size	Relevant Outcome Measures	Findings
Denz-Penhey H, Murdoch JC [31]	1993	New Zealand	Action research in a general practice	10	What patients expected of their GPs.	Patients primarily sought legitimation, and acknowledgement of the illness (i.e., acceptance, diagnosis, support), symptom control, recommendations regarding health behaviours, and relapse prevention. There was much dissatisfaction with GPs' perceived failure to meet patients' needs.

Table 7. Cont.

Authors	Year of Publication	Location	Methodology	Patient Sample Size	Relevant Outcome Measures	Findings
Ax S; Gregg VH; Jones D. [41]	1997	London, U.K.	Semi-structured interviews	18	Illness beliefs, meaning of the diagnosis and satisfaction with medical support.	Most participants found that GP emotional and informational support was inadequate, and they felt unsupported. This was coupled with the rejection of medical and health professionals and an increased sense of self-reliance.
Saltzstein BJ, Wyshak G, Hubbuch JT, Perry JC [42]	1998	U.S.A.	Semi-structured interviews	15	Self-report v. perception of physician's prognosis	Improvement in health appeared associated with early diagnosis and a physician optimistic about prognosis
Chew-Graham CA; Cahill G; Dowrick C; Wearden A; Peters S [43]	2008	NW England	Semi-structured interviews with patients participating in a primary care-based randomised controlled trial (the FINE Trial)	24	Key emergent themes: (1) understanding CFS/ME and management, and (2) accessing alternative sources of evidence.	Patients were aware of the risk to their credibility from GPs who may not have accepted that ME/CFS even existed as a genuine diagnosis, and were also aware of the limitations of many GPs' knowledge of the condition.
Chew-Graham C; Brooks J; Wearden A; Dowrick C; Peters S [44].	2011	NW England	Semi-structured interviews with patients participating in a primary care-based randomised controlled trial (the FINE Trial)	19	Emergent themes: feeling accepted and believed by the therapist, their own acceptance of the diagnosis, and accepting the model of illness presented by the therapist.	Engagement of patients with pragmatic rehabilitation in primary care depends on whether they feel accepted and believed, accept the diagnosis, and have an illness model consistent with the treatment.
Gilje AM; Soderlund A; Malterud K. [45].	2008	Norway	Questionnaire and follow-up meeting	12	Exploration of patients' views about the impact of negative opinions held by doctors.	Lack of GP belief in or acknowledgement of the reality of the illness can be worse for patients than the illness itself. Participants wanted doctors to question, listen and take them seriously. GPs were perceived as knowing little about ME/CFS, and therefore unable to give advice.

Table 7. *Cont.*

Authors	Year of Publication	Location	Methodology	Patient Sample Size	Relevant Outcome Measures	Findings
Hannon K, Peters S, Fisher L, Riste L, Wearden A, Lovell K, Turner P, Leech Y, Chew-Graham C [34]	2012	NW England	Semi-structured interviews with patients, 9 of whom were from BME communities.	16	Key themes identified were the need to be believed, the importance of a positively framed diagnosis, defining, prioritising, and managing symptoms, maximising the benefit of consultation, and the role of carers.	Patients expressed frustration when GPs challenged the legitimacy of the condition, and failed to recognise its seriousness, or how it can affect articulateness and memory. Patients felt a need for signposting, but GPs lacked knowledge of the condition and relevant contacts.
Bayliss K; Riste L; Fisher L; Wearden A; Peters S; Lovell K; Chew-Graham C [35]	2014	NW England	Semi-structured interviews with key stakeholders (11 BME patients, 2 carers, 9 GPs, 5 practice nurses, 4 ME/CFS specialists, 5 BME community leaders)	11	Themes raised by patients included: GPs' perceptions; patients' lack of awareness of ME/CFS; community pressures.	Patients perceived a lack of focus by GPs on non-specific symptoms, lack of continuity among city-centre GPs, negative experiences with GPs (e.g., seeing some BME people as 'work shy'). BME GPs seen as less likely to diagnose ME/CFS. Community pressures include language barriers; family pressures, e.g., to be a high achiever; the influence of religion, so that some would turn to religion or spiritual healers rather than primary care. GPs considered unaware of this.
Bayliss K, Riste L, Band R, Peters S, Wearden A, Lovell K, Fisher L, Chew-Graham CA [36]	2016	NW England	Semi-structured interviews with GPs taking part in an ME/CFS training programme	57	The enquiry centres on the extent of agreement between patients and GPs about how and by whom ME/CFS should be managed in primary care, what is needed to be done to achieve collaboration between patients and GPs, and how the training programme should be assessed.	Patients felt that ME/CFS should be managed within primary care, but wanted to be believed and to receive a positive diagnosis. Where this did not happen, patients disengaged from primary care, illustrating the tension between their needs and barriers to care perceived by GPs, including the inadequacy of a ten-minute consultation for such a complex illness.

4. Discussion

The quantitative surveys of GPs were carried out over a fourteen-year period, and are consistent in demonstrating that a substantial proportion of GPs, which changed little over that time, did not accept ME/CFS as a genuine clinical entity. In addition, it is clear that many GPs, even when they accept that ME/CFS is real, lack confidence in diagnosing or managing it. There is a similar degree of consistency in the surveys of patients with clinically confirmed ME/CFS. Despite differences in geographical location, they again report degrees of criticism of aspects of GP care which are similar in magnitude. Other reviewed quantitative studies suggested that diagnostic fashion played a part in GP diagnosis, that there were substantial delays in diagnosing ME/CFS in primary care in children, and that the problem of lack of recognition of ME/CFS was geographically widespread despite cultural differences between different countries.

Similarly, the qualitative studies of GPs, despite differences in geographical location and methodology, were consistent in demonstrating marked gaps in GPs' knowledge and the understanding of ME/CFS. The extremely heterogeneous studies of patients all came to similar conclusions: that there were problems for patients over legitimation of the illness, and over lack of sympathy and knowledge among GPs. The reviewed overview papers acknowledged that ME/CFS was poorly understood in primary care, but that ME/CFS was best managed by GPs, who needed to show respect for patients and humility.

The strengths of the study are firstly that we were able to perform a wide-ranging review of the literature, including qualitative, quantitative and mix-methods research, from both the GP and the patient perspectives. Secondly, we were able to take a methodologically rigorous approach, following the SWiM methodology. The weakness of the study was that, because of the heterogeneity of the literature identified, we were not able to perform a systematic review, and we were unable to carry out a meta-synthesis of the qualitative papers, or a meta-analysis of the quantitative papers. It is also possible that some papers may have been missed by our search.

The studies of both GPs and patients all point in the same direction. Many doctors display uncertainty about whether ME/CFS is a real illness, either not having been trained in it or refusing to recognise ME/CFS as a genuine clinical entity, with consequent delays in diagnosis and treatment for patients. Patients with ME/CFS, for their part, often experience suspicion from healthcare professionals and resultant marginalisation, which represents professional failure, with ethical and practical consequences for care and treatment [46]. There are other pointers in the research literature, in addition to those papers identified in our MEDLINE search, which lead to the same conclusions. For example, a Dutch study of the prevalence of ME/CFS-like illness in the working population concluded that such illness may be under-detected in the working population and perhaps in other populations as well [47]. An English study assessing the feasibility of a randomised controlled trial of an early intervention for ME/CFS in primary care concluded that this was not feasible, partly because of evidence of GPs' difficulties in diagnosing ME/CFS and managing the condition [48].

The factors underlying under-ascertainment of ME/CFS are complex and multiple. The mistaken conclusion [49,50] that an early recorded manifestation of epidemic ME/CFS, Royal Free disease, was epidemic hysteria [51] has coloured thinking for half a century, with its insistence on the biopsychosocial hypothesis that ME/CFS can be totally explained away as being due to faulty illness beliefs combined with deconditioning. This has been important in creating disbelief and uncertainty among healthcare professionals in respect of diagnosis, living with ME/CFS, treatment and management, professional values, and support for people with ME/CFS, with insufficient importance attached to listening skills and to establishing a therapeutic relationship [52]. Such controversies surrounding the diagnosis have led to tension between patients and healthcare professionals [53], and the helplessness many GPs feel because of their lack of knowledge of ME/CFS leads to avoidance and neglect [54].

The consequences of under-ascertainment, and the lack of services to treat ME/CFS, contributes to patient stress and depression, which is frequently associated with fatigue [55]. Diagnostic delay is a risk factor for severe disease (i.e., rendering the patient housebound or bedbound) [56], and such patients may lie at home without having seen a doctor for many years. Furthermore, diagnostic failures in primary care affect outcomes adversely; for example, it has been shown that failure to diagnose primary sleep disorders in individuals with ME/CFS may be implicated in the development of psychological disturbances [57].

Many of the papers in this review were published some years ago, but there is evidence in the grey literature that very little has changed. A survey of members of the Oxfordshire ME supporters' group in England (OMEGA) in 2012 reported that, of the 56 who responded, all had been diagnosed with ME/CFS, half of them (28) by a GP. However, only 10 had seen their GP in the month prior to completing the questionnaire. Only 27% of OMEGA members surveyed found their GP to be either helpful or most helpful. The report's author commented that "listening to the patient, believing what they say and coming to an accurate diagnosis would seem to be the most basic starting point for any effective treatment or help. However, this is not the case for many ME/CFS patients. 39% mentioned lack of diagnosis and belief as the most unhelpful thing". Uninformed, negative or hostile attitudes from healthcare professionals are very stressful and detrimental to the health and well-being of people with ME/CFS, and could deter them from seeking treatment. Patients had low expectations of their GPs, and frequently failed to receive good advice or effective symptom control because of a lack of information on the part of GPs. They themselves have identified this as a problem, although most GPs (93%) recognised ME/CFS as a genuine clinical entity. Three-quarters (74%) of GPs recognised the need for better information and training about diagnosis and treatment, and the availability of local services. Uninformed, negative, or hostile attitudes to people with ME/CFS from healthcare professionals were very stressful and detrimental to health and well-being, and could deter them from seeking treatment [58].

An unpublished survey was conducted in 2018 in the U.K. of 44 hospital doctors attending a regional training event. They completed a questionnaire, the responses to which showed that 72% did not know how to diagnose ME, while 76% lacked confidence in dealing with ME patients. Eighty-two percent of respondents believed ME to be at least in part a psychological or psychosomatic problem, while 39% did not realise that post exertional malaise is an essential requirement for the diagnosis of ME [59].

Other evidence has been provided in a report from the European Federation of Neurological Associations (EFNA), which published a survey on stigma and neurological disorder. There were 1373 responses to the survey; 402 of these were received from people with ME/CFS, many of whom felt stigmatised in their interactions with medical professionals. A total of 74% felt that a medical professional did not believe the extent or severity of their symptoms, and the same percentage felt that they did not receive adequate or appropriate treatment because a medical professional did not take them seriously. Stigma was also widespread within families and in social situations. Forty-nine percent said that their families sometimes make them feel that they exaggerate their condition and, sadly, 32% of respondents with children have been made to feel that they are inadequate parents. Almost half of respondents who lived with a neurological disorder during childhood found it difficult to make friends or maintain friendships at school, and a similar number were excluded from school events on account of their condition [60].

Finally, in an Australian survey of 1055 people with ME, 70% expressed a wish for better-informed GPs, and 48% of respondents said their GPs were poorly or very poorly informed, compared with 44% in 2015. Only 29% of respondents stated that their GPs were well or very well informed, and only 31% regarded health professionals as a key source of information about ME/CFS [61].

The quantitative studies of GP attitudes in the U.K., which demonstrated a considerable degree of scepticism about ME/CFS, were undertaken in the aftermath of the publication of the report of the U.K. Chief Medical Officer's working party on ME/CFS, which had confirmed its existence as a genuine clinical entity [62]. This suggests that the impact of that report on a substantial body of medical opinion was minimal, which is disappointing. The qualitative studies, and studies involving patients, from a wider time scale and range of geographical locations, suggest that such attitudes are by no means confined to the U.K., and remain widespread. The lack of undergraduate and postgraduate teaching on ME/CFS for medical students and doctors may account in large measure for the persistence of such attitudes, and, in a parallel study, we have investigated the current status of medical education on ME/CFS across Europe, as well as possible solutions to the problem.

5. Conclusions

Between a third and a half of GPs lack confidence in diagnosing or managing ME/CFS, or dispute its existence as a genuine clinical entity. A similar proportion of ME/CFS patients express dissatisfaction with the primary medical care they have received, and experienced marked diagnostic delay when they first fell ill. These proportions have changed little over recent years, and similar conclusions have been reached across the range of geographical locations where these matters have been investigated. This conclusion renders problematic attempts to determine the prevalence of ME/CFS, and hence its economic impact. In addition, diagnostic delay is associated with severe disease and poor prognosis, and the likelihood of increased costs.

Author Contributions: Conceptualisation, all authors; methodology, D.A.H. and D.F.H.P.; validation, all authors.; formal analysis, D.F.H.P.; investigation, D.A.H., D.F.H.P. and X.W.-S.; resources, D.A.H., D.F.H.P. and X.W.-S.; writing—original draft preparation, D.F.H.P.; writing—review and editing, J.C., D.F.H.P., J.-D.d.K., D.A.H. and L.G.; visualization, all authors.; project administration, D.F.H.P. All authors have read and agreed to the published version of the manuscript.

Funding: This research received no external funding. EUROMENE receives funding for networking activities from the COST programme (COST Action 15111), via the COST Association.

Institutional Review Board Statement: Not applicable.

Informed Consent Statement: Not applicable.

Data Availability Statement: No new data were created or analysed in this study. Data sharing is not applicable to this article.

Conflicts of Interest: The authors declare no conflict of interest.

References

1. Lindan, R. Benign Myalgic Encephalomyelitis. *Can. Med. Assoc. J.* **1956**, *75*, 596–597.
2. Acheson, E.D. The clinical syndrome variously called myalgic encephalomyelitis, Iceland disease and epidemic neuromyasthenis. *Am. Med.* **1959**, *26*, 589–595. [CrossRef]
3. Carruthers, B.M.; Jain, A.K.; De Meirleir, K.L.; Peterson, D.L.; Klimas, N.G.; Lerner, A.M.; Sherkey, J.A. Myalgic encephalomyelitis/chronic fatigue syndrome: Clinical working case definition, diagnostic and treatment protocols. *J. Chronic Fatigue Syndr.* **2003**, *11*, 7–116. [CrossRef]
4. Johnstone, S.C.; Staines, D.R.; Marshall-Gradisnik, S.M. Epidemiological characteristics of chronic fatigue syndrome/myalgic encephalomyelitis in Australian patients. *Clin. Epidemiol.* **2016**, *8*, 97–107. [CrossRef]
5. Pheby, D.; Lacerda, E.; Nacul, L.; de Lourdes Drachler, M.; Campion, P.; Howe, A.; Sakellariou, D. A disease register for ME/CFS: Report of a pilot study. *BMC Res. Notes* **2011**, *4*, 139–146. [CrossRef]
6. Lloyd, A.R.; Hickie, I.; Boughton, C.R.; Wakefield, D.; Spencer, O. Prevalence of chronic fatigue syndrome in an Australian population. *Med. J. Aust.* **1990**, *153*, 522–528. [CrossRef]
7. Action for ME. Available online: https://actionforme.org.uk/what-is-me/introduction/. (accessed on 6 January 2020).
8. EUROMENE. Available online: http://euromene.eu/ (accessed on 13 October 2020).
9. Pheby, D.F.; Arāja, D.; Berkis, U.; Brenna, E.; Cullinan, J.; De Korwin, J.-D.; Gitto, L.; Hughes, D.; Hunter, R.; Trepel, D.; et al. The development of a consistent Europe-wide approach to investigating the economic impact of myalgic encephalomyelitis (ME/CFS): A report from the European Network on ME/CFS (EUROMENE). *Healthcare* **2020**, *8*, 88. [CrossRef]
10. COST Action 15111—EUROMENE (European ME/CFS Research Network), Working Group 3: Socio-Economics. Deliverable 10—Common consensus protocol for economic loss calculation due to ME/CFS. Brussels. September 2019. Available online: http://euromene.eu/workinggroups/deliverables/deliverable.html (accessed on 14 October 2020).

11. Bayliss, K.; Goodall, M.; Chisholm, A.; Fordham, B.; Chew-Graham, C.; Riste, L.; Fisher, L.; Lovell, K.; Peters, S.; Wearden, A.J. Overcoming the barriers to the diagnosis and management of chronic fatigue syndrome/ME in primary care: A meta synthesis of qualitative studies. *BMC Fam. Pract.* **2014**, *15*, 44. [CrossRef]
12. Campbell, M.; McKenzie, J.E.; Sowden, A.; Katikireddi, S.V.; Brennan, S.E.; Ellis, S.; Hartmann-Boyce, J.; Ryan, R.; Shepperd, S.; Thomas, J.; et al. Synthesis without meta-analysis (SWiM) in systematic reviews: Reporting guideline. *BMJ* **2020**, *368*, l6890. [CrossRef]
13. Saidi, G.; Haines, L. The management of children with chronic fatigue syndrome-like illness in primary care: A cross-sectional study. *Brit. J. Gen. Pract.* **2006**, *56*, 43–47.
14. Thomas, M.; Smith, A.P. Primary healthcare provision and Chronic Fatigue Syndrome: A survey of patients' and General Practitioners' beliefs. *BMC Fam. Pract.* **2005**, *6*, 49. [CrossRef]
15. Ho-Yen, D.O.; McNamara, I. General practitioners' experience of the chronic fatigue syndrome. *Brit. J. Gen. Pract.* **1991**, *41*, 324–326.
16. Bowen, J.; Pheby, D.; Charlett, A.; McNulty, C. Chronic Fatigue Syndrome: A survey of GPs' attitudes and knowledge. *Fam. Pract.* **2005**, *22*, 389–393. [CrossRef]
17. Steven, I.D.; McGrath, B.; Qureshi, F.; Wong, C.; Chern, I.; Pearn-Rowe, B. General practitioners' beliefs, attitudes and reported actions towards chronic fatigue syndrome. *Aust. Fam. Physician* **2000**, *29*, 80–85.
18. Bazelmans, E.; Vercoulen, J.; Swanink, C.; Fennis, J.; Galama, J.; Van Weel, C.; Van Der Meer, J.; Bleijenberg, G. Chronic Fatigue Syndrome and Primary Fibromyalgia Syndrome as recognized by GPs. *Fam. Pract.* **1999**, *16*, 602–604. [CrossRef]
19. FitzGibbon, E.J.; Murphy, D.; O'Shea, K.; Kelleher, C. Chronic debilitating fatigue in Irish general practice: A survey of general practitioners' experience. *Br. J. Gen. Pract.* **1997**, *47*, 618–622.
20. Van Hoof, E. The doctor-patient relationship in chronic fatigue syndrome: Survey of patient perspectives. *Qual. Prim. Care* **2009**, *17*, 263–270.
21. Vandenbergen, J.; Vanheule, S.; Desmet, M.; Verhaeghe, P. Unexplained chronic fatigue and interpersonal problems: A study in a primary care population. *Int. J. Psychiatry Med.* **2009**, *39*, 325–340. [CrossRef]
22. Cathébras, P.; Jacquin, L.; Le Gal, M.; Fayol, C.; Bouchou, K.; Rousset, H. Correlates of somatic causal attributions in primary care patients with fatigue. *Psychother. Psychosom.* **1995**, *63*, 174–180. [CrossRef]
23. Hansen, A.H.; Lian, O.S. Experiences of general practitioner continuity among women with chronic fatigue syndrome/myalgic encephalomyelitis: A cross-sectional study. *BMC Health Serv. Res.* **2016**, *16*, 1–8. [CrossRef]
24. Hansen, A.H.; Lian, O.S. How do women with chronic fatigue syndrome/myalgic encephalomyelitis rate quality and coordination of healthcare services? A cross-sectional study. *BMJ Open* **2016**, *6*, e010277. [CrossRef] [PubMed]
25. Lian, O.S.; Hansen, A.H. Factors facilitating patient satisfaction among women with medically unexplained long-term fatigue: A relational perspective. *Health Interdiscip. J. Soc. Study Health Illn. Med.* **2015**, *20*, 308–326. [CrossRef] [PubMed]
26. Jason, L.A.; Ferrari, J.R.; Taylor, R.R.; Slavich, S.P.; Stenzel, C.L. A national assessment of the service, support, and housing preferences by persons with chronic fatigue syndrome. Toward a comprehensive rehabilitation program. *Eval. Health Prof.* **1996**, *19*, 194–207. [CrossRef] [PubMed]
27. Gallagher, A.M.; Thomas, J.M.; Hamilton, W.T.; White, P.D. Incidence of fatigue symptoms and diagnoses presenting in UK primary care from 1990 to 2001. *JRSM* **2004**, *97*, 571–575. [CrossRef] [PubMed]
28. Bakken, I.J.; Tveito, K.; Aaberg, K.M.; Ghaderi, S.; Gunnes, N.; Trogstad, L.; Magnus, P.; Stoltenberg, C.; Håberg, S.E. Comorbidities treated in primary care in children with chronic fatigue syndrome / myalgic encephalomyelitis: A nationwide registry linkage study from Norway. *BMC Fam. Pract.* **2016**, *17*, 128. [CrossRef]
29. Cho, H.J.; Menezes, P.R.; Hotopf, M.; Bhugra, D.; Wessely, S. Comparative epidemiology of chronic fatigue syndrome in Brazilian and British primary care: Prevalence and recognition. *Br. J. Psychiatry* **2009**, *194*, 117–122. [CrossRef]
30. Brimmer, D.J.; McCleary, K.K.; A Lupton, T.; Faryna, K.M.; Hynes, K.; Reeves, W.C. A train-the-trainer education and promotion program: Chronic fatigue syndrome-a diagnostic and management challenge. *BMC Med. Educ.* **2008**, *8*, 49. [CrossRef]
31. Denz-Penhey, H.; Murdoch, J.C. Service delivery for people with chronic fatigue syndrome: A pilot action research study. *Fam. Pract.* **1993**, *10*, 14–18. [CrossRef]
32. Bayliss, K.; Riste, L.; Band, R.; Peters, S.; Wearden, A.; Lovell, K.; Fisher, L.; A Chew-Graham, C. Implementing resources to support the diagnosis and management of Chronic Fatigue Syndrome/Myalgic Encephalomyelitis (CFS/ME) in primary care: A qualitative study. *BMC Fam. Pract.* **2016**, *17*, 1–11. [CrossRef]
33. Chew-Graham, C.; Dowrick, C.; Wearden, A.; Richardson, V.; Peters, S. Making the diagnosis of Chronic Fatigue Syndrome/Myalgic Encephalitis in primary care: A qualitative study. *BMC Fam. Pract.* **2010**, *11*, 16. [CrossRef]
34. Hannon, K.L.; Peters, S.; Fisher, L.; Riste, L.; Wearden, A.J.; Lovell, K.; Turner, P.; Leech, Y.; Chew-Graham, C. Developing resources to support the diagnosis and management of Chronic Fatigue Syndrome/Myalgic Encephalitis (CFS/ME) in primary care: A qualitative study. *BMC Fam. Pract.* **2012**, *13*, 93. [CrossRef] [PubMed]
35. Bayliss, K.; Riste, L.; Fisher, L.; Wearden, A.; Peters, S.; Lovell, K.; Chew-Graham, C. Diagnosis and management of chronic fatigue syndrome/myalgic encephalitis in black and minority ethnic people: A qualitative study. *Prim. Health Care Res. Dev.* **2013**, *15*, 143–155. [CrossRef] [PubMed]
36. Raine, R.; Carter, S.; Sensky, T.; Black, N. General practitioners' perceptions of chronic fatigue syndrome and beliefs about its management, compared with irritable bowel syndrome: Qualitative study. *BMJ* **2004**, *328*, 1354–1357. [CrossRef] [PubMed]

37. Bansal, A.S. Investigating unexplained fatigue in general practice with a particular focus on CFS/ME. *BMC Fam. Pract.* **2016**, *17*, 81. [CrossRef] [PubMed]
38. Wearden, A.J.; Chew-Graham, C. Managing chronic fatigue syndrome in U.K. primary care: Challenges and opportunities. *Chronic Illn.* **2006**, *2*, 143–153. [CrossRef]
39. Murdoch, J.C. Chronic fatigue syndrome. The patient centred clinical method–a guide for the perplexed. *Aust. Fam. Physician* **2003**, *32*, 883–887.
40. Campion, P. Chronic fatigue syndrome: Is the biopsychosocial model responsible for patient dissatisfaction and harm? (letter). *Br. J. Gen. Pract.* **2016**, *66*, 511. [CrossRef]
41. Ax, S.; Gregg, V.H.; Jones, D. Chronic Fatigue Syndrome: Sufferers' Evaluation of Medical Support. *J. R. Soc. Med.* **1997**, *90*, 250–254. [CrossRef]
42. Saltzstein, B.J.; Wyshak, G.; Hubbuch, J.T.; Perry, J.C. A naturalistic study of the chronic fatigue syndrome among women in primary care. *Gen. Hosp. Psychiatry* **1998**, *20*, 307–316. [CrossRef]
43. Chew-Graham, C.A.; Cahill, G.; Dowrick, C.; Wearden, A.; Peters, S. Using Multiple Sources of Knowledge to Reach Clinical Understanding of Chronic Fatigue Syndrome. *Ann. Fam. Med.* **2008**, *6*, 340–348. [CrossRef]
44. Chew-Graham, C.; Brooks, J.; Wearden, A.; Dowrick, C.; Peters, S. Factors influencing engagement of patients in a novel intervention for CFS/ME: A qualitative study. *Prim. Health Care Res. Dev.* **2010**, *12*, 112–122. [CrossRef] [PubMed]
45. Gilje, A.M.; Söderlund, A.; Malterud, K. Obstructions for quality care experienced by patients with chronic fatigue syndrome (CFS)—A case study. *Patient Educ. Couns.* **2008**, *73*, 36–41. [CrossRef] [PubMed]
46. Blease, C.; Carel, H.; Geraghty, K. Epistemic injustice in healthcare encounters: Evidence from chronic fatigue syndrome. *J. Med. Ethics.* **2017**, *43*, 549–557. [CrossRef]
47. Huibers, M.J.H.; Kant, I.J.; Swaen, G.M.H.; Kasl, S.V. Prevalence of chronic fatigue syndrome-like caseness in the working population: Results from the Maastricht cohort study. *Occup. Environ. Med.* **2004**, *61*, 464–466. [CrossRef] [PubMed]
48. O'Dowd, H.; Beasant, L.; Ingram, J.; A Montgomery, A.; Hollingworth, W.W.; Gaunt, D.; Collin, S.M.; Horne, S.; Jones, B.; Crawley, E. The feasibility and acceptability of an early intervention in primary care to prevent chronic fatigue syndrome (CFS) in adults: Randomised controlled trial. *Pilot Feasibility Stud.* **2020**, *6*, 65. [CrossRef] [PubMed]
49. Kermack, W.O.; McKendrick, A.G. Contribution to the mathematical theory of epidemics. *Proc. R. Soc. London* **1927**, *772*, 701–721.
50. Waters, F.G.; McDonald, G.J.; Banks, S.; Waters, R.A. Myalgic Encephalomyelitis (ME) outbreaks can be modelled as an infectious disease: A mathematical reconsideration of the Royal Free Epidemic of 1955. *Fatigue: Biomed. Health Behav.* **2020**, *8*, 70–83. [CrossRef]
51. McEvedy, C.P.; Beard, A.W. Royal Free Epidemic of 1955: A Reconsideration. *BMJ* **1970**, *1*, 7–11. [CrossRef]
52. Horton, S.; Poland, F.; Kale, S.; Drachler, M.D.L.; Leite, J.C.D.C.; McArthur, M.; Campion, P.; Pheby, D.; Nacul, L. Chronic fatigue syndrome/myalgic encephalomyelitis (CFS/ME) in adults: A qualitative study of perspectives from professional practice. *BMC Fam. Pract.* **2010**, *11*, 89. [CrossRef]
53. Nacul, L.; Lacerda, E.M.; Kingdon, C.C.; Curran, H.; Bowman, E.W. How have selection bias and disease misclassification undermined the validity of myalgic encephalomyelitis/chronic fatigue syndrome studies? *J. Health Psychol.* **2019**, *24*, 1765–1769. [CrossRef]
54. Speight, N. Severe ME in Children. *Healthcare* **2020**, *8*, 211. [CrossRef]
55. Stadje, R.; Dornieden, K.; Baum, E.; Becker, A.; Biroga, T.; Bösner, S.; Haasenritter, J.; Keunecke, C.; Viniol, A.; Donner-Banzhoff, N. The differential diagnosis of tiredness: A systematic review. *BMC Fam. Pract.* **2016**, *17*, 147. [CrossRef]
56. Pheby, D.; Saffron, L. Risk factors for severe ME/CFS. *Biol. Med.* **2009**, *1*, 50–74.
57. Fossey, M.; Libman, E.; Bailes, S.; Baltzan, M.; Schondorf, R.; Amsel, R.; Fichten, C.S. Sleep quality and psychological adjustment in chronic fatigue syndrome. *J. Behav. Med.* **2004**, *27*, 581–605. [CrossRef]
58. Oxfordshire ME Group for Action (OMEGA). OMEGA Membership Survey on Local NHS Services for ME/CFS (April 2013). Available online: http://omegaoxon.org/publications (accessed on 22 July 2020).
59. Hng, K.N. Doctors' Knowledge and Understanding of Myalgic Encephalomyelitis—United Kingdom. 2018. Available online: https://bit.ly/2yFAtY8 or https://bit.ly/3byfwga (accessed on 14 October 2020).
60. European Federation of Neurological Associations [EFNA] 2020—Survey on Stigma and Neurological Disorder. Available online: https://www.efna.net/survey2020/ (accessed on 22 July 2020).
61. Anon. Lifelong Lockdown: Lessons Learned from the Health and Wellbeing Survey of Australians Living with ME/CFS 2019. Emerge Australia, October 2020. Available online: https://www.emerge.org.au/health-and-wellbeing-survey-2019 (accessed on 14 October 2020).
62. CFS/ME Working Group. *Report to the Chief Medical Officer of an Independent Working Group*; Department of Health: London, UK, 2001.

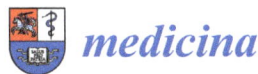

Article

Perceptions of European ME/CFS Experts Concerning Knowledge and Understanding of ME/CFS among Primary Care Physicians in Europe: A Report from the European ME/CFS Research Network (EUROMENE)

John Cullinan [1,*], Derek F. H. Pheby [2,†], Diana Araja [3], Uldis Berkis [3], Elenka Brenna [4], Jean-Dominique de Korwin [5,6], Lara Gitto [7], Dyfrig A. Hughes [8], Rachael M. Hunter [9], Dominic Trepel [10,11,12] and Xia Wang-Steverding [13]

1. School of Business & Economics, National University of Ireland Galway, University Road, H91 TK33 Galway, Ireland
2. Society and Health, Buckinghamshire New University, High Wycombe HP11 2JZ, UK; derekpheby@btinternet.com
3. Department of Dosage Form Technology, Faculty of Pharmacy, Institute of Microbiology and Virology, Riga Stradins University, Dzirciema Street 16, LV-1007 Riga, Latvia; diana.araja@rsu.lv (D.A.); Uldis.Berkis@rsu.lv (U.B.)
4. Department of Economics and Finance, Università Cattolica del Sacro Cuore, Largo Agostino Gemelli 1, 20123 Milan, Italy; elenka.brenna@unicatt.it
5. Internal Medicine Department, University of Lorraine, 34, Cours Léopold, CS 25233, 54052 Nancy CEDEX, France; jean-dominique.dekorwin@univ-lorraine.fr
6. University Hospital of Nancy, Rue du Morvan, 54511 Vandoeuvre-Lès-Nancy CEDEX, France
7. Department of Economics, University of Messina, Piazza Pugliatti 1, 98122 Messina, Italy; lara.gitto@unime.it
8. Centre for Health Economics & Medicines Evaluation, Bangor University, Bangor LL57 2PZ, UK; d.a.hughes@bangor.ac.uk
9. Research Department of Primary Care and Population Health, Royal Free Medical School, University College London, London NW3 2PF, UK; r.hunter@ucl.ac.uk
10. School of Medicine, Trinity College Dublin, College Green, D02 PN40 Dublin, Ireland; trepeld@tcd.ie
11. Global Brain Health Institute, Trinity College Dublin, D02 PN40 Dublin, Ireland
12. Global Brain Health Institute, University of Califonia, San Francisco, CA 94143, USA
13. Warwick Medical School and Zeeman Institute, University of Warwick, Coventry CV4 7AL, UK; xiasteverding@gmail.com
* Correspondence: john.cullinan@nuigalway.ie
† Retired.

Abstract: *Background and Objectives*: We have conducted a survey of academic and clinical experts who are participants in the European ME/CFS Research Network (EUROMENE) to elicit perceptions of general practitioner (GP) knowledge and understanding of myalgic encephalomyelitis/chronic fatigue syndrome (ME/CFS) and suggestions as to how this could be improved. *Materials and Methods*: A questionnaire was sent to all national representatives and members of the EUROMENE Core Group and Management Committee. Survey responses were collated and then summarized based on the numbers and percentages of respondents selecting each response option, while weighted average responses were calculated for questions with numerical value response options. Free text responses were analysed using thematic analysis. *Results*: Overall there were 23 responses to the survey from participants across 19 different European countries, with a 95% country-level response rate. Serious concerns were expressed about GPs' knowledge and understanding of ME/CFS, and, it was felt, about 60% of patients with ME/CFS went undiagnosed as a result. The vast majority of GPs were perceived to lack confidence in either diagnosing or managing the condition. Disbelief, and misleading illness attributions, were perceived to be widespread, and the unavailability of specialist centres to which GPs could refer patients and seek advice and support was frequently commented upon. There was widespread support for more training on ME/CFS at both undergraduate and postgraduate levels. *Conclusion*: The results of this survey are consistent with the existing scientific literature. ME/CFS experts report that lack of knowledge and understanding of ME/CFS among GPs is a major cause of missed and delayed diagnoses, which renders problematic attempts to determine

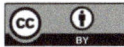

Citation: Cullinan, J.; Pheby, D.F.H.; Araja, D.; Berkis, U.; Brenna, E.; de Korwin, J.-D.; Gitto, L.; Hughes, D.A.; Hunter, R.M.; Trepel, D.; et al. Perceptions of European ME/CFS Experts Concerning Knowledge and Understanding of ME/CFS among Primary Care Physicians in Europe: A Report from the European ME/CFS Research Network (EUROMENE). *Medicina* **2021**, *57*, 208. https://doi.org/10.3390/medicina57030208

Academic Editor: Edgaras Stankevičius

Received: 8 January 2021
Accepted: 22 February 2021
Published: 26 February 2021

Publisher's Note: MDPI stays neutral with regard to jurisdictional claims in published maps and institutional affiliations.

Copyright: © 2021 by the authors. Licensee MDPI, Basel, Switzerland. This article is an open access article distributed under the terms and conditions of the Creative Commons Attribution (CC BY) license (https://creativecommons.org/licenses/by/4.0/).

the incidence and prevalence of the disease, and to measure its economic impact. It also contributes to the burden of disease through mismanagement in its early stages.

Keywords: ME/CFS; myalgic encephalomyelitis; chronic fatigue syndrome; primary care; GP knowledge and understanding

1. Introduction

Myalgic encephalomyelitis/chronic fatigue syndrome (ME/CFS) is a complex multi-system disorder that is characterised by a range of symptoms that can fluctuate in severity and change over time. These symptoms include post-exertional malaise, incapacitating fatigue that is not alleviated by rest, cognitive dysfunction, sleep disturbances, and muscle pain, while the condition can cause severe diminution in functioning and in quality of life [1].

It is estimated that there are around two million people with ME/CFS in the European Union and the United Kingdom combined, with an economic impact in the region of €40 billion per annum [2]. However, there are considerable difficulties in determining accurate prevalence and cost estimates, for a number of reasons. These include differences in case definitions, lack of empirical information in much of Europe about incidence and prevalence, natural variation between populations in, for example, the proportion of severely affected people, the heterogeneity of national economies and health care systems and, perhaps most importantly, the unwillingness of many doctors, particularly in primary care, either to recognise the condition as a genuine clinical entity or to diagnose it [2,3].

A recent literature review, covering studies from a wide variety of geographical locations world-wide over a 14-year period, found that between a third and a half of general practitioners (GPs) were unwilling to recognise or diagnose ME/CFS, that a similar proportion of patients were dissatisfied with the quality of primary care they had received, and that these proportions varied little over time [4]. In order to investigate this further, and to assess how knowledge and understanding of ME/CFS is perceived by experts in the condition across Europe, we conducted a survey of participants in the European ME/CFS Research Network (EUROMENE) project. EUROMENE was established to promote collaborative research on ME/CFS across Europe and is currently in receipt of EU funding from the COST Association (COST Action 15111) to support network activities. The aims of EUROMENE include reviewing the current state of the art and identifying gaps in knowledge about ME/CFS.

2. Materials and Methods

A survey questionnaire was sent to national representatives and members of the EUROMENE Core Group and Management Committee in September 2020—see Supplementary Materials. The questionnaire included a number of separate questions relating to: (i) the existence of GP patient lists and national guidance on treatment pathways; (ii) percentages of people with ME/CFS undiagnosed and presenting to a GP; (iii) percentages of GPs recognising, confident to diagnose, and confident to manage ME/CFS; (iv) percentages of patients diagnosed by GP, referred by GP to specialist care, and self-referring to specialist services; and (v) views on needs for teaching, training, reference literature, and referral centres. Responses to these questions were collated and summarized based on the numbers and percentages of respondents selecting each available option and these summary statistics were then used to generate a range of charts to clearly illustrate our main findings. Where options given in questions were in the form of percentages (e.g., 20–40%), weighted averages were calculated assuming the mid-points of the presented percentage ranges.

The questionnaire also included four questions seeking free text responses. The first such question sought purely factual information concerning the existence or otherwise of official guidance in respondents' countries on the management of ME/CFS. The other three questions requested opinions on what constitutes specialist care in respondents' countries, ways to increase knowledge and understanding among GPs, and other comments. The responses to these three questions were analysed using thematic analysis [5].

3. Results

3.1. Survey Question Responses

In total there were 23 responses received from EUROMENE members across 19 countries, namely: Austria, Belgium, Bulgaria, Denmark, Finland, France, Germany (3 responses), Greece, Ireland, Italy, Latvia, Netherlands, Norway, Poland, Romania, Serbia, Slovenia, Spain (3 responses), and the UK. With 20 member countries in EUROMENE, this represents a 95% country-level response rate. Where multiple responses were received from a country (namely Germany and Spain), we first examined the consistency of responses at a country level. Since there were some differences in responses for these countries for some questions, we chose to use data from all 23 responses in our analysis. Overall, however, our key results and findings do not alter significantly if we instead use a measure of the average response for these countries (results available on request).

In terms of the professional roles of respondents, 9 indicated that they were academics, 8 that they were medical consultants (e.g., neurology, internal medicine, infectious disease, psychology), 8 that they were GPs, 2 that they were retired, while 2 did not specify. Some respondents reported dual roles e.g., consultant and academic positions.

To start, Figure 1 presents a summary of survey responses relating to the existence of GP patient lists and national guidance on treatment pathways. Overall 16 respondents (70%) reported there are no GP lists of registered patients in their country, while 15 (65%) reported no specific national guidance on treatment pathways.

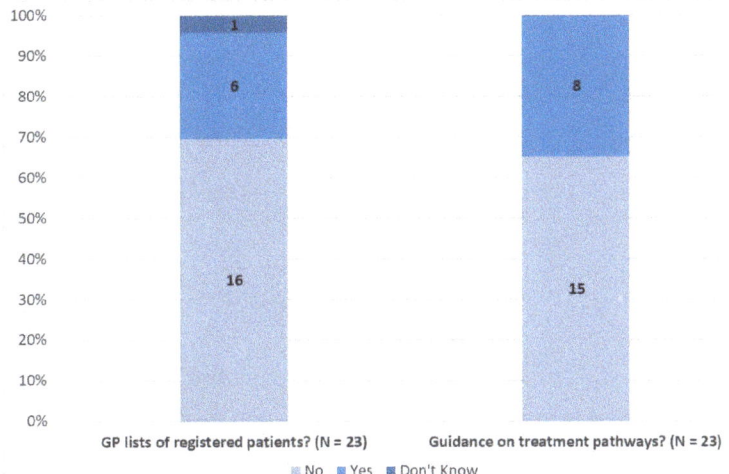

Figure 1. Existence of GP Patient Lists and National Guidance on Treatment Pathways (% Respondents). Note: Data labels indicate number of respondents per category. Source: EUROMENE Survey of Diagnosis and Management of ME/CFS in Primary Care in Europe, 2020.

Figure 2 presents results relating to the percentage of people with ME/CFS that remain undiagnosed and the percentage that present to a GP. In relation to the former, there is considerable variation across respondents, with 4 respondents (18%) reporting between 0% and 20% remain undiagnosed, 6 (27%) that the proportion is 40–60%, 5 (23%) that it is 60% and 80%, and 7 (32%) that between 80% and 100% remain undiagnosed. It should be noted that one respondent did not answer this question. Taking a weighted average of all responses, and assuming a mid-point value for each option, gives an estimated average of 60% of people with ME/CFS remaining undiagnosed across our survey responses. Figure 2 also includes responses relating to the percentage of people with ME/CFS that present to a GP. Here 3 respondents (13%) reported that 0–20% do so, 3 (13%) that it is 20–40%, 10 (44%) that it is 60–80%, and 7 (30%) reported that between 80% and 100% of people with ME/CFS present to a GP. The weighted average is 66%, implying the majority present to a GP.

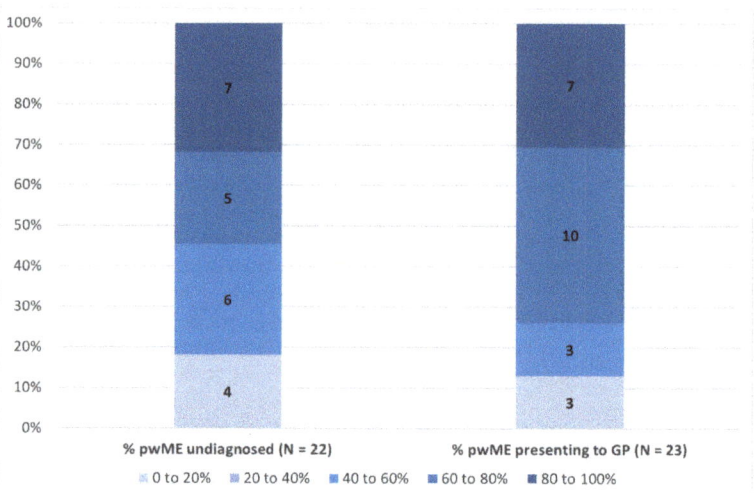

Figure 2. Percentage of People with ME/CFS Undiagnosed and Percentage Presenting to a GP (% Respondents). Note: Data labels indicate number of respondents per category. pwME denotes person with ME/CFS. Source: EUROMENE Survey of Diagnosis and Management of ME/CFS in Primary Care in Europe, 2020.

Responses to the questions relating to GP recognition, confidence in diagnosing, and confidence in managing ME/CFS are presented in Figure 3. For GP recognition of the condition, 14 respondents (61%) chose the 0–20% option, while 5 (22%) reported 20–40%. Only a small number of respondents selected the other options and the weighted average estimate of the percentage of GPs recognising ME/CFS as a genuine clinical entity was 23%. Similar yet more pronounced patterns are evident for the diagnosis and management of ME/CFS. For example, 18 respondents (78%) reported that between 0% and 20% of GPs are confident of their ability to diagnose ME/CFS, with a weighted average of 17%. For management, 21 respondents (91%) reported that between 0% and 20% of GPs are confident of their ability to manage ME/CFS patients, with a weighted average of just 14%.

Figure 4 presents an overview of responses to the questions relating to the percentages of patients that are diagnosed by their GP, that are referred by their GP to specialist care, and that self-refer to specialist services. Overall, 14 respondents (61%) reported that between 0% and 20% of patients with ME/CFS who consult with their GP are in fact diagnosed by them, with 4 (18%) reporting the proportion to be 20–40% and 40–80%. The weighted average estimate from these respondents is 26%. There was more variation across responses to the question relating to GP referral to specialist care. For example, 5 respondents (23%) reported this to be 0–20% in their country, 5 (23%) that it is 20–40%, 3 (14%) that it is 40–60%, 7 (32%) that it is 60–80%, and 2 (9%) that 80–100% of patients that present to a GP are referred by the GP to specialist care. The weighted average response is 46%. Finally, Figure 4 also shows the responses relating to self-referral to specialist services. Again there is quite a lot of variation across respondents for this question, possibly due to variability in how this question was interpreted by ME/CFS specialists versus other specialists, and the weighted average percentage of patients self-referring is an estimated 51%.

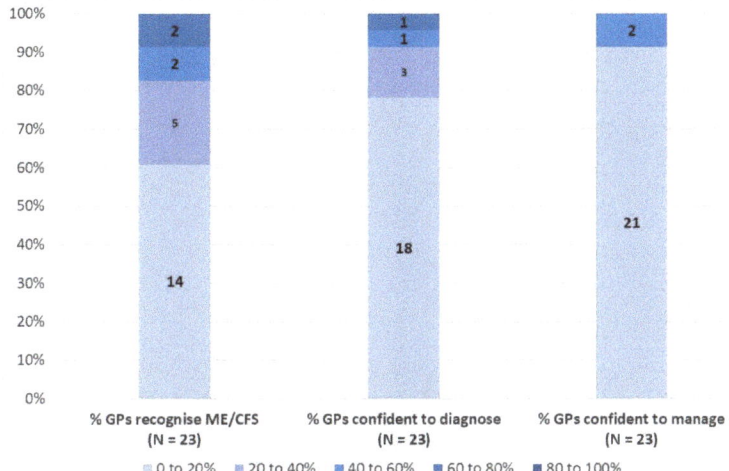

Figure 3. Percentage of GPs Recognising, Confident to Diagnose, and Confident to Manage ME/CFS (% Respondents). Note: Data labels indicate number of respondents per category. Source: EUROMENE Survey of Diagnosis and Management of ME/CFS in Primary Care in Europe, 2020.

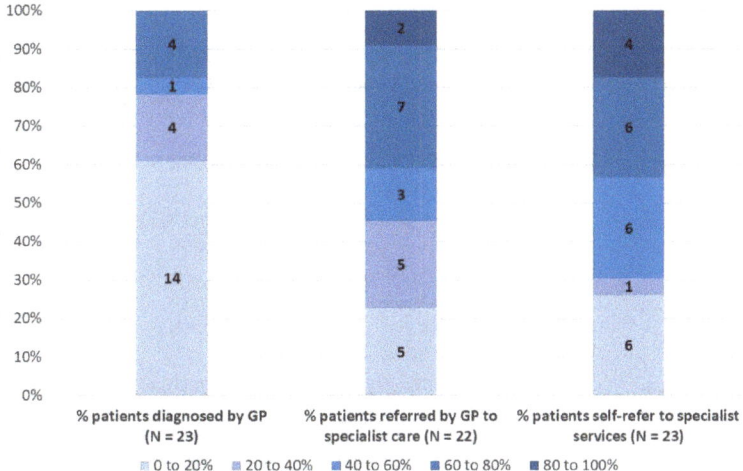

Figure 4. Percentage of Patients Diagnosed by GP, Referred by GP to Specialist Care, and Self-Referring to Specialist Services (% Respondents). Note: Data labels indicate number of respondents per category. Source: EUROMENE Survey of Diagnosis and Management of ME/CFS in Primary Care in Europe, 2020.

Responses to the questions relating to the needs for teaching, training, reference literature, and referral centres are presented in Figure 5. Given the very high levels of consistency in responses across these responses, there is little need to discuss them in detail. Nonetheless, it is important to note that 21 respondents (91%) strongly agreed that there should be more teaching about ME/CFS in undergraduate medical curricula, while 21 respondents (91%) strongly agreed that postgraduate training about ME/CFS should be available for doctors and other healthcare professionals. For the latter question, the remaining survey respondents agreed with the statement. In addition, all respondents either strongly agreed or agreed that there is a need for succinct reference literature on ME/CFS for doctors and other healthcare professionals in primary care and that there is a need to ensure the existence of adequate secondary and tertiary referral centres for ME/CFS, from which primary care doctors could seek help and advice when necessary.

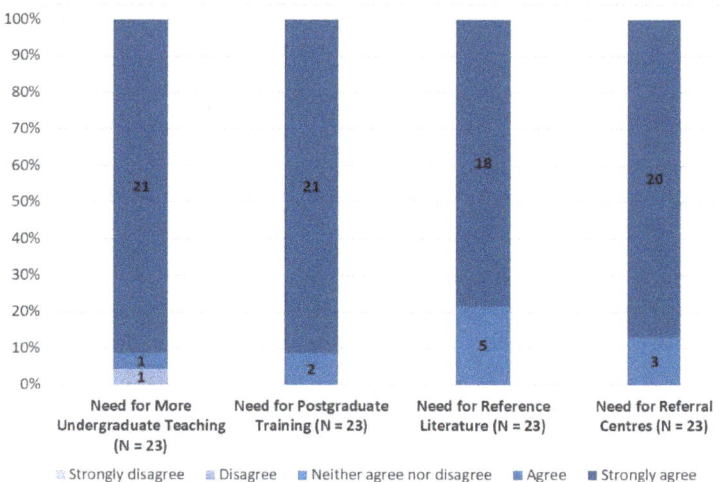

Figure 5. Views on Needs for Teaching, Training, Reference Literature, and Referral Centres (% Respondents). Note: Data labels indicate number of respondents per category. Source: EUROMENE Survey of Diagnosis and Management of ME/CFS in Primary Care in Europe, 2020.

3.2. Analysis of Free Text Responses

3.2.1. Official Guidance on ME/CFS

Respondents were asked to indicate whether official guidance on ME/CFS for healthcare professionals existed in their countries. Their free text responses indicated that such guidance was available and accessible, or under development, in Belgium, Germany, Italy, the Netherlands, Norway, Slovenia, Spain, the United Kingdom, and Finland. In Ireland, while there were no guidelines, clinicians tended to follow the UK NICE guidelines. The responses are summarised below.

Belgium has guidelines on diagnosis and clinical pathways from the government's illness insurance programme. In Germany, there is a guideline on fatigue in general, which also covers ME/CFS, but it is said to be quite superficial and to lack understanding of the disease, and is therefore unhelpful. In Italy, a document was published in 2014 on behalf of AGENAS (the National Agency for Regional Health Services), which is part of the Health Ministry. It promotes a multidisciplinary approach to ME/CFS, with advice on aetiology, physiopathology, clinical features, diagnosis, and treatment. Practice in the Netherlands was reported to be based on American guidance from 2015. This likely refers to guidance published by the Institute of Medicine (IOM), now the National Academy of Medicine (NAM), entitled "Beyond Myalgic Encephalomyelitis/ Chronic Fatigue Syndrome: Redefining an Illness", and summarised in a guide for healthcare providers [6]. Norway published guidance in 2014, and this was revised in 2015. It covers interdisciplinary investigation, diagnosis, treatment, rehabilitation and care, in various care locations (outpatients, inpatients, rehabilitation institutions, and self-management programmes) [7].

In Slovenia, EULAR recommendations for the management of fibromyalgia are followed [8]. In Spain, the public health system published a guide in 2019, but this guide was withdrawn, and patient associations and doctors who treat patients with ME/CFS have requested a complete review. It is also suggested that AQUAS 2017 is followed. AQUAS (Aggregated Quality Assurance for Systems) is an EU supported project promoting a holistic approach to safety, security, and performance in system development, medicine being one of the priority areas [9]. However, this appears rather remote from the diagnosis and management of patients with ME/CFS. In the United Kingdom, the NICE (National Institute for Health and Care Excellence) guidelines for ME/CFS are currently being revised [10]. Finland has official guidance in preparation. While it includes little on treatment pathways, there will be confirmation that pacing has a role in management, and that graded exercise therapy (GET) and cognitive behaviour therapy (CBT) will not be considered as effective treatment, which is very much in line with the current UK draft guideline from NICE.

3.2.2. Specialist Care

Themes identified in the responses included the inadequacy of specialist care, the nature of the illness, specialties involved in care, multidisciplinary approaches, GP involvement, psychiatric involvement in care, the content of therapy, and the role of specialist centres. Emergent sub-themes regarding the nature of the illness included reporting of widespread disbelief in ME/CFS, as well as concern that it was regarded as a psychiatric, functional, or psychosomatic disease. On the content of therapy, emergent sub-themes were the use of CBT and GET, the involvement of rehabilitation institutions, and the role of laboratory investigations and psychological examination. A detailed examination of sub-themes is summarised below.

The central role of dedicated specialists was reported from Latvia and of specialised centres from Spain. There was one such dedicated specialist cluster in Latvia, and certain specific centres in Spain, with a role in diagnosis and management. Widespread disbelief in the existence of ME/CFS was reported as a factor limiting provision of specialist care in Greece. There was reported to be no specialist care available in Austria, Denmark, the Netherlands or Rumania, and little available in France, Germany, Ireland, or Poland. However, since specialist was not defined explicitly in the survey, it is possible that respondents may be referring to a lack of ME/CFS specialists, rather than saying that people with ME/CFS don't have access to internal medicine and rehabilitation medicine specialists, neurologists, etc. Collaboration with GPs was seen as important in specialist care delivery in Belgium and Slovenia, but seen as problematic in Italy. In Ireland and the UK, GP referral is important as the gateway to specialist care, though this may be verging on non-existent or involve prolonged delays. The two specialist centres in Germany are involved in teaching GPs.

Psychiatric involvement in specialist care was widespread. ME/CFS was perceived to be seen as a functional or psychiatric disease in Austria and Finland, and in Belgium psychiatrists were involved in care. In Italy and the UK, multidisciplinary care involved psychiatrists and psychologists, and psychologists were also involved in care in Serbia. A variety of clinical specialties are involved in the specialist care of people with ME/CFS, though are few in number in most countries. Neurologists are most frequently mentioned, in France, Greece, Italy, Latvia, Slovenia, and Spain. In the UK, various specialties are involved, which would include neurology. Internal medicine specialists are mentioned as being involved in Belgium, France, Italy, Latvia, and Spain. In France and Italy, the involvement of immunologists was mentioned. In Italy and Latvia, the involvement of infectious disease specialists was mentioned. Physical medicine involvement was reported from Italy, rehabilitation medicine from Norway, exercise physiology from Poland, and rheumatology from Slovenia and Spain. There was little information volunteered regarding the content of therapy delivered in specialist care, though CBT and GET were reported from Belgium. The involvement of rehabilitation institutions was reported from Norway, and the role of laboratory investigations and psychological examination from Serbia. A multidisciplinary approach was reported as important in specialist care in Italy, Norway, Slovenia and the UK.

3.2.3. Increasing GP Knowledge and Understanding

Respondents were asked if they had any other suggestions as to possible ways to increase the knowledge and understanding of ME/CFS among primary care doctors and/or other healthcare professionals in primary care. Emergent themes from the responses were the inadequacy of current approaches, the need for top-down action to improve the situation, the importance of centres of excellence, the question of who needed training, the content of curricula, and communications strategies. The inadequacy of current approaches was reported from Austria, where it was stated that few healthcare professionals were involved in the care of people with ME/CFS and interest in the topic was largely down to chance. In Finland similarly, the approach was seen as inadequate because it reinforced the belief that ME/CFS was a functional disorder.

Suggested top-down approaches to improve the situation included the suggestion from Austria that such an approach was needed to establish specialist centres, while from the Netherlands there was seen to be a need for consensus and advice in order to establish such centres. From Germany, it was suggested that standard operating procedures were needed Europe-wide or even world-wide. A similar approach was suggested from Latvia through the development of clinical algorithms, while from Poland financial support for diagnosis and therapy was seen as a priority. In France also, the development of specialist centres was seen as a priority, and in Germany such a centre provided information and education for physicians and patients.

The need for education and training about ME/CFS in undergraduate curricula was raised in Greece, and for Belgium it was suggested that curricula should include the neurophysiology of chronic pain and fatigue. The question of who required training was addressed from Germany, and it was suggested that not only GPs but also neurologists, psychiatrists, cardiologists, endocrinologists, rheumatologists, oncologists, infectious disease specialists, and other specialists required training. Suggestions for possible communications strategies included video-talks, flyers in all general practice premises, health 'passports' with basic information on ME/CFS, local and national meetings involving patients' associations, webinars, on-line short courses and Massive Open Online Courses (MOOCs), and information for the general public on overlapping syndromes like fibromyalgia.

3.2.4. Final Comments

Final comments were ventured from six countries. In Austria, the lack of a systematic plan for ME/CFS was stressed, as was the difficulty patients experienced in medical care and also as regards social insurance through dismissal of their illness. From Denmark it was pointed out that the history of ME/CFS could aid understanding of Covid and its sequelae. In Finland, it was felt that, despite current unhelpful attitudes and official opposition, the healthcare system was on the threshold of a change in attitudes, and patience, more research, and effective treatments were needed to bring this about. However, in Slovenia there was less optimism about the future. Finally, the French contribution was philosophical, quoting William 1st of Orange-Nassau: *"Il n'est pas nécessaire d'espérer pour entreprendre, ni de réussir pour persévérer"* ("*It is not necessary to hope to embark on a course of action, nor to succeed in order to persevere*").

4. Discussion

This survey has identified serious concerns among academic and clinical experts on ME/CFS about the state of knowledge and understanding among primary care physicians across a large number of European countries. Overall, based on respondents' experience, it was estimated that around 60% of patients went undiagnosed, and while about two-thirds of patients were estimated to have consulted their GPs and around a quarter were diagnosed by them, the vast majority of GPs were perceived to lack confidence in either diagnosing or managing the condition. About half of patients diagnosed by their GPs were not referred for specialist care, which is not surprising since many countries lack specialist care facilities to which patients could be referred. Disbelief on the part of doctors, or misleading illness attributions, are seen as major factors impeding patients' access to care. There was almost unanimous support for proposed solutions to the problem, in particular including more teaching about ME/CFS in undergraduate medical curricula and in postgraduate training programmes, as well as providing accessible reference material in primary care, and making advice and support available from specialist centres. In order for this to happen, though, there was a perceived need to develop specialist ME/CFS centres in the majority of countries where they currently do not exist at all or only on a very small scale. To achieve this, there was a prior need to develop consensus about their role and their modus operandi, and to identify the necessary resources.

The strength of this study is that, for the first time, it has been possible to conduct a Europe-wide study to elicit the views of ME/CFS experts on the problem of apparent lack of knowledge and understanding of ME/CFS among primary care physicians. Its weakness is that we were unable to survey GPs directly in the participating countries, though there were 8 GP respondents in our sample, and further research is needed to remedy this deficiency. A further weakness is that since our respondents work in the ME/CFS area there may be some bias in responses, particularly given that the survey questions relate mainly to opinions. In addition, it is important to acknowledge that depending on the specific question, respondents may have varied first-hand knowledge/experience on which to base their responses, given that they have different backgrounds and roles with respect to ME/CFS.

Surveys of GPs on this topic have been confined to Ireland [11] and the UK [12–14], and it has been assumed by inference that similar conclusions could be applied more widely across European countries. In all four studies, large minorities of GPs did not accept the existence of ME/CFS as a genuine clinical entity. In the Irish study published in 1997 [11], this proportion was 42% of respondents. The UK studies were from in Scotland in 2005 [12], South Wales in 1991 [13] and South-West England in 2005 [14], and the proportions of respondents not accepting the genuineness of ME/CFS as a diagnosis were 29%, 46% and 28% respectively. We recently carried out a literature review, looking more widely at the question and took into consideration qualitative reports, patient surveys and grey literature, which covered a wider time span and a more extensive geographical area [4]. In particular, our review covered the period from 1946 until 20 August 2020 and included studies from more than 10 countries. It concluded that between a third and a half of GPs lack confidence in diagnosing or managing ME/CFS, with many disputing its existence, while a similar proportion of ME/CFS patients express dissatisfaction with the primary medical care they have received. This has implied an important role for ME/CFS patient associations in the provision of assistance to patients and the dissemination of knowledge about the disease [15]. The findings of our survey are thus broadly in line with the pre-existing scientific literature.

The problem of deficiencies in GP knowledge and understanding of ME/CFS, and an apparent high level of missed and delayed diagnoses, not only impedes attempts to quantify both the prevalence and incidence of the disease, as well as the economic impact of ME/CFS, but is also likely to increase the economic burden attributable to it, since mismanagement of the early stages of the illness is a known risk factor for severe, prolonged disease [16]. Further work to be undertaken should therefore focus, not only on surveys designed to quantify the scale of the problem in different European countries, but also on developing initiatives to improve GP knowledge and understanding, and to facilitate the diagnostic process in primary care.

5. Conclusions

A group of academic and clinical experts on ME/CFS, from nineteen European countries, were strongly of the opinion that lack of knowledge and understanding of the illness among primary care physicians, including disbelief in the very existence of the condition as a genuine clinical entity, was very widespread. As a result, they believed a high proportion had gone undiagnosed. There were seen to be inadequacies in both undergraduate and postgraduate teaching about the illness, and a lack of sources of advice and information for primary care. To address this, ME/CFS specialist centres for referral, support, and advice were needed, but in a majority of countries these either did not exist, or where present, existed only in certain restricted geographical locations. Further research is needed to survey GPs' attitudes in participating countries, and to develop programmes to inform and support healthcare professionals in the primary care sector.

Supplementary Materials: The following are available online at https://www.mdpi.com/article/10.3390/medicina57030208/s1, Questionnaire: Survey of Diagnosis and Management of ME/CFS in Primary Care in Europe.

Author Contributions: Conceptualisation, all authors; methodology, D.F.H.P. and J.C.; validation, all authors.; formal analysis, J.C. and D.F.H.P.; investigation, D.F.H.P. and J.C.; writing—original draft preparation, D.F.H.P. and J.C.; writing—review and editing, J.C., D.F.H.P., J.-D.d.K., U.B., D.A., L.G., E.B., D.A.H., D.T., X.W.-S., and R.M.H.; project administration, D.F.H.P. All authors have read and agreed to the published version of the manuscript.

Funding: This article/publication is based upon work from COST Action "European Network on Myalgic Encephalomyelitis/Chronic Fatigue Syndrome", EUROMENE, supported by COST (European Cooperation in Science and Technology). COST (European Cooperation in Science and Technology) is a funding agency for research and innovation networks. Its actions help connect research initiatives across Europe and enable scientists to grow their ideas by sharing them with their peers. This boosts their research, career and innovation. This research received no external funding. EUROMENE receives funding for networking activities from the COST programme (COST Action 15111), via the COT Association. www.cost.eu. Accessed 25 February 2021.

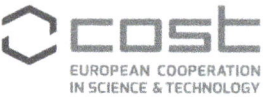
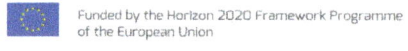

Institutional Review Board Statement: Not applicable.

Informed Consent Statement: Not applicable.

Data Availability Statement: De-identified responses to the survey questions are available on request from the corresponding author.

Conflicts of Interest: The authors declare no conflict of interest.

References

1. Carruthers, B.M.; Jain, A.K.; De Meirleir, K.L.; Peterson, D.L.; Klimas, N.G.; Lerner, A.M.; Bested, A.C.; Flor-Henry, P.; Joshi, P.; Powles, A.P.; et al. Myalgic encephalomyelitis/ chronic fatigue syndrome: Clinical working case definition, diagnostic and treatment protocols. *J. Chronic Fatigue Syndr.* **2003**, *11*, 7–116. [CrossRef]
2. Pheby, D.F.H.; Araja, D.; Berkis, U.; Brenna, E.; Cullinan, J.; de Korwin, J.-D.; Gitto, L.; Hughes, D.A.; Hunter, R.M.; Trepel, D.; et al. The development of a consistent Europe-wide approach to investigating the economic impact of myalgic encephalomyelitis (ME/CFS): A Report from the European Network on ME/CFS (EUROMENE). *Healthcare* **2020**, *8*, 88. [CrossRef] [PubMed]
3. Cullinan, J.; Ni Chomrai, O.; Kindlon, T.; Black, L.; Casey, B. Understanding the economic impact of myalgic encephalomyelitis/chronic fatigue syndrome (ME/CFS) in Ireland: A qualitative study. *HRB Open Res.* **2020**, *3*, 88. [CrossRef]
4. Pheby, D.F.H.; Araja, D.; Berkis, U.; Brenna, E.; Cullinan, J.; de Korwin, J.-D.; Gitto, L.; Hughes, D.A.; Hunter, R.M.; Trepel, D.; et al. A Literature Review of GP Knowledge and Understanding of ME/CFS: A Report from the Socioeconomic Working Group of the European Network on ME/CFS (EUROMENE). *Medicina* **2021**, *57*, 7. [CrossRef] [PubMed]
5. Braun, V.; Clarke, V. Using thematic analysis in psychology. *Qual. Res. Psychol.* **2006**, *3*, 77–101. [CrossRef]
6. The National Academies Press. Available online: https://www.nap.edu/resource/19012/MECFScliniciansguide.pdf (accessed on 17 November 2020).
7. Department of Rehabilitation and Rare Conditions. *National Guidance—Patients with CFS/ME: Investigation, Diagnosis, Treatment, Rehabilitation and Care*; Norwegian Directorate of Health: Oslo, Norway, 2014; (updated 2015).

8. European Alliance of Associations for Rheumatology. Available online: https://www.eular.org (accessed on 17 November 2020).
9. Aggregated Quality Assurance for Systems. Available online: http://aquas-project.eu/ (accessed on 17 November 2020).
10. National Institute for Health and Care Excellence. Available online: https://www.nice.org.uk/guidance/GID-NG10091/documents/draft-guideline (accessed on 17 November 2020).
11. Fitzgibbon, E.J.; Murphy, D.; O'Shea, K.; Kelleher, C. Chronic debilitating fatigue in Irish general practice: A survey of general practitioners' experience. *Br. J. Gen. Pract.* **1997**, *47*, 618–622. [PubMed]
12. Thomas, M.; Smith, A.P. Primary healthcare provision and chronic fatigue syndrome: A survey of patients' and general practitioners' beliefs. *BMC Fam. Pract.* **2005**, *6*, 1–6. [CrossRef] [PubMed]
13. Ho-Yen, D.O.; McNamara, I. General practitioners' experience of the chronic fatigue syndrome. *Br. J. Gen. Pract.* **1991**, *41*, 324–326. [PubMed]
14. Bowen, J.; Pheby, D.; Charlett, A.; McNulty, C. Chronic Fatigue Syndrome: A survey of GPs' attitudes and knowledge. *Fam. Pract.* **2005**, *22*, 389–393. [CrossRef] [PubMed]
15. Ardino, R.B.; Lorusso, L. La sindrome da affaticamento cronico/encefalomielite mialgica: Le caratteristiche della malattia e il ruolo dell'Associazione Malati CFS. *Politiche Sanit.* **2018**, *2*, 91–95.
16. Pheby, D.; Saffron, L. Risk factors for severe ME/CFS. *Biol. Med.* **2009**, *1*, 50–74.

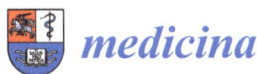

Article

Medical School Education on Myalgic Encephalomyelitis

Nina Muirhead [1,*], John Muirhead [2], Grace Lavery [3] and Ben Marsh [4]

1. Buckinghamshire Healthcare NHS Trust, Amersham Hospital, Whielden Street, Amersham HP7 0JD, UK
2. Boston Consultants Ltd., Solihull, West Midlands B93 8PG, UK; john.muirhead@btinternet.com
3. School of Medicine, Cardiff University Medical School, Neuadd Meirionnydd, Cardiff CF14 4YS, UK; LaveryGE@Cardiff.ac.uk
4. University Hospitals Plymouth NHS Trust, Derriford Hospital, Derriford Road, Plymouth, Devon PL6 8DH, UK; bmarsh@doctors.org.uk
* Correspondence: nina.muirhead@btinternet.com

Abstract: *Background and objectives:* Myalgic Encephalomyelitis/Chronic Fatigue Syndrome (ME/CFS) is a complex multi-system disease with a significant impact on the quality of life of patients and their families, yet the majority of ME/CFS patients go unrecognised or undiagnosed. For two decades, the medical education establishment in the UK has been challenged to remedy these failings, but little has changed. Meanwhile, there has been an exponential increase in biomedical research and an international paradigm shift in the literature, which defines ME/CFS as a multisystem disease, replacing the psychogenic narrative. This study was designed to explore the current UK medical school education on ME/CFS and to identify challenges and opportunities relating to future ME/CFS medical education. *Materials and methods*: A questionnaire, developed under the guidance of the Medical Schools Council, was sent to all 34 UK medical schools to collect data for the academic year 2018–2019. *Results:* Responses were provided by 22 out of a total of 34 medical schools (65%); of these 13/22 (59%) taught ME/CFS, and teaching was led by lecturers from ten medical specialties. Teaching delivery was usually by lecture; discussion, case studies and e-learning were also used. Questions on ME/CFS were included by seven schools in their examinations and three schools reported likely clinical exposure to ME/CFS patients. Two-thirds of respondents were interested in receiving further teaching aids in ME/CFS. None of the schools shared details of their teaching syllabus, so it was not possible to ascertain what the students were being taught. *Conclusions:* This exploratory study reveals inadequacies in medical school teaching on ME/CFS. Many medical schools (64% of respondents) acknowledge the need to update ME/CFS education by expressing an appetite for further educational materials. The General Medical Council (GMC) and Medical Schools Council (MSC) are called upon to use their considerable influence to bring about the appropriate changes to medical school curricula so future doctors can recognise, diagnose and treat ME/CFS. The GMC is urged to consider creating a registered specialty encompassing ME/CFS, post-viral fatigue and long Covid.

Keywords: ME/CFS; education; medical school; teaching; patient safety; NICE Guidelines; Health Act 1983; General Medical Council; GMC; Medical Schools Council; MSC; long Covid

Citation: Muirhead, N.; Muirhead, J.; Lavery, G.; Marsh, B. Medical School Education on Myalgic Encephalomyelitis. *Medicina* **2021**, *57*, 542. https://doi.org/10.3390/medicina57060542

Academic Editors: Derek FH Pheby, Kenneth J. Friedman, Modra Murovska and Pawel Zalewski

Received: 27 March 2021
Accepted: 25 May 2021
Published: 28 May 2021

Publisher's Note: MDPI stays neutral with regard to jurisdictional claims in published maps and institutional affiliations.

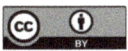

Copyright: © 2021 by the authors. Licensee MDPI, Basel, Switzerland. This article is an open access article distributed under the terms and conditions of the Creative Commons Attribution (CC BY) license (https://creativecommons.org/licenses/by/4.0/).

1. Introduction

Myalgic Encephalomyelitis/Chronic Fatigue Syndrome (ME/CFS) affects around 250,000 patients in the United Kingdom (UK); it is twice as common as other diseases that feature in undergraduate curricula, such as Human Immunodeficiency Virus (HIV) and Multiple Sclerosis (MS). In a recent survey of 4038 ME/CFS patients, 62% stated they are not confident their General Practitioner (GP) understands the condition, and 18% of patients wait longer than six years for a diagnosis [1]. The impact of this disease on patients' wellbeing [2] and quality of life is significant compared with other diseases [3]; yet, between a third and half of GPs lack confidence in acknowledging, diagnosing and managing ME/CFS [4], and the disease is often incorrectly dismissed as psychosomatic [5].

Davenport et al. note that up to 90% of patients are undercounted, undiagnosed and under-treated [6].

ME/CFS is a complex, multi-system disease, diagnosed on a history of significant fatigue impairing function, post exertional malaise, unrefreshing sleep, orthostatic intolerance and/or cognitive impairment [7]. Unlike any other illness and disease, advice to exercise is contraindicated. Exercise in ME/CFS has been shown to result in symptom exacerbation, deterioration of cellular bioenergetics and increased disability. A growing number of recent studies demonstrate abnormalities in cognition, brain changes on spectroscopy scans, lower metabolic energy generation and altered immune system response as well as neuroinflammation following repeated exercise [8].

In 1998, The Chief Medical Officer (CMO) of the UK appointed an Independent Working Group (IWG) to investigate divergent clinical views of ME/CFS and dissatisfaction among patients and patient support groups about the paucity of medical services to deal with this disease [9]. The IWG, which was first to acknowledge the importance of the patient voice, published their report in 2002, recommending that: "improvements are needed in the education and training of doctors, nurses and healthcare professionals, especially in primary care; ME/CFS should be considered as a differential diagnosis and GPs and medical specialists should be able to provide basic guidance after diagnosing this condition".

Given that, 20 years later, patients and patient support groups continue to be dissatisfied with the healthcare community's response to ME/CFS, this study was undertaken to establish the extent to which medical schools are covering this subject in their curricula and, if possible, why healthcare professionals still seemingly struggle to understand ME/CFS or, in some cases, deny the existence of this disease other than as a mental health condition [4,5].

In November 2020, the UK's National Institute for Health and Care Excellence (NICE) issued new draft guidelines [10] on ME/CFS. These acknowledge that ME/CFS is a chronic multi-system medical condition with distinct clinical diagnostic criteria. Echoing the 2002 CFS/ME IWG report, NICE calls for significant improvements in the education of healthcare professionals with greater emphasis on the delivery of evidence-based training to represent current knowledge and the experiences of people with ME/CFS.

The fact that NICE in 2020 makes virtually the same recommendations as the IWG in 2002 demonstrates serious failures in medical education in ME/CFS over the past almost 20 years. European ME/CFS experts have expressed serious concerns about knowledge and understanding among primary care physicians, and survey responses demonstrated that 91% strongly agreed there should be more teaching about ME/CFS in undergraduate medical curricula [11].

This study establishes a baseline of how and to what extent the subject of ME/CFS is being taught in UK medical schools and reveals an exciting opportunity to research the pedagogy surrounding a paradigm shift in a disease narrative. Knowledge of this complex multi-system disease has been hindered by a failure to "move on". We can no longer describe ME/CFS as a figment of patients' unhelpful beliefs, and the burden of ME/CFS in the wake of COVID is an opportunity to learn [12]. Improved medical education on the topic of ME/CFS is urgently required to improve patient safety.

2. Materials and Methods

Approval of the UK Medical Schools Council was obtained before this study was undertaken. The study was advocated by Forward ME, Cardiff University and the CFS/ME research collaborative (CMRC).

A questionnaire comprising ten questions was developed to ascertain the extent of current teaching ME/CFS in all UK medical schools. The Medical Schools Council circulated a request to all 34 schools in the UK in October 2018, this invited schools to participate voluntarily in the study and providing them with a link to the online questionnaire (using

Survey Monkey). E-mail reminders were sent in February and March 2019. Not all schools responded, and some responded anonymously.

3. Results

Out of a total of 34 schools, 22 responded (65%), of which 13 schools taught ME/CFS in their syllabuses (59%), leaving nine schools (41%) that did not.

3.1. Teaching Methodology

As Figure 1 shows, nine schools out of 13 (69%) taught by lecture, five used discussion and/or case study methods and some stated that the "Unrest" video [13] had been shown and formed a part of their discussions. E-Learning, tutorial and handouts were less frequently used. Some schools use more than one method; a single method was used by seven schools, two methods were used by five schools, and four methods were used by one school.

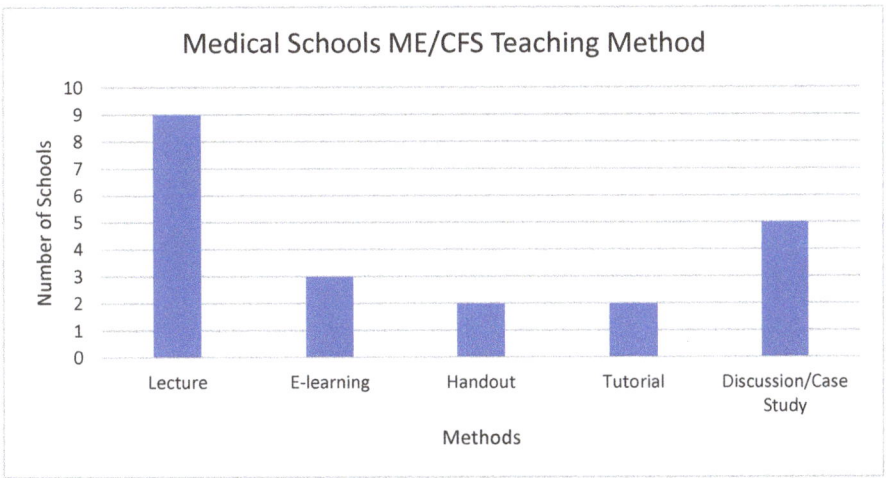

Figure 1. Teaching Methodology. ME/CFS, Myalgic Encephalomyelitis/Chronic Fatigue Syndrome.

3.2. Teaching Duration

The nine medical schools who responded that they do not teach this subject are included here as zero hours (h). Eight schools devoted between 1 and 2 h to teaching ME/CFS; two schools devoted more than 3 h while one school devoted less than 1 h to the subject; one school was unable to quantify teaching duration. See Figure 2.

3.3. Part of Curriculum Covering ME/CFS Teaching

On average, ME/CFS was taught within two parts of the curriculum, described here as medical disciplines. Figure 3 shows that ME/CFS across the 13 schools was taught by at least six different medical disciplines. The most common was General Practice ($n = 5$); followed by Chronic Disease, Neurology and Psychiatry (all $n = 4$), Rheumatology ($n = 3$) and Paediatrics ($n = 1$), details were not provided for 'other'.

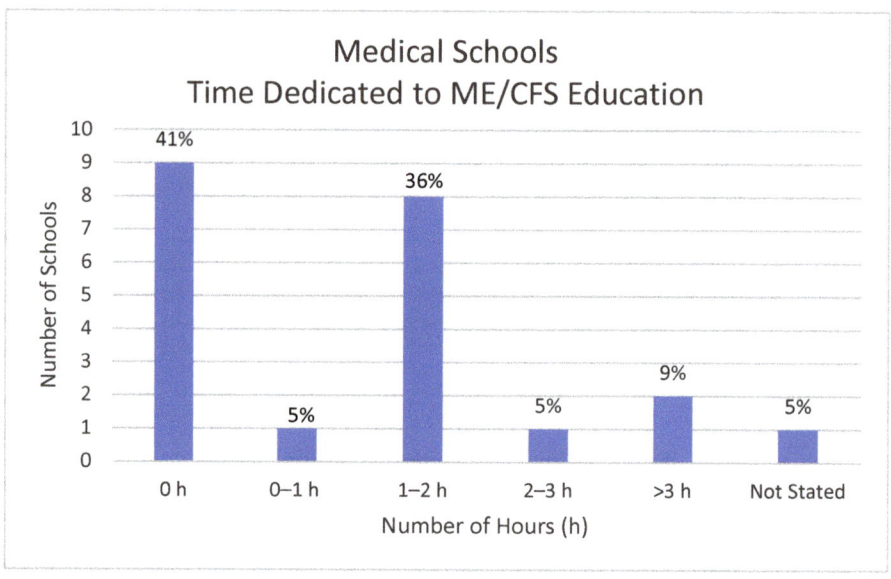

Figure 2. Teaching Duration.

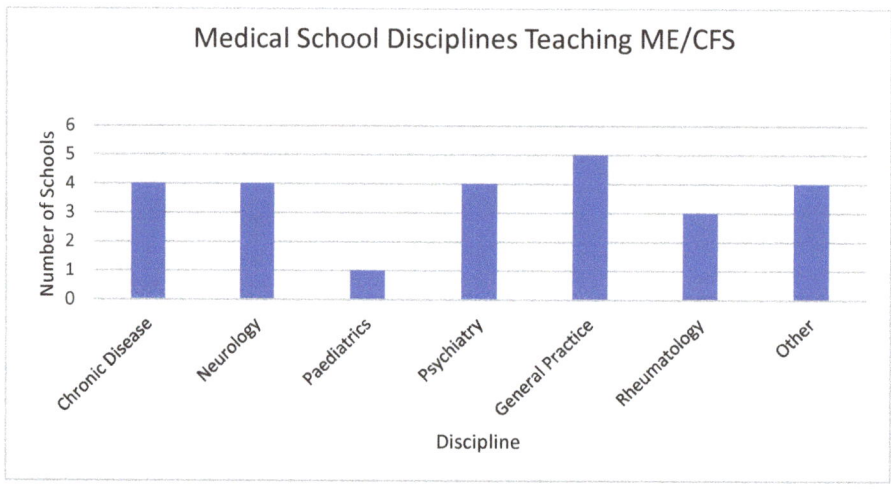

Figure 3. Disciplines Providing ME/CFS Teaching.

3.4. Medical Specialists Leading Teaching of ME/CFS

Various specialists provided the core of teaching for ME/CFS, as shown in Figure 4. Some supplied more than one specialist to teach the subject, seven schools referred to professors or senior teaching fellows without stating their area of expertise, and ten different specialists were listed. Psychiatrists ($n = 5$) and general practitioners ($n = 4$) were the dominant specialists in ME/CFS teaching, followed by rheumatologists ($n = 3$) and neurologists, general medicine and public health specialists ($n = 2$). ME/CFS teaching was also delivered by behavioural scientists, infectious disease specialists, ophthalmologists and clinical communicators (each $n = 1$).

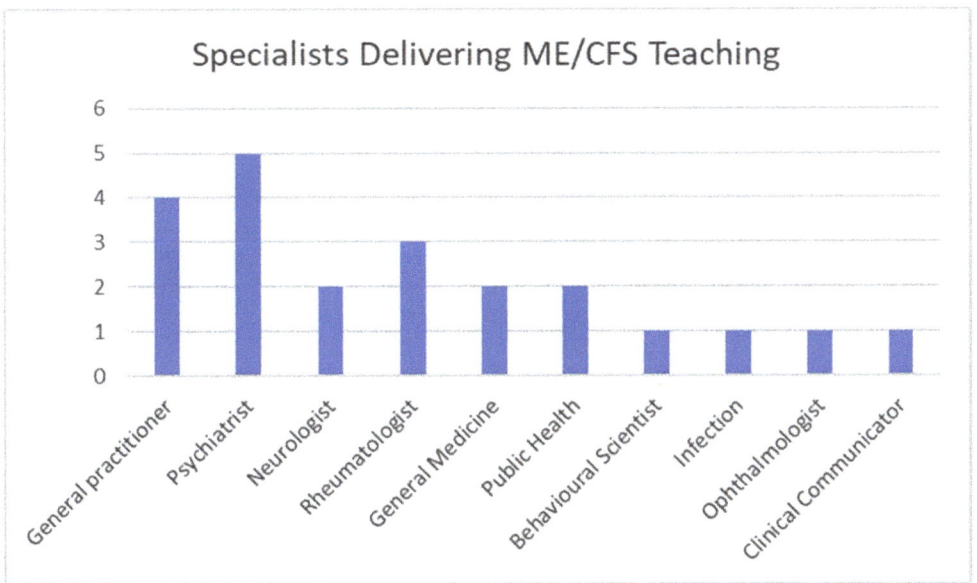

Figure 4. Medical Specialists Leading Teaching of ME/CFS.

3.5. Clinical Contact with ME/CFS Patients

Only three schools out of 13 (23%) responded affirmatively to the inclusion of contact with ME/CFS patients as part of their curriculum.

3.6. Examination Practices

The following results relate to all 22 respondents irrespective of whether they taught ME/CFS in their curriculum. Seven schools out of 22 (32%) stated that they set questions on the subject in their examinations.

3.7. Interest in Further Teaching Aids

Fourteen schools out of 22 (64%) stated that they were interested in receiving further teaching aids on the subject of ME/CFS. Of the nine schools that do not teach ME/CFS, seven schools (78%) said they were interested in receiving further teaching aids or materials.

The most common teaching aid of interest was educational videos of 20–30 min duration, followed by e-learning module of 30–60 min duration or lecture with patient volunteers of 30–60 min duration. Each of these options was preferred by five schools (note: not necessarily by the same five schools). Three schools showed an interest in a lecture of 30–60 min duration. A total of 27 options were chosen by 14 schools, an average of almost two per school; see Figure 5.

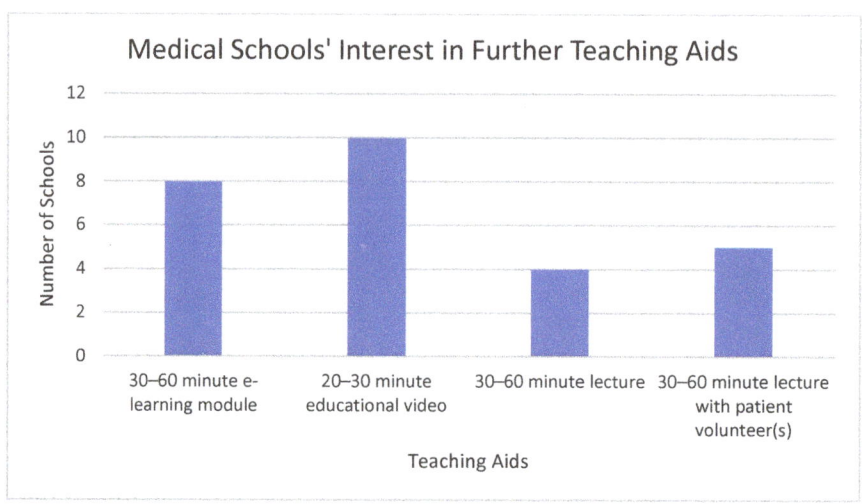

Figure 5. Interest in Further Teaching Aids.

4. Discussion

4.1. Potential Bias

The lack of response from some medical schools could bias the results of this study to over- or under-estimate the current teaching. Given the high level of undiagnosed sufferers with ME/CFS, the low level of confidence among GPs to be able to diagnose this disease [14] and the absence of patient satisfaction in the medical profession [1], it is plausible that 41% of medical schools do not teach ME/CFS. From the data gathered, the actual number of medical schools that cover this topic could lie be between 38% and 73%. This study would be more accurate with more respondents; however, the 64% overall response rate across the UK is greater than the 54% response rate in published research on ME/CFS teaching in medical schools in the United States [15] and other similar UK medical school surveys on ageing [16], neuroanatomy [17] and frailty [18], which had 19/30 (63%), 24/34 (70%) and 25/34 (74%) medical school responses, respectively. Another way of verifying if medical schools have timetabled teaching on ME/CFS would be to explore the existing data, already carried out for the 2014/15 academic year, with 47,258 timetabled teaching events in 25 UK medical schools [19].

4.2. Teaching Time and Methodology

Of the 59% that do cover ME/CFS, teaching duration is usually about one hour, it is not always examinable, and few augment their teaching with exposure to patients with the disease. One to two hours of teaching seems to be very low for a common chronic disease. A typical UK medical student receives 3960 timetabled hours of teaching during their five-year course [19]. Other research showed that the mean amount of core neuroanatomy teaching was 29.3 h [17], and the median time spent on teaching ageing and geriatric medicine was 55.5 h [16].

Another limitation of the study was the lack of information provided on what is being taught, which leaves us unable to comment on the quality and content of the teaching. Indeed, there is a risk that teaching could misrepresent the illness, or categorise it as psychosomatic. Therefore, teaching outdated content could be far worse than not teaching undergraduates about ME/CFS.

Little seems to have changed since a study in 2008 [20], which revealed "Family physicians obtain information about [ME/CFS] from their nonprofessional world which they incorporate into their professional realm". A more recent analysis of ME/CFS teaching in one UK medical school [21] concluded that "Students acquired their knowledge and attitudes largely from informal sources and expressed difficulty understanding [ME/CFS] within a traditional biomedical framework", which is further evidence that education improvements proposed by IWG in 2002 have not been implemented.

4.3. Medical School Curriculum

Respondents were invited to send their syllabuses to enable a more detailed analysis of what is being taught about ME/CFS in their respective schools. A similar study undertaken in the United States revealed only 5.6% of medical schools were judged to deliver sufficient clinical, curricula and research on ME/CFS [15]. However, as no syllabus details were provided by any of the respondents and no explanations given, it was not possible to throw any light on why many healthcare professionals in the UK still struggle to recognise this disease, be able to diagnose it or agree upon suitable management or treatments.

The wide spectrum of medical specialists that are involved in teaching ME/CFS, as revealed by this study, could explain why healthcare professionals remain confused. Whilst ME/CFS is a complex, multi-system disease that will continue to attract a variety of theories at a research level, there is no apparent reason why undergraduate medical students cannot be taught how to recognise and diagnose this disease and be able to make recommendations on its management. The over-riding priority in undergraduate teaching is to improve attitudes towards patients and acknowledgement of genuineness of the patient experience and validity of the disease. Some treatment approaches should have no place in undergraduate teaching; especially those that are shown to cause patient harm, delayed diagnosis and unsafe advice to exercise, as well as outdated assumptions such that dysfunctional beliefs, behaviours or even personality traits that are responsible for causing or perpetuating this illness [22].

4.4. Medical Education Challenges

Despite almost twenty years of stagnation, there is now a substantial need for ME/CFS medical education to "move on", and the 64% interest in further teaching aids is encouraging. It is proposed that the paradigm shift in international understanding of this condition [12], along with a lack of specialists, is an opportunity for medical educators to develop new teaching materials for medical schools to use in a flipped classroom model. Such materials, updated to reflect the latest biomedical science developments and patient perspectives, would transform what is taught. Regarding diagnosis and management of ME/CFS, a recently developed online module [23] has shown that such measures significantly increase confidence in recognising diagnostic criteria. Teaching could be augmented with patient videos [24], webinars and podcast interviews to convey both the complexity and patient experience of this disease. Over the last twenty years, there have been huge strides in online communication, patient support groups on social media and the emergence of the 'patient expert'. The patient voice and perspective are also becoming central to medical education; there is an opportunity for medical schools to work with networks of patients and family members, who have an existing wealth of knowledge, to assist in augmenting future medical education.

This proposal would, furthermore, comply with the new NICE draft guidelines [10], which call for improvements in evidence-based education and training of healthcare professionals and better acknowledgment of the patient experience.

A much broader question arising from this study is why ten different specialties were involved in teaching this subject. Medical education is already moving away from specialty silos, but the secondary care system remains poorly equipped to manage the needs of patients with complex multisystem disease. ME/CFS patients are often cycled through multiple secondary care specialists, with the potential for each hospital visit to exacerbate their symptoms. Apart from the obvious economic drain on resources, the effect on patients and their families may explain why so many patients disconnect from the healthcare system. Clinicians with a knowledge and understanding of ME/CFS could reduce harm, save resources, improve patient care, limit delays to diagnosis and remove misplaced advice to exercise.

Based upon the findings in this study, the UK General Medical Council (GMC), which has statutory responsibilities under the Health Act 1983 for medical education curricula and standards, and the Medical Schools Council (MSC), which represents medical schools in various areas of common interest, are called upon to use their considerable influence to bring about changes in medical schools' undergraduate and postgraduate curricula so that doctors of the future are more capable of recognising, diagnosing and treating ME/CFS. Additionally, the GMC may also wish to consider recognition of ME/CFS as a specialty, which could also encompass post-viral fatigue and the growing subset of long Covid patients who present with ME/CFS.

The authors are not aware of any earlier study into the extent and nature of ME/CFS medical education across UK medical schools. This study therefore provides a baseline as to where UK medical education currently stands in relation to quantity, although it is difficult to comment on the content or quality of teaching in this subject.

4.5. Further Research

While this study is merely exploratory, it provides evidence that further research is required into what is being taught, whether this is evidence based, how it is assessed and how this might affect student knowledge and attitudes towards ME/CFS patients and their families.

Medical students from a variety of UK medical schools could be surveyed on their knowledge and perception of ME/CFS, what they have learned during medical school and how they think the undergraduate curriculum might adapt to improve ME/CFS education. The paradigm shift in ME/CFS literature and guidelines provides new opportunities for medical education research, which could be designed to measure changes in knowledge and/or attitudes and beliefs following updated teaching interventions. The lack of disease recognition and delays to ME/CFS diagnosis are not only a challenge in the UK, but also worldwide; this study and its findings are relevant to international colleagues researching ME/CFS education in other countries.

5. Conclusions

UK medical education in ME/CFS is currently inadequate and appears not to have progressed over the past two decades. Of the medical schools responding, 41% do not teach the subject at all. Data on the 59% of the medical schools that do cover ME/CFS show that education is delivered by multiple medical specialists, mostly by lectures of one-hour duration, which is not always examinable and often takes place without any exposure to patients with the disease.

Differences in beliefs of medical specialists concerning the pathogenesis of ME/CFS need to be set aside in the interest of improving the clarity of what is taught at undergraduate level with renewed focus on diagnosis and management, acknowledging and believing the patient and their families, as well as treating patients with care, empathy and compassion.

Many medical schools (64% of respondents) acknowledge the need to improve education and training of healthcare professionals by expressing a strong appetite for more teaching aids and materials that convey the complexity of this disease. The GMC and MSC are encouraged to use their considerable influence to bring about change in medical schools' curricula in ME/CFS.

Author Contributions: Conceptualization, N.M. and G.L.; methodology, G.L.; software, G.L.; validation, N.M., G.L. and J.M.; formal analysis, G.L.; investigation, N.M.; resources, N.M.; data curation, G.L.; writing—original draft preparation, G.L.; writing—review and editing, N.M., J.M. and B.M.; visualization, J.M.; supervision, J.M.; project administration, N.M. All authors have read and agreed to the published version of the manuscript.

Funding: This research received no external funding. Funds to cover publication costs were received from an anonymous donor.

Institutional Review Board Statement: This study relates to medical education, all answers in relation to Section 4 of the school of medicine board ethics review were 'No' and the data collected do not directly relate to human subjects, material or data (as per the Helsinki Accord) or to living persons (as per the UK Data Protection Act).

Informed Consent Statement: Informed consent was obtained from all schools responding to the study and no respondent has withdrawn informed consent to the Survey Monkey questionnaire.

Data Availability Statement: The anonymous data presented in this study are available on request from the corresponding author.

Acknowledgments: We would like to thank Clare Owen, Jenny Higham and Steve Riley for their interest in this study and the support and guidance of the Medical Schools' Council (MSC) in the creation and dissemination of the questionnaire. We would like to thank Forward ME, the CFS/ME research collaborative (CMRC), Cardiff University, Liz Forty and the medical school's deans and directors who responded to the questionnaire. Finally, we would like to thank the peer reviewers for their time spent giving constructive feedback and support.

Conflicts of Interest: N.M. is a member of Forward ME, chair of the Education working group of the CMRC (CFS/ME research collaborative) and author of the online education module with StudyPRN. B.M. is a patient member of the ME/CFS Priority Setting Partnership steering group. There are no financial conflicts of interest to declare.

References

1. Action for ME Big Survey. Available online: https://www.actionforme.org.uk/uploads/images/2020/02/Big-Survey-Impact-of-ME.pdf (accessed on 24 April 2019).
2. Nacul, L.; Lacerda, E.; Campion, P.; Pheby, D.; Drachler, M.; Leite, J.; Poland, F.; Howe, A.; Fayyaz, S.; Molokhia, M. The functional status and well being of people with myalgic encephalomyelitis/chronic fatigue syndrome and their carers. *BMC Public Health* **2011**, *11*. [CrossRef] [PubMed]
3. Falk Hvidberg, M.; Brinth, L.S.; Olesen, A.V.; Petersen, K.D.; Ehlers, L. The Health-Related Quality of Life for Patients with Myalgic Encephomyelitis / Chronic Fatigue Syndrome (ME/CFS). *PLoS ONE* **2015**, *10*. [CrossRef] [PubMed]
4. Pheby, D.F.H.; Araja, D.; Berkis, U.; Brenna, E.; Cullinan, J.; de Korwin, J.-D.; Gitto, L.; Hughes, D.A.; Hunter, R.M.; Trepel, D.; et al. A Literature Review of GP Knowledge and Understanding of ME/CFS: A Report from the Socioeconomic Working Group of the European Network on ME/CFS (EUROMENE). *Medicina* **2021**, *57*, 7. [CrossRef] [PubMed]
5. Timbol, C.R.; Baraniuk, J.N. Chronic fatigue syndrome in the emergency department. *Open Access Emerg Med.* **2019**, *11*, 15–28. [CrossRef] [PubMed]
6. Davenport, T.E.; Stevens, S.R.; VanNess, J.M.; Stevens, J.; Snellet, C.R. Checking our blind spots: Current status of research evidence summaries in ME/CFS. *Br. J. Sports Med.* **2019**, *53*, 1198. [CrossRef] [PubMed]
7. Strand, E.B.; Nacul, L.; Mengshoel, A.M.; Helland, I.B.; Grabowski, P.; Krumina, A.; Alegre-Martin, J.; Efrim-Budisteanu, M.; Sekulic, S.; Pheby, D.; et al. European Network on ME/CFS (EUROMENE). Myalgic encephalomyelitis/chronic fatigue Syndrome (ME/CFS): Investigating care practices pointed out to disparities in diagnosis and treatment across European Union. *PLoS ONE* **2019**, *14*, e0225995. [CrossRef] [PubMed]
8. Komaroff, A.L. Advances in Understanding the Pathophysiology of Chronic Fatigue Syndrome. *JAMA* **2019**, *322*, 499–500. [CrossRef] [PubMed]
9. CFS/ME Working Group. A Report of the CFS/ME Working Group: Report to the Chief Medical Officer of an Independent Working Group. *London CFS/ME Working Group 2002*. Available online: www.publications.doh.gov.uk/cmo/cfsmereport (accessed on 24 April 2019).
10. Myalgic Encephomyelitis/Chronic Fatigue Syndrome NICE Draft Guidelines (November 2020). Available online: https://www.nice.org.uk/news/article/nice-draft-guidance-addresses-the-continuing-debate-about-the-best-approach-to-the-diagnosis-and-management-of-me-cfs (accessed on 8 December 2020).
11. Cullinan, J.; Pheby, D.F.H.; Araja, D.; Berkis, U.; Brenna, E.; de Korwin, J.-D.; Gitto, L.; Hughes, D.A.; Hunter, R.M.; Trepel, D.; et al. Perceptions of European ME/CFS Experts Concerning Knowledge and Understanding of ME/CFS among Primary Care Physicians in Europe: A Report from the European ME/CFS Research Network (EUROMENE). *Medicina* **2021**, *57*, 208. [CrossRef] [PubMed]
12. Hughes, B.; Lubet, S.; Tuller, D. "Paradigm Lost: Lessons For Long COVID-19 From A Changing Approach To Chronic Fatigue Syndrome, " Health Affairs Blog. *Health Affairs* **2021**. [CrossRef]
13. UNREST. Available online: https://www.unrest.film/ (accessed on 23 May 2021).

14. Thomas, M.A.; Smith, A.P. Primary healthcare provision and Chronic Fatigue Syndrome: A survey of patients' and General Practitioners' beliefs. *BMC Fam. Pract.* **2005**, *6*, 49. [CrossRef] [PubMed]
15. Peterson, T.M.; Peterson, T.W.; Emerson, S.; Regalbuto, E.; Evans, M.A.; Jason, L.A. Coverage of CFS within U.S. Medical Schools. *Univers. J. Public Health* **2013**, *1*, 177–179. [CrossRef]
16. Gordon, A.L.; Blundell, A.; Dhesi, J.K.; Forrester-Paton, C.; Forrester-Paton, J.; Mitchell, H.K.; Bracewell, N.; Mjojo, J.; Masud, T.; Gladman, J.R. UK medical teaching about ageing is improving but there is still work to be done: The Second National Survey of Undergraduate Teaching in Ageing and Geriatric Medicine. *Age Ageing* **2014**, *43*, 293–297. [CrossRef] [PubMed]
17. Edwards-Bailey, A.; Ktayen, H.; Solomou, G.; Bligh, E.; Boyle, A.; Gharooni, A.A.; Lim, G.H.T.; Varma, A.; Standring, S.; Santarius, T.; et al. Neurology and Neurosurgery Students Interest Group (NANSIG). A survey of teaching undergraduate neuroanatomy in the United Kingdom and Ireland. *Br. J. Neurosurg.* **2021**, *8*, 1–6. [CrossRef] [PubMed]
18. Winter, R.; Al-Jawad, M.; Wright, J.; Shrewsbury, D.; Van Marwijk, H.; Johnson, H.; Levett, T. What is meant by "frailty" in undergraduate medical education? A national survey of UK medical schools. *Eur. Geriatr. Med.* **2021**, *12*, 355–362. [CrossRef] [PubMed]
19. Devine, O.P.; Harborne, A.C.; Horsfall, H.L.; Joseph, T.; Marshall-Andon, T.; Samuels, R.; Kearsley, J.W.; Abbas, N.; Baig, H.; Beecham, J.; et al. The Analysis of Teaching of Medical Schools (*AToMS*) survey: An analysis of 47,258 timetabled teaching events in 25 UK medical schools relating to timing, duration, teaching formats, teaching content, and problem-based learning. *BMC Med.* **2020**, *18*, 126. [CrossRef] [PubMed]
20. Carolyn, A. Chew-Graham, Greg Cahill, Christopher Dowrick, Alison Wearden and Sarah Peters. Using Multiple Sources of Knowledge to Reach Clinical Understanding of Chronic Fatigue Syndrome. *Ann. Fam. Med.* **2008**, *6*, 340–348. [CrossRef]
21. Stenhoff, A.L.; Sadreddini, S.; Peters, S.; Wearden, A. Understanding medical students' views of chronic fatigue syndrome: A qualitative study. *J. Health Psychol.* **2015**, *20*, 198–209. [CrossRef] [PubMed]
22. Geraghty, K.J.; Blease, C. Myalgic encephalomyelitis/chronic fatigue syndrome and the biopsychosocial model: A review of patient harm and distress in the medical encounter. *Disabil. Rehabil.* **2019**, *41*, 3092–3102. [CrossRef] [PubMed]
23. Muirhead, N. Myalgic Encephalomyelitis/Chronic Fatigue Syndrome 2020; CPD Module: Published by Diploma MSc in partnership with the University of South. Wales. Available online: https://www.studyprn.com/p/chronic-fatigue-syndrome (accessed on 23 May 2021).
24. Boulton, N.; Biggs, J. Dialogues for a Neglected Illness: Wellcome Public Engagement Award 2018–2021. Collection of Educational Videos on ME/CFS Featuring Medical Professionals, Exercise Scientists, Researchers, Patients and Carers. Available online: https://www.dialogues-mecfs.co.uk/ (accessed on 23 May 2021).

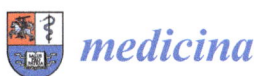

Article

An Audit of UK Hospital Doctors' Knowledge and Experience of Myalgic Encephalomyelitis

Keng Ngee Hng [1,*], Keith Geraghty [2] and Derek F. H. Pheby [3]

[1] ST7 General Internal Medicine and Gastroenterology (Ret), Doctors with M.E., Office 7, 37-39 Shakespeare Street, Southport PR8 5AB, UK
[2] Centre for Primary Care, Division of Population Health, Health Services Research and Primary Care, University of Manchester, Manchester M13 9PL, UK; keithgeraghty2@gmail.com
[3] Society and Health, Buckinghamshire New University, High Wycombe HP11 2JZ, UK; derekpheby@btinternet.com
* Correspondence: hng@doctorswith.me

Abstract: *Background and Objectives:* There is some evidence that knowledge and understanding of ME among doctors is limited. Consequently, an audit study was carried out on a group of hospital doctors attending a training event to establish how much they knew about ME and their attitudes towards it. *Materials and Methods:* Participants at the training event were asked to complete a questionnaire, enquiring about prior knowledge and experience of ME and their approaches to diagnosis and treatment. A total of 44 completed questionnaires were returned. Responses were tabulated, proportions selecting available options determined, 95% confidence limits calculated, and the significance of associations determined by Fisher's exact test. *Results:* Few respondents had any formal teaching on ME, though most had some experience of it. Few knew how to diagnose it and most lacked confidence in managing it. None of the respondents who had had teaching or prior experience of ME considered it a purely physical illness. Overall, 91% of participants believed ME was at least in part psychological. Most participants responded correctly to a series of propositions about the general epidemiology and chronicity of ME. There was little knowledge of definitions of ME, diagnosis, or of clinical manifestations. Understanding about appropriate management was very deficient. Similarly, there was little appreciation of the impact of the disease on daily living or quality of life. Where some doctors expressed confidence diagnosing or managing ME, this was misplaced as they were incorrect on the nature of ME, its diagnostic criteria and its treatment. *Conclusions:* This audit demonstrates that most doctors lack training and clinical expertise in ME. Nevertheless, participants recognised a need for further training and indicated a wish to participate in this. It is strongly recommended that factually correct and up-to-date medical education on ME be made a priority at undergraduate and postgraduate levels. It is also recommended that this audit be repeated following a period of medical education.

Keywords: myalgic encephalomyelitis; chronic fatigue syndrome; ME/CFS; ME; medical education; postgraduate education

1. Introduction

Myalgic encephalomyelitis/chronic fatigue syndrome (ME/CFS) is a complex, multisystem illness defined by its clinical characteristics rather than by its underlying pathology, which remains obscure. These characteristics include severe incapacitating fatigue, post exertional malaise and other symptoms including cognitive dysfunction, orthostatic intolerance, muscle pain and sleep disturbances, with substantial reductions in functional activity and quality of life [1]. The severity, clinical course and duration of the illness are very variable. It most frequently occurs in the 20–50 age group and is more common in women than in men [2–4]. It is frequently asserted that there are some 250,000 sufferers

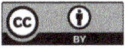

in the UK [5]. If this is correct, there may be in the region of two million patients across Europe and over one million sufferers in the US [6].

A major problem faced by patients with ME/CFS is that many doctors do not recognise the condition as a genuine clinical entity. Disbelief is widespread, and many doctors lack knowledge and understanding of the illness. A recent literature review found that between a third and a half of GPs refused to accept the reality of the condition, that a similar proportion of patients were dissatisfied by the quality of primary care that they had received, and that similar proportions were reported across various geographical locations and had changed little over many years [7]. A study of the perceptions of European ME/CFS specialists concerning GP knowledge and understanding of the illness demonstrated serious misgivings about shortcomings, widely across Europe [8], and this is confirmed by a German paper that reported low satisfaction with medical care and that patients with ME/CFS are medically underserved [9]. It is also consistent with reports that individuals with ME/CFS in the US are medically underserved [10]. It has been argued that ME patients suffer delegitimation of their illness experience through their condition being defined as nonexistent or psychosomatic, leading to their being shamed or stigmatised as having a psychological disorder [11]. A US survey of emergency department attenders with ME/CFS found that 42% of such attenders were dismissed as having psychosomatic problems, and that staff lacked knowledge of the condition [12], while another American survey of patients with ME/CFS and other diseases of the neuro-endocrine-immune system including fibromyalgia and chronic Lyme disease found that 54.4% of respondents reported dissatisfaction with their medical care due to lack of training on the part of their physicians. In total, 71% consulted four or more physicians, and 63% took at least two years, before receiving a correct diagnosis, indicating a need for more education about these conditions in medical school, and for multi-system disease specialty clinics [13].

In this paper, the term ME (myalgic encephalomyelitis) is used in reporting our research findings, rather than the more usual ME/CFS, because that was the term used in the original training session on which this report is based. The term ME/CFS is used in reporting the relevant research literature, as the two terms are effectively synonymous.

As outlined above, it has long been the experience of patients with myalgic encephalomyelitis (ME) that their doctors have little knowledge and understanding of the condition and are largely unable to help. Worse, many report that their doctors do not believe their illness is real, resulting in lack of medical support. Examination of sample medical curricula in 2018 in the UK confirmed that ME was not in the syllabus at either undergraduate or postgraduate levels, and this is consistent with a report demonstrating serious inadequacies in undergraduate teaching about ME/CFS, in which 64% of responding medical schools acknowledged the need for improvement [14], and also with an earlier report from the US in which only 28% of responding medical schools met an adequate standard of coverage in their curricula [15].

It is therefore quite conceivable that patients' widely reported impressions are well founded, so to investigate this, we undertook an ad hoc opportunistic audit of hospital doctors' knowledge and understanding. This study appears to be the first attempt in the United Kingdom to assess knowledge and understanding of ME among a group of hospital doctors.

2. Methods

In 2018, we conducted an audit of hospital doctors attending a training event. Traditionally, response rates from physician-knowledge surveys are often low. As such, approaching doctors in person presented an informal setting and rapid way to gather responses.

All physicians in the region who were training in general internal medicine at ST3-8 level were required to attend this mandatory training day. Only those who were on-call or on leave would have been excused. There were in the region of one hundred attendees. Most of these GIM trainees were also training in another medical specialty, such as cardiology, respiratory medicine, endocrinology, nephrology, gastroenterology, neurology, rheumatology, haematology, dermatology, infectious diseases, palliative care, oncology, geriatrics or acute medicine.

This particular training day was unique in that a short introductory lecture on ME was scheduled. Other lectures were on unrelated topics. We developed a pre-planned questionnaire with input from experts in the field (Appendix A). These were handed out and returned on the same day. It was specified that answers should be based on participants' knowledge before the lecture on ME. The questionnaire asked about prior knowledge and experience of ME, including previous education, confidence in managing the condition, and understanding of its epidemiology and pattern of chronicity. It also enquired about participants' approaches to diagnosis and management, the perceived impact of the illness, and whether or not participants were interested in having additional education on ME.

A total of 44 completed questionnaires were returned. Responses were tabulated, proportions selecting available options determined, and 95% confidence limits calculated. Where relevant, associations between responses were presented in 2 × 2 tables, and the significance of such associations determined by Fisher's exact test.

3. Results

3.1. Prior Teaching and Experience of ME, Doctors' Confidence

Only 27% of respondents reported having previously received formal teaching on ME. Most of this was in the form of undergraduate or postgraduate lectures. 70% reported having had some experience of ME patients. This was in GP clinics, specialty clinics, or in hospitals. Twenty-three percent had had neither formal teaching on ME nor any experience of it.

A total of 89% of respondents admitted not knowing how to diagnose ME, which is very unsatisfactory. 93% did not feel confident dealing with ME patients. Only two respondents (5%) said they knew how to diagnose ME and also felt confident managing ME patients. However, one of them annotated "ish" against the answers indicating he/she was not fully confident, and the other annotated "If by ME chronic fatigue syndrome is meant," indicating he/she did not understand the difference between the terms. These results are summarised in Table 1.

Table 1. Prior teaching and experience of ME, confidence to diagnose and manage it.

	Number of Respondents	Responding 'Yes' Number	Responding 'Yes' % Total	95% Confidence Interval
Have received some formal teaching on ME	44	12	37.9	16.3–41.9
Have seen some ME patients	44	31	70.5	55.8–81,8
I know how to diagnose ME	44	5	11.4	5.0–24.0
I feel confident dealing with ME patients	44	3	6.8	2.4–18.2

There was a significant association between being confident about diagnosing ME and feeling confident about dealing with ME patients ($p = 0.029$). These results are summarised in Table 2.

Table 2. Relationship between confidence in diagnosing ME and confidence in managing it.

	I Feel Confident Dealing with ME Patients		Total
I know how to diagnose ME	Yes	No	
Yes	2	3	5
No	1	38	39
Total	3	41	44

by Fisher's exact test) = 0.029.

Doctors' confidence was cross tabulated against key indicators of understanding, diagnostic ability and management. Of the six respondents who felt they knew how to diagnose ME or felt confident dealing with ME patients (i.e., five who said they knew how to diagnose ME and three who said they felt confident dealing with ME patients, or six in total as two were confident in both), all thought ME was partly or wholly psychological, and none selected the right combination of diagnostic criteria. All thought ME could be treated with graded exercise therapy (GET) and four thought it could be treated with cognitive behavioural therapy (CBT) to help patients get out of the sick role. Therefore, it appears that the greater the doctor's confidence, the worse was his or her understanding of the illness and diagnostic skill. These observations are interesting, though they do not reach statistical significance since numbers were small.

On the central question of whether or not ME was thought to be entirely or in part a psychological or psychosomatic illness, respondents were given the options of psychological/psychosomatic or physical illness, and they were allowed to tick both (i.e., with a substantial psychological element). The correct answer, selected by only four respondents (9.1%), was a physical illness only, while 36 out of the 44 respondents (81.8%) believed ME was partly or entirely psychological.

The responses regarding whether participants had received prior teaching on ME or had seen ME patients were cross tabulated against responses to the question as to whether ME was thought to be a physical illness or at least in part psychological. All four respondents who understood that ME is a real, physical illness are among the ten who had received no formal teaching on ME, nor ever seen any ME patients (i.e., 40%), compared to 0% of respondents who had received previous formal teaching on ME or had seen any ME patients (Table 3). This was a very strong association ($p = 0.0015$). This begs the question as to what they were being taught on ME, and what they were told by their colleagues when they came across ME patients in the clinical setting.

Table 3. Effect of previous teaching or experience on understanding of ME.

	Thinks ME Is at Least in Part Psychological	Knows ME Is Physical	Total
Had received teaching on ME or has seen some ME patients	31	0	34 (3 don't know)
Not had teaching on ME and not seen any ME patients	5	4	10 (1 don't know)
Total	36	4	44

p (by Fisher's exact test) = 0.0002.

3.2. General Epidemiology

Respondents performed fairly well on questions relating to the general epidemiology and chronicity of the illness. A series of propositions were put to respondents, who were asked to identify whether they were true or false. Correct responses ranged from 56.8% to 97.7% (average 82.3%). However, it was a matter of some concern that around a third of respondents considered the statement "children with ME miss school because their parents support their sick role and this should be discouraged" to be correct (Table 4).

Table 4. Responses to propositions regarding the nature and epidemiology of ME.

Proposition	Correct Answer	Number of Respondents	Respondents Giving Correct Answer		95% Confidence Interval (%)
			Number	% Total	
We have national guidelines on ME.	True	44	25	56.8	42.2–70.3
ME is rare.	False	44	31	70.5	55.8–82.8
ME affects more women than men.	True	44	40	90.9	78.8–96.4
ME can affect children.	True	44	36	81.8	68.0–90.4
ME resolves within 6 months.	False	44	41	93.2	81.8–97.7
ME causes chronic disability.	True	44	42	95.5	84.9–98.7
If they do not improve it's because they are not trying hard enough.	False	44	40	90.9	78.8–96.4
Children with ME can miss long periods of school.	True	44	43	97.7	88.2–99.6
Children with ME miss school because their parents support their sick role and this should be discouraged.	False	44	28	63.6	48.9–76.2

3.3. Definitions and Clinical Understanding

Respondents performed poorly on overall categorisation, with 66% of them wrongly believing that ME belonged in the class of illness called medically unexplained symptoms and 59% of them not knowing the difference between ME, chronic fatigue syndrome and post viral fatigue syndrome. On the manifestations and impact of the illness, there was widespread appreciation that the illness was painful, but it was not generally appreciated that ME could affect all body systems and could be lethal. Nor was it appreciated that ME can be severely disabling. The approach to management was equally misguided, with only two respondents (4.5%) disagreeing with the false proposition that "patients need to think positive and build up their strength with exercise or gradually increasing activity." (Table 5).

3.4. Diagnostic Process and Diagnostic Criteria

Respondents were asked which part of the process was the most important in making a diagnosis of ME, which is a careful history. In answer to "ME is mainly diagnosed with ... ", 40 (90.9%) of our 44 participants selected a careful history, of which 31 (70.5%) also selected physical examination and/or investigations, and 17 (39%) also selected a psychiatric history. Thus, only 23 (52.3%) participants selected the correct combination of a careful history without a psychiatric history, with or without physical examination or investigations. (Table 6).

Respondents were then presented with a number of propositions regarding clinical features required for a diagnosis of ME to be made. Some of these propositions were true and some were false. Thus, 38 participants (86.3%; 95% confidence interval: 73.3–93.6%) believed, erroneously, that six months of fatigue was necessary for diagnosis. A significant 39% of respondents did not realise that post exertional malaise is an essential requirement for the diagnosis of ME. Psychiatric features are not part of the diagnosis, but only 24 of 44 respondents recognised this (54.5%; 95% confidence interval 40.1–68.3). A total of 17 participants selected psychiatric symptoms, signs of anxiety or depression, or both, and three participants failed to select any answer. Only six of 44 respondents selected the correct combination of features (i.e., post exertional malaise and symptoms from multiple systems, without psychiatric features (i.e., 13.6%; 95% confidence interval 6.4–26.7). The results are detailed in Table 7.

3.5. Disability, Impact and Clinical Manifestations of ME

When asked about the level of disability suffered by ME patients, 64% of respondents under-estimated the level of disability compared to other common or serious illnesses (Table 8). Only 36% of respondents correctly recognised that ME patients can be as disabled as patients with all seven of the other conditions named. These are multiple sclerosis, cancer, advanced HIV, chronic respiratory disease, end stage renal failure, heart failure and a broken leg. In total, 45% of respondents over-estimated the ability of ME patients to stay in work (Table 5). The vast majority (97.7%, 43 out of 44, 95% confidence interval 88.2–99.6%) did, however, recognise that children with ME can miss long periods of school (Table 4). The majority of respondents (79.6%, 35 out of 44, 95% confidence interval 65.5–88.9%) indicated that ME is painful but only a quarter of respondents (25.0%, 11 out of 44, 95% confidence interval 14.6–39.4%) knew that ME can kill (Table 5).

Table 5. Respondents' knowledge of definitions and clinical understanding.

Question	Correct Answer	Number of Respondents	Respondents Giving Correct Answer		95% Confidence Interval (%)
			Number	% Total	
Is ME is a physical illness or psychological?	Physical	44	4	9.1	3.6–21.1
ME belongs in the class of illness called Medically Unexplained Symptoms. True or false?	False	44	12	27.3	16.3–41.9
Myalgic Encephalomyelitis, Chronic Fatigue Syndrome and Post Viral Fatigue Syndrome all mean the same thing. True or false?	False	44	18	18.2	27.7–55.6
ME is painful. True or false?	True	44	35	79.5	65.5–88.9
ME is as disabling as: MS, cancer, advanced HIV, chronic respiratory disease, end stage renal failure, heart failure, broken leg. True or false?	All 7 conditions	44	16	36.4	23.7–51.3
Which of the following body systems can ME affect? Nervous system, cardiovascular system, endocrine system, musculoskeletal system, gastrointestinal system, immune system, cellular metabolism.	All 7 body systems	44	13	29.5	18.2–44.2
What proportion of ME patients is able to work?	Less than half	44	22	50.0	35.8–64.2
ME doesn't kill. True or false?	False	44	11	25.0	14.6–39.4
Patients need to think positive and build up their strength with exercise or gradually increasing activity. True or false?	False	44	2	4.5	1.2–15.4

Table 6. Respondents' views on diagnostic methods.

	Correct Answer	Number of Respondents	Respondents Making Correct Choice		95% Confidence Interval
			Number	% Total	
ME is mainly diagnosed with: (multiple options allowed)					
Careful history	Yes	44	40	90.9	78.8–96.4
Psychiatric history	No	44	27	61.4	46.6–74.3
Right combination (careful history without psychiatric history)		44	23	52.3	37.9–67.3

Table 7. Diagnostic requirements.

Proposition	True or False?	Number of Respondents	Correct Answer Selected?		95% Confidence Interval
			Number	% Total	
The diagnosis of ME requires:					
• Fatigue lasting at least 6 months	False	44	3	6.8	2.4–18.2
• Psychiatric symptoms (i)	False	44	30	68.2	53.4–80.9
• Post Exertional Malaise (PEM)	True	44	27	61.4	46.6–74.3
• Symptoms from multiple systems	True	44	31	70.5	55.8–81.8
• Signs of anxiety or depression (ii)	False	44	26	59.1	44.4–72.3
• Physical signs	False	44	28	63.6	48.9–76.2
Combination		Number of Respondents	This Combination Selected?		95% Confidence Interval
			Number	% Total	
Don't know (i.e., no feature selected)		44	3	6.8	2.4–18.2
Any psychiatric feature-(i) or (ii) selected		44	17	38.6	25.7–53.4
Correct combination (PEM, symptoms from multiple systems, no psychiatric features)		44	6	13.6	6.4–26.7

Table 8. The impact of ME—Perceived level of disability.

	Total Respondents	Respondents Selecting:		95% Confidence Interval
		Number	% Total	
Question: Patients with ME can be as disabled as patients with (viz. multiple sclerosis, cancer, advanced HIV, chronic respiratory disease, end stage renal failure, heart failure, broken leg).				
Number of conditions in respect of which ME is regarded as being as disabling or more so:				
0	44	4	9.1	3.6–21.2
1	44	11	25.0	14.6–39.4
2	44	3	6.8	2.4–18.2
3	44	4	9.1	3.6–21.2
4	44	3	6.8	2.4–18.2
5	44	0	0.0	-
6	44	3	6.8	2.4–18.2
All 7 (correct answer)	44	16	36.4	23.8–52.3
<7 (incorrect)	44	28	63.6	48.9–76.2

Of our respondents, 70% did not realise the breadth of manifestations and symptoms of ME (Tables 5 and 9). Seven body systems very commonly affected in ME were listed, and only 30% of respondents indicated that ME can affect all seven body systems, i.e., the nervous system, the cardiovascular system, the endocrine system, the musculoskeletal system, the gastrointestinal system, the immune system and cellular metabolism. These results are summarised in Table 9 below:

Table 9. The Impact of ME—Perceived extent of involvement of body systems.

	Total Respondents	Respondents Selecting:		95% Confidence Interval
		Number	% Total	
Question: ME can affect . . . (nervous system, cardiovascular system, endocrine system, musculoskeletal system, gastrointestinal system, immune system, cellular metabolism)				
Number of body systems thought to be capable of being affected by ME:				
0	44	4	9.1	3.6–21.2
1	44	1	2.3	0.4–11.8
2	44	3	6.8	2.4–18.2
3	44	7	15.9	7.9–29.4
4	44	4	9.1	3.6–21.2
5	44	4	9.1	3.6–21.2
6	44	8	18.2	9.5–32.0
All 7 (correct answer)	44	13	29.6	18.2–44.2
<7 (incorrect)	44	31	70.5	55.8–81.8

3.6. Treatment

Almost all (98%) respondents believed that graded exercise therapy (GET) is a suitable treatment for ME. In addition, 61% believed that cognitive behavioural therapy (CBT), designed to assist patients to rethink their illness attributions and abandon the sick role, is also a suitable treatment. These results are summarised in Table 10.

Table 10. Respondents' opinions regarding specific therapies for ME.

Treatment Options (Not Mutually Exclusive)	Number of Respondents	Respondents Selecting Treatment		95% Confidence Interval
		Number	% Total	
Inappropriate therapies:				
Graded exercise therapy	44	43	97.7	88.2–99.6
Cognitive behaviour therapy	44	27	62.8	47.9–75.6
Any harmful treatment selected (GET or CBT)	44	43	97.7	88.2–99.6
Other therapies:				
Antivirals	44	3	7.0	2.4–18.6
Vitamin supplements	44	7	16.3	8.1–30.0

3.7. Interest in Further Education on ME

The response to this was very positive. Participants were asked to respond to the statement: "After today's introductory lecture, I would like further more in-depth teaching on Myalgic Encephalomyelitis." A total of 36 doctors answered this question. The lower response rate may relate to having had to wait until after they had had the lecture before answering. Of those who responded, 20 said Yes, 3 said No, and 13 were Neutral. Therefore, only a very small minority (8%) did not want further teaching on ME. Over half of the respondents (56%) would welcome further education on ME, and the rest (36%) are presumably amenable to it, making a total of 92% who would be amenable to further education on ME. These results are summarised in Table 11.

Table 11. Interest in further education on ME.

	Answer Options	Total Respondents	Number of Respondents Selecting Response		95% Confidence Interval (%)
			Number	% Total	
Participants requesting further in-depth teaching on Myalgic Encephalomyelitis	Yes	36	20	55.6	39.6–70.5
	Undecided	36	13	36.1	22.5–52.4
	No	36	3	8.3	2.9–23.6

3.8. Summary of Results

Overall, there was little knowledge of definitions of ME, or of its clinical manifestations and impact, and equally little knowledge of appropriate management of the condition, with the consequence that patients with ME were likely to have imposed on them treatment that is at best ineffective and at worst damaging, like graded exercise therapy. Diagnosis was equally problematic, with little understanding of required clinical features, in particular the essential symptom of post exertional malaise.

The effect of all this ignorance is to put patients at risk, but a saving grace is the very positive response of participants to the prospect of further education on ME.

This audit study captures baseline data, which sadly confirms patients' perception that their doctors know little about ME and that many do not even believe it is real. By measuring participants' responses against the reasonable expectation that all participants should get all answers correct, it enables us to highlight errors in basic fundamental understanding, such as the misconception that ME is partly or wholly psychological or psychosomatic. It also enables the highlighting of large deficiencies in education and clinical knowledge on ME, as well as dangerous prevailing ideas on treatment.

4. Discussion

4.1. Prior Teaching, Experience and Confidence Level

A minority of respondents had had formal teaching on ME, though most had had some experience of ME patients. Despite this, few knew how to diagnose ME, and nearly all lacked confidence in dealing with ME patients.

The majority of participants (82%) believed that ME is at least in part psychological, and it is a matter of concern that 91% of respondents who had had teaching or experience of ME thought this, when only 50% of those without such experience thought so. This places a considerable question mark over the content of such teaching and experience, since those who had received it more frequently expressed erroneous views about ME than those who had not.

It is also of particular note that doctors who expressed confidence in diagnosing ME or in dealing with ME patients were universally wrong in their understanding of the nature of ME, its diagnostic criteria, and its treatment. All six of them (100%) thought ME was at least in part psychological/psychosomatic, failed to select the right combination of diagnostic features, and thought ME could be treated with extremely hazardous graded exercise therapy.

4.2. Making the Diagnosis

Myalgic encephalomyelitis is mainly diagnosed with a careful and thorough history. Physical examination and appropriate investigations are performed to rule out other pathology, but the diagnosis is made on the presence of post exertional malaise (PEM) and other symptoms, as identified in the history. While certain physical signs can be present, such as orthostatic changes in blood pressure or heart rate, pallor, and a multitude of neurological signs including tremor, incoordination, ataxia, photophobia, muscle weakness, fatiguability, fasciculations and myopathic facies, they are, like everything else in ME, variable and fluctuating.

On diagnostic criteria, 38 participants (86.3%; 95% confidence interval: 73.3–93.6%) believed six months of fatigue is necessary for diagnosis. This is contrary to the MYAL-GIC ENCEPHALOMYELITIS—Adult and Paediatric: International Consensus Primer for Medical Practitioners, which allows one to make a positive diagnosis based on symptom constellation, without having to wait six months [16]. This is important as it allows timely diagnosis and management. Diagnostic delay and lack of crucial medical advice in the early part of the illness frequently results in significant harm and increased severity of illness.

A total of 39% of respondents incorrectly believed that psychiatric symptoms, or signs of anxiety or depression, were necessary for a diagnosis of ME, in line with the misconception that ME is a psychological or psychosomatic problem. None of the respondents were in fact psychiatrists, psychologists or psychotherapists. These doctors could misdiagnose depression or other mental health problems as ME, depriving patients of necessary treatment. They could also miss the diagnosis of ME, depriving patients of crucial recognition, medical advice and support. Of course, where ME and depression coexist, both need to be recognised and appropriately managed. It should be noted that comorbid depression is as common in other chronic diseases such as multiple sclerosis as it is in ME [17].

The same proportion did not realise that an essential requirement for diagnosis is post exertional malaise, which is an exacerbation of the symptoms of ME/CFS after exertion, which may be physical or cognitive [16,18]. It is recognised as the defining characteristic of ME/CFS [19], can persist for prolonged periods [20], and is unrelieved by sleep or rest [21]. These doctors could erroneously diagnose ME while missing other pathologies. Only 13.6% of participants chose the correct combination of post exertional malaise and symptoms from multiple systems, without psychiatric features, as being necessary to make the diagnosis.

4.3. Clinical Understanding

Most participants responded correctly to a series of propositions on the general epidemiology of ME, and nearly all respondents recognised that children with ME can miss long periods of school. However, it is a matter of concern that around a third of respondents considered the statement "children with ME miss school because their parents support their sick role and this should be discouraged" to be correct. ME/CFS is the single most common cause of long-term school absence for medical reasons in England [22], and this has been shown to be due to physical incapacity rather than anxiety [23]. Given the high incidence of unjustified child protection and safeguarding proceedings instigated against families of children with ME, often with disastrous consequences to the health of these children, this misconception is of grave concern [24].

On the overall categorization of ME, most respondents thought that ME belonged in the class of illness called medically unexplained symptoms. This is an umbrella term that encompasses many conditions once thought to be "functional", or without a pathological basis, and for which psychological treatments were advised [25]. However, the underlying pathology is steadily being elucidated, so the condition can no longer be regarded as being medically unexplained [26].

There were also considerable misapprehensions among the participants regarding the level of disability suffered by ME patients, with approximately two-thirds of all respondents under-estimating the level of disability among people with ME, compared to other common or serious illnesses. Only just over a third of participants correctly recognised that ME patients can be as disabled as patients with all seven of the other conditions named. These are multiple sclerosis, cancer, advanced HIV, chronic respiratory disease, end stage renal failure, heart failure and a broken leg. All these conditions have previously been identified in the literature or described by expert clinicians as having comparable levels of disability to ME, both in adults [18,27–29] and in children [30–32].

Similarly, nearly half of the respondents over-estimated the ability of ME patients to stay in work, even though research indicates that loss of employment among people with ME/CFS is widespread. A Spanish community-based study found that 63% of ME/CFS patients were unable to work [33], while the comparable percentage in a large UK study, using data from the UK CFS/ME National Outcomes Database, was 50.1% [34]. This British study found that 998 (50.1%) of 1991 patients had lost employment because of illness. Extrapolation suggested the impact of ME/CFS on employment was responsible for UK annual productivity costs of £102.2 million (range £75.5–£128.9 million) [23]. Another Spanish report from the same research group found that 636 of 1116 people with ME/CFS were unemployed (58.6%) [35], while a Norwegian study of hospital patients [36] found that 43 (45%) of 92 were unemployed. Vink and Vink-Niese in a wide-ranging review of the literature on employment in ME/CFS reported both these studies. They also reported a series of studies by national patient organisations that came to similar conclusions, and additionally demonstrated that where patients were able to continue to work, most had to make adjustments to the nature and duration of the work that they undertook [37].

Most participants appreciated that ME is painful. However, only 25% knew that ME can kill, though research indicates increased mortality from cardiovascular disease, cancer and suicide [38,39], the latter being particularly tragic [40,41]. A recent paper has pointed out that there is a considerable risk to life from malnutrition among patients with very severe ME [42]. About two-thirds of participants did not appreciate the wide range of symptoms occurring in ME patients (Tables 5 and 9). Seven body systems very commonly affected in ME were listed, and only 30% of respondents indicated that ME can affect all seven body systems (see Table 9). These are the nervous system, the cardiovascular system, the endocrine system, the musculoskeletal system, the gastrointestinal system, the immune system and cellular metabolism [20]. The International Consensus Panel made clear the multi-system nature of the condition in 2012 [16], and this was reiterated in the IACFS/ME (International Association for CFS/ME) Primer for Clinical Practitioners in 2014 [19] and the Institute of Medicine case definition of 2015 [18]. This is applicable to children and adolescents [21] as well as adults.

4.4. Hazardous Treatments

The responses regarding treatment were a matter of great concern, with nearly all participants (98%) believing that graded exercise therapy (GET) is a suitable treatment for ME (Table 10), while 61% believed that cognitive behavioural therapy (CBT), designed to help patients get out of the sick role and to rethink their illness beliefs, is also an appropriate treatment. It is salutary to reflect on why such misconceptions have become so widespread. Much of this may have been shaped by previous research on ME, particularly that promoting the cognitive-behavioural model of ME/CFS. Thus, one study concluded that behavioural, cognitive and affective factors had a role in prolonging fatigue and that therefore these factors should be the focus of treatment [43], but later work concluded that this model lacked credibility as it had inadequate supporting evidence and did not address the increasing evidence of pathophysiological changes in ME/CFS [44].

As outlined above, ME is a serious and debilitating multi-system neuro-immune condition. As such, CBT, attempting to convince patients that they are not actually sick, is no more a useful treatment than it is for cancer [45,46]. Instead, by convincing patients that they are not ill, it is likely to cause harm, for patients who over-exert themselves may suffer a deterioration in their illness. Even without the behavioural effects, just travelling to and sitting through unhelpful CBT sessions can be harmful to ME patients, whose energy is in short supply and who already struggle to manage minimum essential daily activities. Patient evidence suggest adverse outcomes occur in 20% of cases treated with CBT [47].

Many of the participants (98%) believed that graded exercise therapy (GET) was a suitable treatment for ME, perhaps not a surprise given that NICE UK included it as a recommended treatment in 2007. However, many doctors may not be aware of how unpopular this treatment is among ME patients [48], or that it can lead to worsening of symptoms for some patients with ME, and there is in any event increasing evidence that such treatment is ineffective and can be damaging in patients of all levels of severity [19]. The evidence base for GET use has revealed that exercise therapy is not an effective treatment for ME. Reanalysis of the largest GET trial, the PACE trial, revealed recovery rates close to just 10% (little above natural recovery rates), rather than the 22% recovery rate reported by the PACE trial authors [49]. Adverse effects in the trial were dismissed as a consequence of inappropriate implementation by inexperienced practitioners [45]. A 2019 Cochrane review considered eight reports on the use of exercise therapy on ME in adults and concluded that such treatment probably had a positive effect on fatigue [50]. However, a subsequent reanalysis found that this analysis was flawed due to the non-reporting of harms in the reports initially studied, and that in fact GET appeared to not only be ineffective but also unsafe [47].

Similarly, a 2011 review of eight surveys found that 51% of survey respondents had reported that GET had made their health worse [51]. An analysis of primary and secondary surveys found that 54–74% of patients responded negatively to GET [52]. The UK ME Association reported this finding, and advised that GET should play no part in activity management advice in ME. They also recommended that CBT, which also impacted negatively on outcomes, should be avoided in ME/CFS [53]. An American report by experienced clinicians concluded that not only did GET fail to improve function, but that it could provoke the hallmark ME symptom of post exertional malaise (PEM) [48]. CBT, similarly, was found to be of benefit to only 8–35% of patients [48], which supports the earlier view of the authors of the IACFS/ME *Primer for Clinical Practitioners* that the belief that CBT and GET can cure ME "is not supported by post-intervention outcome data" [19].

A report from the Centers for Disease Control and Prevention concluded that patients with ME cannot tolerate vigorous aerobic exercise regimes [54], and the evidence on

GET continues to accumulate. A recent survey of the experience of ME patients in Italy, Latvia and the UK found that, while none of the Italian or Latvian participants reported having experienced GET, in the UK out of 70 respondents who had had GET, only 1 (1.4%) reported that it had been effective [55]. For these reasons, of ineffectiveness, distress to patients, and risk of harmful sequelae, the National Academy of Medicine in the US no longer recommends GET for ME [18], and it is noteworthy that the draft guideline from NICE in the UK on ME/CFS recommends that GET, or indeed any therapy based on fixed incremental increases in physical activity or exercise, or any programme founded on the supposition that deconditioning is the cause of ME, should no longer be offered to patients [56].

4.5. The Urgent Need and Appetite for Medical Education

The results of this study make a strong case for putting Myalgic Encephalomyelitis into formal medical education in the UK. We would argue that with ME being more than twice as common as multiple sclerosis [4] and as debilitating or worse than most other chronic illnesses such as heart failure or end stage renal disease [18,27–29] and being the single greatest cause of long term school absence in children [22], the medical profession cannot afford to be so ignorant, and so misinformed, about ME. This becomes even more evident when considering the hazards of currently favoured therapies, as outlined above, in conjunction with the rising costs of clinical negligence [52]. The costs to the UK economy are also considerable, with direct costs estimated at £3.3 billion per annum to the country [57] and productivity costs at £102.2 million per annum [34].

Doctors need to be able to recognise ME regardless of their specialty, as it has such a wide range of symptoms and presentations. Not only does this audit demonstrate the great and urgent need for medical education on ME, which must be scientifically accurate and up-to-date, responses also demonstrate the appetite for it. More than half the respondents (56%) who answered this question wished to have more in-depth teaching on ME, and a total of 92% were amenable to it. Medical royal colleges and medical schools should take heed.

4.6. Strengths and Weaknesses

The main strength of this study is that it is one of the few studies in the United Kingdom to make a formal appraisal of doctors' knowledge and understanding of myalgic encephalomyelitis. It also conducted an investigation into the beliefs regarding ME of a group of hospital doctors. The weakness of the study is that it was relatively small-scale, ad hoc and may not be representative of all doctors' views. Furthermore, the small size of the study meant that only relatively large effects could be detected. However, our findings do appear to be consistent with other studies [58,59], and such findings of poor knowledge and negative attitudes appear persistent over decades. These may be linked to how doctors are taught and trained in UK medical schools [59], with both doctors and medical students developing their ideas about ME from lay and informal sources rather than scientific knowledge and evidence on the disease. Although attendance at the training event was mandatory, the participants were self-selected, since returning the survey was not obligatory and participants opted to take part in the survey, which may reflect a self-selection bias. Clearly, future research is needed, with larger samples, the involvement of doctors from different specialties, and the use of a pre-post design in any future training event in order to assess the impact of the event on participants' knowledge of ME.

5. Conclusions and Recommendations

ME suffers from being a Cinderella topic within the medical profession, largely ignored by the research community, as is evidenced by very low levels of institutional research funding over many years [60], as well as by high levels of ignorance and disbelief among doctors. This clinical audit has sought to investigate the beliefs about ME of a group of hospital doctors attending a training event and their knowledge and understanding of the condition. It has demonstrated areas of ignorance so considerable that patients treated on the basis of this would be put very much at risk. Nevertheless, it was encouraging that participants recognised a need for further training and indicated a wish to participate in this. It is strongly recommended that scientifically accurate and up-to-date medical education on ME be made a priority at undergraduate and postgraduate levels. It is also recommended that this audit be repeated following a period of medical education.

Author Contributions: Conceptualisation, K.N.H.; methodology, K.N.H.; validation, K.N.H.; formal analysis, K.N.H. and D.F.H.P.; investigation, K.N.H. and D.F.H.P.; resources, K.N.H.; writing—original draft preparation, K.N.H.; writing—review and editing, K.N.H., K.G. and D.F.H.P.; visualization, K.N.H. and D.F.H.P.; project administration, K.N.H. All authors have read and agreed to the published version of the manuscript.

Funding: This research received no external funding.

Institutional Review Board Statement: Not applicable.

Informed Consent Statement: Respondents took part in this audit voluntarily on the basis of informed consent. All responses were completely anonymous.

Data Availability Statement: Tabulations of the original data are available from the corresponding author.

Conflicts of Interest: The authors declare no conflict of interest. Geraghty has no financial conflicts of interest to declare but declares that he has previously received research grants from ME charities, UK non-governmental bodies, and crowdfunding. All of this funding has supported research on ME/CFS.

Appendix A. Doctors' Knowledge and Understanding of ME, UK 2018

Myalgic Encephalomyelitis-please base answers on your knowledge before today's lecture.

Education on ME, Prior Experience, Confidence	
I have received formal teaching on ME in:	Undergraduate lectures Yes ☐ No ☐
	Undergraduate e-learning or PBL Yes ☐ No ☐
	Postgraduate lectures Yes ☐ No ☐
I have seen ME patients in:	GP clinics Yes ☐ No ☐
	Specialty clinics Yes ☐ No ☐ If yes, which _____
	In hospital Yes ☐ No ☐ (tick no if it was just an item on the GP summary list)
I know how to diagnose ME:	Yes ☐ No ☐
I feel confident dealing with ME patients:	Yes ☐ No ☐
Knowledge on ME: (tick all that apply)	
ME is a:	psychological/psychosomatic illness ☐ physical illness ☐
ME is rare:	Yes ☐ No ☐
ME affects more:	Men ☐ Women ☐
ME can affect children:	Yes ☐ No ☐
ME resolves within 6 months:	Yes ☐ No ☐
ME belongs in the class of illness called Medically Unexplained Symptoms.	True ☐ False ☐

Education on ME, Prior Experience, Confidence	
Myalgic Encephalomyelitis (ME), Chronic Fatigue Syndrome (CFS) and Postviral Fatigue Syndrome (PVFS) all mean the same thing.	True ☐ False ☐
ME is mainly diagnosed with:	A careful history ☐
	A thorough physical examination ☐
	Investigations ☐
	A psychiatric history ☐
The diagnosis of ME requires:	Six months of fatigue ☐
	Symptoms from multiple systems ☐
	Psychiatric symptoms ☐
	Signs of anxiety or depression ☐
	Post exertional malaise ☐
	Certain physical signs ☐
Patients with ME can be as disabled as patients with:	MS ☐
	Advanced HIV ☐
	Heart failure ☐
	Cancer ☐
	Chronic respiratory disease ☐
	A broken leg ☐
	End stage renal failure ☐
ME doesn't kill	True ☐ False ☐
ME causes chronic disability	True ☐ False ☐
ME is painful	True ☐ False ☐
Children with ME can miss long periods of school	True ☐ False ☐
How many ME patients are able to work?	Most of them ☐
	About half ☐
	Less than half ☐
ME can affect:	The cardiovascular system ☐
	The musculoskeletal system ☐
	The nervous system ☐
	The immune system ☐
	The endocrine system ☐
	Cellular metabolism ☐
	The gastrointestinal system ☐
ME can be treated with:	Antivirals ☐
	Graded Exercise Therapy ☐
	Vitamin supplements ☐
	CBT to help patients get out of the sick role ☐
Patients need to think positive and build up their strength with exercise or gradually increasing activity.	True ☐ False ☐

Education on ME, Prior Experience, Confidence	
If they do not improve it's because they're not trying hard enough	True ☐ False ☐
Children with ME miss school because their parents support their sick role and this should be discouraged.	True ☐ False ☐
We have national guidelines on ME.	True ☐ False ☐
After today's introductory lecture, I would like further more in-depth teaching on Myalgic Encephalomyelitis:	Yes ☐
	No ☐
	Neutral ☐

References

1. Carruthers, B.M.; Jain, A.K.; De Meirleir, K.L.; Peterson, D.L.; Klimas, N.G.; Lerner, A.M.; Bested, A.C.; Flor-Henry, P.; Joshi, P.; Powles, A.P.; et al. Myalgic encephalomyelitis/chronic fatigue syndrome: Clinical working case definition, diagnostic and treatment protocols. *J. Chronic Fatigue Syndr.* **2003**, *11*, 7–115. [CrossRef]
2. Johnstone, S.C.; Staines, D.R.; Marshall-Gradisnik, S.M. Epidemiological characteristics of chronic fatigue syndrome/myalgic encephalomyelitis in Australian patients. *Clin. Epidemiol.* **2016**, *8*, 97–107. [CrossRef] [PubMed]
3. Pheby, D.; Lacerda, E.; Nacul, L.; de Lourdes Drachler, M.; Campion, P.; Howe, A.; Poland, F.; Curran, M.; Featherstone, V.; Fayyaz, S.; et al. A disease register for ME/CFS: Report of a pilot study. *BMC Res. Notes* **2011**, *4*, 139–146. [CrossRef] [PubMed]
4. Lloyd, A.R.; Hickie, I.; Boughton, C.R.; Wakefield, D.; Spencer, O. Prevalence of chronic fatigue syndrome in an Australian population. *Med. J. Aust.* **1990**, *153*, 522–528. [CrossRef] [PubMed]
5. Action for ME. Available online: https://actionforme.org.uk/what-is-me/introduction/ (accessed on 6 January 2020).
6. Pheby, D.F.H.; Araja, D.; Berkis, U.; Brenna, E.; Cullinan, J.; de Korwin, J.-D.; Gitto, L.; Hughes, D.A.; Hunter, R.M.; Trepel, D.; et al. The development of a consistent Europe-wide approach to investigating the economic impact of myalgic encephalomyelitis (ME/CFS): A report from the European Network on ME/CFS (EUROMENE). *Healthcare* **2020**, *8*, 88. [CrossRef]
7. Pheby, D.F.H.; Araja, D.; Berkis, U.; Brenna, E.; Cullinan, J.; de Korwin, J.-D.; Gitto, L.; Hughes, D.A.; Hunter, R.M.; Trepel, D.; et al. A Literature Review of GP Knowledge and Understanding of ME/CFS: A Report from the SocioeconomicWorking Group of the European Network on ME/CFS (EUROMENE). *Medicina* **2021**, *57*, 7. [CrossRef]
8. Cullinan, J.; Pheby, D.F.H.; Araja, D.; Berkis, U.; Brenna, E.; de Korwin, J.-D.; Gitto, L.; Hughes, D.A.; Hunter, R.M.; Trepel, D.; et al. Perceptions of European ME/CFS specialists concerning knowledge and understanding of ME/CFS among primary care physicians in Europe: A report from the European ME/CFS Research Network (EUROMENE). *Medicina* **2021**, *57*, 208. [CrossRef]
9. Froehlich, L.; Hattesohl, D.B.R.; Jason, L.A.; Scheibenbogen, C.; Behrends, U.; Thoma, M. Medical care situation of people with myalgic encephalomyelitis/chronic fatigue syndrome in Germany. *Medicina* **2021**, *57*, 646. [CrossRef]
10. Sunnquist, M.; Nicholson, L.; Jason, L.A.; Friedman, K.J. Access to medical care for individuals with myalgic encephalomyelitis and chronic fatigue syndrome: A call for centers of excellence. *Mod. Clin. Med. Res.* **2017**, *1*, 28–35. [CrossRef]
11. Ware, N.C. Suffering and the social construction of illness: The delegitimation of illness experience in chronic fatigue syndrome. *Med. Anthropol. Q.* **1992**, *6*, 347–361. [CrossRef]
12. Timbol, C.R.; Baraniuk, J.N. Chronic fatigue syndrome in the emergency department. *Open Access Emerg. Med.* **2019**, *11*, 15–28. [CrossRef] [PubMed]
13. Tidmore, T.M.; Jason, L.A.; Chapo-Kroger, L.; So, S.; Brown, A.; Silverman, M.C. Lack of knowledgeable healthcare access for patients with neuro-endocrine-immune diseases. *Front. Clin. Med.* **2015**, *2*, 46–54.
14. Muirhead, N.; Muirhead, J.; Lavery, G.; Marsh, B. Medical school education on myalgic encephalomyelitis. *Medicina* **2021**, *57*, 542. [CrossRef] [PubMed]
15. Peterson, T.M.; Peterson, T.W.; Emerson, S.; Regalbuto, E.; Evans, M.; Jason, L.A. Coverage of cfs within U.S. Medical textbooks. *Univers. J. Public Health* **2013**, *1*, 177–179. [CrossRef]
16. Carruthers, B.M.; van de Sande, M.I.; De Meirleir, K.L.; Klimas, N.G.; Broderick, G.; Mitchell, T.; Staines, D.; Powles, A.C.P.; Speight, N.; Vallings, S.; et al. Myalgic Encephalomyelitis–Adult and Paediatric: International Consensus Primer for Medical Practitioners. 2012. Available online: http://hetalternatief.org/ICC%20primer%202012.pdf (accessed on 30 March 2021).
17. Patten, S.B.; Marrie, R.A.; Carta, M.G. Depression in multiple sclerosis. *Int. Rev. Psychiatry* **2017**, *29*, 463–472. [CrossRef]
18. Institute of Medicine. *Beyond Myalgic Encephalomyelitis/Chronic Fatigue Syndrome: Redefining an Illness*; The National Academies Press: Washington, DC, USA, 2015; Available online: https://www.nap.edu/catalog/19012/beyond-myalgic-encephalomyelitisvhronic-fatigue-syndrome-redefining-an-illness (accessed on 28 June 2021).
19. Friedberg, F.; Bateman, L.; Bested, A.C.; Davenport, T.; Friedman, K.J.; Gurwitt, A.; Jason, L.A.; Lapp, C.W.; Stevens, S.R.; Underhill, R.A.; et al. *Chronic Fatigue Syndrome Myalgic Encephalomyelitis Primer for Clinical Practitioners*; International Association for IACFS/ME: Chicago, IL, USA, 2014; Available online: https://www.massmecfs.org/images/pdf/Primer_2014.pdf (accessed on 13 May 2021).

20. Kaufman, D. Diagnosing and Managing Myalgic Encephalomyelitis and Chronic Fatigue Syndrome (YouTube Video). Available online: http://bit.ly/D-KaufmanMEcfs2018 (accessed on 28 June 2021).
21. Rowe, P.C.; Underhill, R.A.; Friedman, K.J.; Gurwitt, A.; Medow, M.S.; Schwartz, M.S.; Speight, N.; Stewart, J.M.; Vallings, R.; Rowe, K.S.; et al. Myalgic Encephalomyelitis/Chronic Fatigue Syndrome Diagnosis and Management in Young People: A Primer. *Front. Paediatr.* **2017**, *5*, 121. [CrossRef]
22. Dowsett, E.G.; Colby, J. Long-Term Sickness Absence Due to ME/CFS in UK Schools: An epidemiological study with medical and educational implications. *J. Chronic Fatigue Syndr.* **1997**, *3*, 29–42. [CrossRef]
23. Crawley, E.; Sterne, J.A.C. Association between school absence and physical functiiningon in paediatric chronic fatigue syndrome/myalgic encephalopathy. *Arch. Dis. Child.* **2009**, *94*, 752–756. [CrossRef]
24. Colby, J. False Allegations of Child Abuse in Cases Childhood Myalgic Encephalomyelitis (ME). Argument and Critique, July 2014. Available online: http://bit.ly/TTChildAbuse (accessed on 28 June 2021).
25. Wessely, S.; Nimnuan, C.; Sharpe, M. Functional somatic syndromes: One or many? *Lancet* **1999**, *354*, 936–939. [CrossRef]
26. Komaroff, A.L. Advances in Understanding the Pathophysiology of Chronic Fatigue Syndrome. *JAMA* **2019**, *322*, 499–500. [CrossRef]
27. Kingdon, C.C.; Bowman, E.W.; Curran, H.; Nacul, L.; Lacerda, E.M. Functional Status and Well-Being in People with Myalgic Encephalomyelitis/Chronic Fatigue Syndrome Compared with People with Multiple Sclerosis and Healthy Controls. *Pharm. Open* **2018**, *2*, 381–392. [CrossRef] [PubMed]
28. Hvidberg, M.F.; Schouborg, B.L.; Olesen, A.V.; Petersen, K.D.; Ehlers, L. The Health-Related Quality of Life for Patients with Myalgic Encephalomyelitis/Chronic Fatigue Syndrome (ME/CFS). *PLoS ONE* **2015**, *10*, e0132421. [CrossRef]
29. Nacul, L.C.; Lacerda, E.M.; Campion, P.; Pheby, D.; de Drachler, M.L.; Leite, J.C.; Poland, F.; Howe, A.; Fayyaz, S.; Molokhia, M. The functional status and wellbeing of people with myalgic encephalomyelitis/chronic fatigue syndrome and their carers. *BMC Public Health* **2011**, *11*, 402. Available online: http://www.biomedcentral.com/1471-2458/11/402 (accessed on 28 June 2021). [CrossRef] [PubMed]
30. Rowe, P.; Marden, C.; Flaherty, M.; Johns, A.; Fontaine, K.R.; Violand, R. Impact of adolescent chronic fatigue syndrome. In Proceedings of the IACFS/ME Biennial Conference, San Francisco, CA, USA, 20–23 March 2014.
31. Ingerski, L.M.; Modi, A.C.; Hood, K.K.; Pai, A.L.; Zeller, M.; Piazza-Waggoner, C.; Driscoll, K.A.; Rothenberg, M.E.; Franciosi, J.; Hommel, K.A. Health-related quality of life across pediatric chronic conditions. *J. Pediatr.* **2010**, *156*, 639–644. [CrossRef]
32. Varni, J.W.; Limbers, C.A.; Burwinkle, T.M. Impaired health-related quality of life in children and adolescents with chronic conditions: A comparative analysis of 10 disease clusters and 33 disease categories/severities utilizing the PedsQL 4.0 generic core scales. *Health Qual. Life Outcomes* **2007**, *5*, 43. [CrossRef]
33. Castro-Marrero, J.; Faro, M.; Aliste, L.; Sáez-Francàs, N.; Calvo, N.; Martínez-Martínez, A.; de Sevilla, T.F.; Alegre, J. Comorbidity in Chronic Fatigue Syndrome/Myalgic Encephalomyelitis: A Nationwide Population-Based Cohort Study. *Psychosomatics* **2017**, *58*, 533–543. [CrossRef] [PubMed]
34. Collin, S.M.; Crawley, E.; May, M.T.; Sterne, J.A.C.; Hollingworth, W.; For UK CFS/ME National Outcomes Database. The impact of CFS/ME on employment and productivity in the UK: A cross-sectional study based on the CFS/ME national outcomes database. *BMC Health Serv. Res.* **2011**, *11*, 217. Available online: http://www.biomedcentral.com/1472-6963/11/217 (accessed on 28 June 2021). [CrossRef] [PubMed]
35. Jesús Castro-Marrero, J.; Mónica Faro, M.; Zaragozá, M.; Aliste, L.; Fernández de Sevilla, T.; Alegre, J. Unemployment and work disability in individuals with chronic fatigue syndrome/myalgic encephalomyelitis: A community based cross-sectional study from Spain. *BMC Public Health* **2019**, *19*, 840. [CrossRef]
36. Nyland, M.; Naess, H.; Birkeland, J.S.; Nyland, H. Longitudinal follow-up of employment status in patients with chronic fatigue syndrome after mononucleosis. *BMJ Open* **2014**, *4*, e005798. [CrossRef]
37. Vink, M.; Vink-Niese, F. Work Rehabilitation and Medical Retirement for Myalgic Encephalomyelitis/Chronic Fatigue Syndrome Patients. A Review and Appraisal of Diagnostic Strategies. *Diagnostics* **2019**, *9*, 124. [CrossRef]
38. McManimen, S.L.; Devendorf, A.R.; Brown, A.A.; Moore, B.C.; Moore, J.H.; Jason, L.A. Mortality in Patients with Myalgic Encephalomyelitis and Chronic Fatigue Syndrome. *Fatigue* **2016**, *4*, 195–207. [CrossRef] [PubMed]
39. Jason, L.A.; Corradi, K.; Gress, S.; Williams, S.; Torres-Harding, S. Causes of death among patients with chronic fatigue syndrome. *Health Care Women Int.* **2006**, *27*, 615–626. Available online: https://www.ncbi.nlm.nih.gov/pubmed/16844674 (accessed on 3 May 2021). [CrossRef]
40. Siddle, J. Inquest Ruling: Young Drama Student Merryn Crofts Killed by ME. ME Association. 18 May 2018. Available online: http://bit.ly/MerrynCroftsMEA (accessed on 3 May 2021).
41. Kregloe, K. In Remembrance of Sophia Mirza on Severe M.E. Awareness Day. Solve ME/CFS Initiative. 8 August 2019. Available online: https://solvecfs.org/in-remembrance-of-sophia-mirza-on-severe-m-e-awareness-day/ (accessed on 3 May 2021).
42. Baxter, H.; Speight, N.; Weir, W. Life-Threatening Malnutrition in Very Severe ME/CFS. *Healthcare* **2021**, *9*, 459. [CrossRef]
43. Vercoulen, J.; Swanink, C.; Galama, J.; Fennis, J.; Jongen, P.; Hommes, O.; van der Meer, J.; Bleijenberg, G. The persistence of fatigue in chronic fatigue syndrome and multiple sclerosis. *J. Psychosom. Res.* **1998**, *45*, 507–517. [CrossRef]
44. Geraghty, K.; Jason, L.; Sunnquist, M.; Tuller, D.; Blease, C.; Adeniji, C. The 'cognitive behavioural model' of chronic fatigue syndrome: Critique of a flawed model. *Health Psychol Open* **2019**, *6*, 2055102919838907. [CrossRef] [PubMed]

45. Bavinton, J.; Darbishire, L.; White, P.D. *Manual For Therapists-Graded Exercise Therapy for CFS/ME*; PACE Trial Management Group: London, UK, 2004; Available online: https://www.qmul.ac.uk/wolfson/media/wolfson/current-projects/5.get-therapist-manual.pdf (accessed on 14 May 2021).
46. Vink, M.; Vink-Niese, A. Cognitive behavioural therapy for myalgic encephalomyelitis/ chronic fatigue syndrome is not effective. Re-analysis of a Cochrane review. *Health Psychol. Open* **2019**, *6*, 1–23. [CrossRef]
47. Vink, M.; Vink-Niese, A. Graded exercise therapy for myalgic encephalomyelitis/chronic fatigue syndrome is not effective and unsafe. Re-analysis of a Cochrane review. *Health Psychol. Open* **2018**, *5*, 1–12. Available online: http://bit.ly/GET-crit-rv-MarkVink (accessed on 28 June 2021). [CrossRef]
48. VanNess, J.M.; Davenport, T.E.; Snell, C.R.; Stevens, S. *Opposition to Graded Exercise Therapy (GET) for ME/CFS Workwell Foundation, 1st May 2018*; Workwell Foundation: Ripon, CA, USA, 2018; Available online: https://workwellfoundation.org/wp-content/uploads/2019/07/MECFS-GET-Letter-to-Health-Care-Providers-v4-30-2.pdf (accessed on 14 May 2021).
49. White, P.D.; Goldsmith, K.A.; Johnson, A.L.; Potts, L.; Walwyn, R.; De Cesare, J.C.; Baber, H.L.; Burgess, M.; Clark, L.V.; Cox, D.L.; et al. Comparison of adaptive pacing therapy, cognitive behaviour therapy, graded exercise therapy, and specialist medical care for chronic fatigue syndrome (PACE): A randomised trial. *Lancet* **2011**, *377*, 823–836. [CrossRef]
50. Larun, L.; Brurberg, K.G.; Odgaard-Jensen, J.; Price, J.R. Exercise therapy for chronic fatigue syndrome. *Cochrane Database Syst. Rev.* **2019**, CD003200. [CrossRef]
51. Kindlon, T. Reporting of Harms Associated with Graded Exercise Therapy and Cognitive Behavioural Therapy in Myalgic Encephalomyelitis/Chronic Fatigue Syndrome. *Bull. IACFS/ME* **2011**, *19*, 59–111. Available online: https://www.ncf-net.org/library/Reporting%20of%20Harms.pdf (accessed on 14 May 2021).
52. Geraghty, K.; Hann, M.; Kurtev, S. Myalgic encephalomyelitis / chronic fatigue syndrome patients' reports of symptom changes following cognitive behavioural therapy, graded exercise therapy and pacing treatments: Analysis of a primary survey compared with secondary surveys. *J. Health Psychol.* **2017**, *24*, 1318–1333. [CrossRef] [PubMed]
53. ME Association. *ME/CFS Illness Management Survey Results "No Decisions about Me without Me"*; The ME Association: Buckingham, UK, 2015; Available online: http://bit.ly/MEAssSurvey2015 (accessed on 14 May 2021).
54. Centers for Disease Control and Prevention. *Myalgic Encephalomyelitis/Chronic Fatigue Syndrome. Treatment of ME/CFS*; Centers for Disease Control, CDC: Atlanta, GA, USA, 2021. Available online: https://www.cdc.gov/me-cfs/treatment/index.html (accessed on 5 July 2021).
55. Brenna, E.; Araja, D.; Pheby, D.F.H. Comparative Survey of People with ME/CFS in Italy, Latvia, and the UK: A Report on Behalf of the Socioeconomics Working Group of the European ME/CFS Research Network (EUROMENE). *Medicina* **2021**, *57*, 300. [CrossRef] [PubMed]
56. National Institute for Health and Care Excellence. Guideline: Myalgic Encephalomyelitis (or Encephalopathy)/Chronic Fatigue Syndrome: Diagnosis and Management. Draft for Consultation, November 2020. Para. 1.11.16. Available online: https://www.nice.org.uk/guidance/GID-NG10091/documents/draft-guideline (accessed on 15 February 2021).
57. Hunter, R.M.; James, M.; Paxman, J. *Chronic Fatigue Syndrome/Myalgic Encephalomyelitis: Counting the Cost—Full Report*; 2020 Health: London, UK, 2017; Available online: https://2020health.org/wp-content/uploads/2020/11/Counting-the-Cost-CFS-ME.pdf (accessed on 14 May 2021).
58. Raine, R.; Carter, S.; Sensky, T.; Black, N. General practitioners' perceptions of chronic fatigue syndrome and beliefs about its management, compared with irritable bowel syndrome: Qualitative study. *BMJ* **2004**, *328*, 1354–1357. [CrossRef] [PubMed]
59. Stenhoff, A.L.; Sadreddini, S.; Peters, S.; Wearden, A. Understanding medical students' views of chronic fatigue syndrome: A qualitative study. *J. Health Psychol.* **2015**, *20*, 198–209. [CrossRef] [PubMed]
60. Radford, G.; Chowdhury, S. *ME/CFS Research Funding—An Overview of Activity by Major Institutional Funders Included on the Dimensions Database*; Action for ME: Bristol, UK, 2016; Available online: https://www.meassociation.org.uk/wp-content/uploads/mecfs-research-funding-report-2016.pdf (accessed on 14 May 2021).

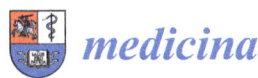
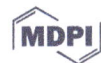

Review

Long COVID and Myalgic Encephalomyelitis/Chronic Fatigue Syndrome (ME/CFS)—A Systemic Review and Comparison of Clinical Presentation and Symptomatology

Timothy L. Wong * and Danielle J. Weitzer

Department of Psychiatry, Rowan University School of Osteopathic Medicine, Mt. Laurel, NJ 08054, USA; Weitzer@rowan.edu
* Correspondence: Wongt@rowan.edu; Tel.: +1-609-941-5486

Abstract: *Background and Objectives:* Long COVID defines a series of chronic symptoms that patients may experience after resolution of acute COVID-19. Early reports from studies with patients with long COVID suggests a constellation of symptoms with similarities to another chronic medical illness—myalgic encephalomyelitis/chronic fatigue syndrome (ME/CFS). A review study comparing and contrasting ME/CFS with reported symptoms of long COVID may yield mutualistic insight into the characterization and management of both conditions. *Materials and Methods:* A systemic literature search was conducted in MEDLINE and PsycInfo through to 31 January 2021 for studies related to long COVID symptomatology. The literature search was conducted in accordance with PRISMA methodology. *Results:* Twenty-one studies were included in the qualitative analysis. Long COVID symptoms reported by the included studies were compared to a list of ME/CFS symptoms compiled from multiple case definitions. Twenty-five out of 29 known ME/CFS symptoms were reported by at least one selected long COVID study. *Conclusions:* Early studies into long COVID symptomatology suggest many overlaps with clinical presentation of ME/CFS. The need for monitoring and treatment for patients post-COVID is evident. Advancements and standardization of long COVID research methodologies would improve the quality of future research, and may allow further investigations into the similarities and differences between long COVID and ME/CFS.

Keywords: long-haul COVID-19; COVID-19; ME/CFS; myalgic encephalomyelitis; chronic fatigue syndrome; systemic review

Citation: Wong, T.L.; Weitzer, D.J. Long COVID and Myalgic Encephalomyelitis/Chronic Fatigue Syndrome (ME/CFS)—A Systemic Review and Comparison of Clinical Presentation and Symptomatology. *Medicina* **2021**, *57*, 418. https://doi.org/10.3390/medicina57050418

Academic Editor: Woojae Myung

Received: 26 March 2021
Accepted: 21 April 2021
Published: 26 April 2021

Publisher's Note: MDPI stays neutral with regard to jurisdictional claims in published maps and institutional affiliations.

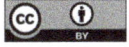

Copyright: © 2021 by the authors. Licensee MDPI, Basel, Switzerland. This article is an open access article distributed under the terms and conditions of the Creative Commons Attribution (CC BY) license (https://creativecommons.org/licenses/by/4.0/).

1. Introduction

Coronavirus disease 2019 (COVID-19), a highly contagious respiratory disease caused by the severe acute respiratory syndrome coronavirus 2 (SARS-COV-2), was declared a pandemic by the World Health Organization in March 2020 [1]. As of 7 March 2021, there are over 100 million cumulative cases, with over 2.5 million deaths worldwide [2]. Within the United States alone, there have been almost 30 million cumulative cases, with over half a million deaths as of mid-March [3].

In terms of clinical profile and disease symptomatology, individuals afflicted with COVID-19 vary greatly in terms of clinical presentation [4,5]. While some individuals remain asymptomatic, others experience symptoms generally associated with other viral respiratory diseases, such as fever, cough, dyspnea, headache, and sore throat [6–8]. During the acute phase of COVID-19, various other systemic impacts including gastrointestinal, renal, hepatological, rheumatological, and neurological symptoms and complications have been reported [9,10]. While there continues to be significant public concern and research centered around the acute course and presentation of COVID-19, there is increasing public and academic interest in the chronic sequelae of the disease [11–13].

There is currently no uniform terminology for this so-called long COVID [14], or, as it has also been termed, long-haul COVID-19 [15,16], post-COVID syndrome [17], chronic

COVID syndrome [18], and more recently, post-acute sequelae of SARS-COV-2 infection (PASC) [19]. There is no established case definition or diagnostic criteria, but some have suggested long COVID as being defined by persistent signs and symptoms more than four weeks after initial infection with SARS-COV-2 [20,21]. Research into the prevalence of long COVID is ongoing, but one study has estimated that over 87% of COVID patients continue to experience at least one symptom, two months after COVID symptom onset [22]. The risk for developing long COVID does not appear to be correlated with the severity of acute illness [23]. The etiologies of long COVID are uncertain, with some linking it to autoimmune condition or hyperinflammatory states after resolution of acute COVID [24–26].

The characteristics and mysterious nature of long COVID led some to suggest a connection to a debilitating but lesser-known chronic medical condition: myalgic encephalomyelitis/chronic fatigue syndrome (ME/CFS) [27–29]. ME/CFS is a long-term complicated illness characterized by at least six months of fatigue and exhaustion. This illness is estimated to account for USD 18–51 billion dollars in economic costs. In total, 2.5 million Americans suffer from chronic fatigue syndrome, with one quarter of those diagnosed being house or bed bound [30]. Within the general population, the prevalence of chronic fatigue ranges between ten and forty percent. Despite this, due to a lack in diagnostic testing without consistent and established treatments, there has been disputes regarding the actual existence of chronic fatigue syndrome. As the diagnosis is mostly based upon patient's subjective feedback, this has sparked stigma that has led to dismissive behaviors in the medical community. The misconception regarding chronic fatigue syndrome may have been started because of how it was initially characterized. For example, early reports of chronic fatigue were described as a derogatory term known as the Yuppie Flu, which initially characterized the illness among young workers, with the implication of individuals trying to get out of their job responsibilities. However, since this time, the illness has come to be understood to rather affect a broader array of populations, but with a predominance of women being more affected than men [31]. To better understand this illness, improved knowledge of the research and definitions surrounding the illness is needed.

One of the most recent definitions of the illness was formed by the Institute of Medicine in 2015 to avoid further stigma and to promote more knowledge of chronic fatigue syndrome. At that time, the illness was redefined as systemic exertion intolerance disease, with criteria stating that a patient must have significant impairment in the ability to engage in pre-illness levels of educational, occupational, personal, or social activities. This must be due to fatigue that persists for more than 6 months, in addition to post-exertional malaise and unrefreshing sleep, which are other key features of the illness. In addition, the criteria state that a patient must have at least one of the following symptoms: orthostatic intolerance or cognitive decline. As there may be a significant impairment in overall functioning, symptoms should be present with moderate, substantial, or severe intensity with a high frequency of occurrence. These symptoms in chronic fatigue syndrome have been shown to have common onset factors and course. It has been found that during the initial duration of the illness, the most common symptoms were fatigue, pain, cognitive and sleep changes, and flu-related symptoms. As the illness progressed, other medical illnesses tended to worsen the overall course, and few patients had full remission after years of struggle, but rather remained disabled with functional impairments. The most common pattern of onset was following an infectious event, which was followed by gradual progression to consistent sickness. While there have been many theories on the causes of ME/CFS, the three most common precipitating factors have been demonstrated to be infectious illness, stress or major life event, and exposure to an environmental toxin [32]. Several studies have shown that chronic fatigue syndrome patients also react to stressors in an abnormal way, including an abnormal rise in serum cortisol and heart rate in response to the stress of waking up [33].

Over the years, there have been various proposed models for the pathophysiology of ME/CFS. One of the most prominent potential causes of chronic fatigue syndrome includes infection with Epstein–Barr virus (EBV), being highly studied in this setting. A subset of severe chronic fatigue patients exhibit upregulation of EBV-induced gene 2, which serves as a critical gene in immune and central nervous system function. Induction of this gene by EBV could explain the variance of neurological and immune-related symptoms encountered, which has been seen in 38–55% of patients with the illness and has been associated with a variety of autoimmune diseases [34]. Studies have found many other infectious organisms to be associated with chronic fatigue syndrome, including enterovirus, cytomegalovirus, human herpesvirus-6, human parvovirus B19, hepatitis C, *Chlamydophila pneumoniae* and *Coxiella burnetii* [35]. When considering an infectious cause, it will also be important to determine how the human microbiome of persistent pathogens may drive chronic symptoms by interfering with host metabolism, gene expression and immunity. One example of this occurs as bacterial microbes modulate natural killer activity, which has been shown to be reduced in chronic fatigue patients [36]. In terms of immunological explanations, the most consistently reported are increased numbers of activated cytotoxic CD8+T cells and poorly functioning natural killer cells, increased immune activation markers, greater numbers of CD16+/CD3− natural killer cells, and the presence of interferon gamma in serum and cerebrospinal fluid [37]. Other etiologies may include metabolic and endocrine abnormalities, where the body lacks energy and drive because the cells have a problem generating and using energy from oxygen, sugars, lipids, and amino acids. In terms of metabolism, studies have revealed that patients with chronic fatigue syndrome have metabolites including sphingolipids and phospholipids that resemble a hibernation state with significantly lower than normal levels [38].

There exists a large volume of research on the pathogenesis and management of ME/CFS. If long COVID is demonstrated to be a similar chronic medical illness with overlaps in clinical features and symptomatology, it may be conjectured that the existing knowledge on ME/CFS may benefit patients of long COVID. Given the statistics on disease prevalence reported by early studies into long COVID, millions of patients will stand to benefit from insights into the treatment and management of their conditions. Conversely, the increasing public interest in long COVID and an outpouring of research efforts into this condition may yield additional research findings that can benefit patients suffering from ME/CFS. There is an urgent need for studies on the similarities and differences of the symptomatology and pathophysiology of long COVID and ME/CFS. To the authors' knowledge, there has been no comparative review study into the clinical profiles of long COVID and ME/CFS. Therefore, we conducted a systemic review of the research available thus far into the symptomatology of long COVID, and compared them with known symptoms of ME/CFS based on multiple, widely accepted case definitions.

2. Materials and Methods

2.1. Search Strategy

We searched MEDLINE and PsycInfo for articles with studies into clinical profiles and symptoms of long COVID, published up to 31 January 2021. As noted in the introduction, due to the lack of uniformed terminologies for long COVID, we used broad, general search terms with the intention of capturing the widest possible array of articles in our literature search.

For MEDLINE, we used the following search terms: (Long COVID) OR (long haul covid) OR (Chronic COVID) OR (Post-COVID) OR (("Coronavirus Infections/complications" [Mesh]) AND "COVID-19" [Mesh] AND "Symptom Assessment" [Mesh]). For PsycInfo, we used the following search terms: (Long COVID) OR (long haul covid) OR (Chronic COVID) OR (Post-COVID). The titles and abstracts of the identified articles were reviewed, and the full texts of the selected studies were further examined according to the eligibility criteria. The search and review process are illustrated in Figure 1, following the PRISMA guideline for systemic reviews [39].

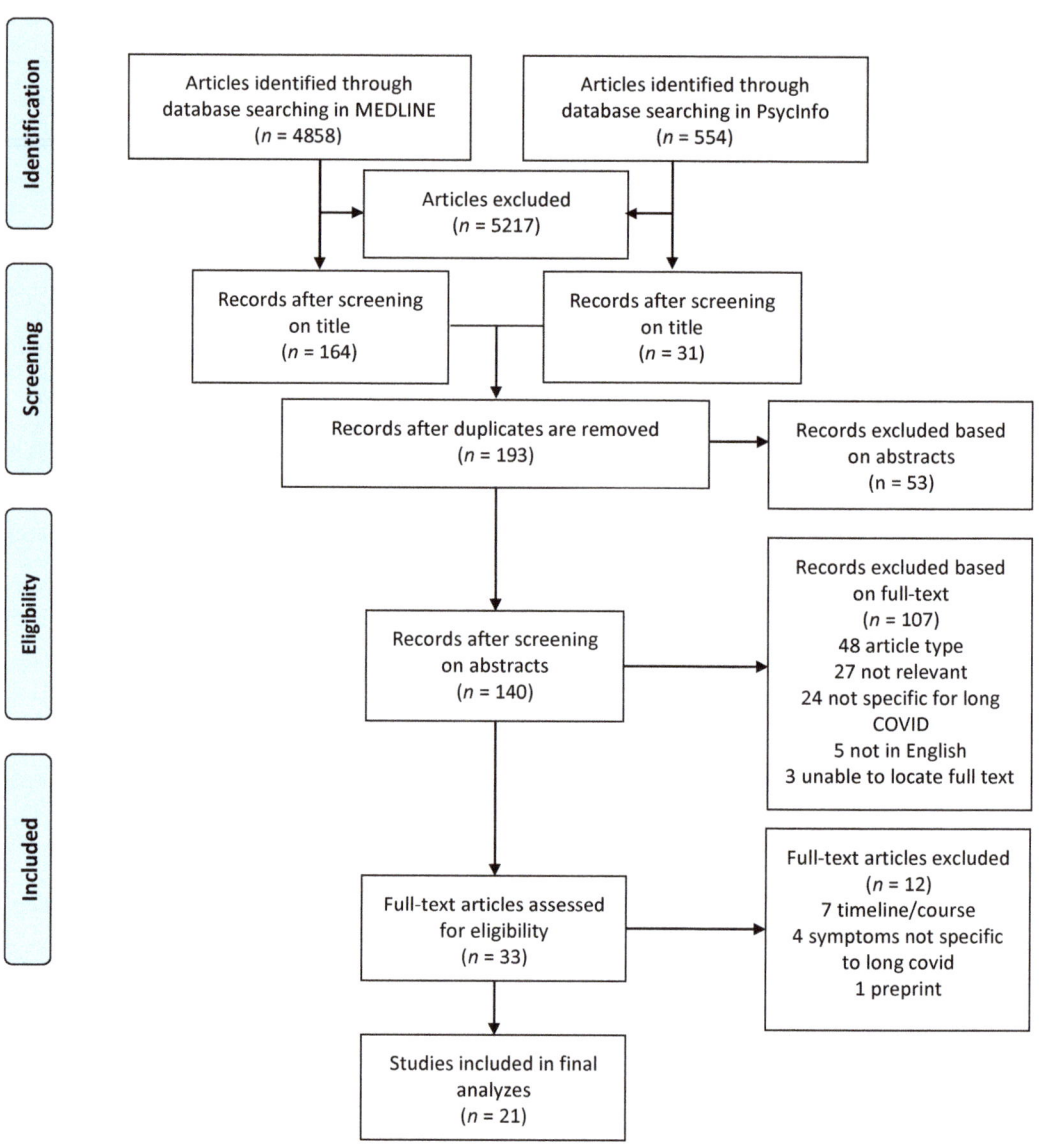

Figure 1. PRISMA flowchart.

2.2. Eligibility Criteria

For the purpose of this review article, we required studies with original research data into symptoms of COVID-19, with a clearly defined timeline of at least 4 weeks after the respective study's reference beginning point, typically time of symptom onset or time of positive COVID test. The reported symptoms must be ongoing at the time of measurement. The symptoms must not be the result of known or identified disease processes that are either self-resolving or resolved with treatment.

2.3. Synthesis of Results

We performed qualitative compilation and analysis of data reported by the selected studies. Research into the clinical profile and symptomatology of long COVID is still in its infancy, and there is currently no established methodology or protocol for studying patients with long COVID. Due to the heterogeneity in many aspects of the selected studies, including study populations, data gathering methodologies, and study timelines, a quantitative analysis of the data would be mistaken and inappropriate.

Another consequence of the heterogeneity of long COVID studies and the lack of uniform case definition of long COVID is that the selected studies utilize different terminologies for signs/symptoms that are similar or even identical. As part of the analysis process of study data, we attempted to standardize the terminologies of findings and symptoms by examining the methodologies and measurement methods as described by the corresponding studies, and then further comparing those terminologies to those utilized by ME/CFS case definitions. At times, certain findings and symptoms required further research and interpretation for data analysis. One example would be the 6 min walking test (6MWT) [40], an assessment tool that has been used previously in ME/CFS studies [41,42] and is classified under post-exertional malaise for the purpose of this study.

All long COVID symptoms reported by the selected studies are mapped onto a comparison chart with known ME/CFS criteria. The ME/CFS criteria is adopted from a study by Lim et al. [43] comparing known case definitions of ME/CFS. We selected this compilation of ME/CFS case definitions for our analysis to capture the widest possible array of known ME/CFS symptoms.

3. Results

Initially, a total of 5412 articles were identified through database searches through MEDLINE and PsycInfo. After examining the titles and available abstracts of articles, and removing duplicate articles, 140 articles remained. The full texts of the 140 articles were examined and evaluated based on article type and content relevance, and distilled down to 33 articles. The articles were further evaluated based on the eligibility criteria, and 21 articles were selected for the final analysis.

The included long COVID studies are shown in Table 1. The chart further specifies the number of patients included in the studies, patient populations, location, median time at the time of symptom assessment, methodology of assessment, key findings, and other additional findings. The studies are ranked in the chart in descending order according to the number of patients included. As noted in the methods section, the heterogeneity of study methods meant the impracticality of quantitative analysis of the studies; the studies are ranked in this order for the purpose of clarity and qualitative interpretations of the studies. When applicable, the percentage of study patients experiencing long COVID symptoms was provided with the key findings of each study.

Table 1. Studies included in analysis.

	# of Patients	Patient Population	Location	Median Time at Assessment	Methodology	Key Findings	Other Findings
Goertz et al. [44]	2113	Adult; hospitalized + nonhospitalized	Netherlands	79 days after symptom onset	Online questionnaire	Fatigue (87%), dyspnea (71%), chest tightness (44%)	Headache, muscle pain, heart palpitations, cough, sore throat, etc.
Huang et al. [45]	1733	Adult; discharged from hospital	China	186 days after symptom onset	Ambidirectional cohort; questionnaires, etc.	Fatigue/muscle weakness (63%), sleep difficulties (26%)	Anxiety/depression, hair loss, smell disorder, etc.
Mandal et al. [23]	384	Adult; discharged from hospital	U.K.	54 days after discharge	Questionnaire	Fatigue (69%), Breathlessness (53%)	Cough (34%), depression (15%)

Table 1. Cont.

	# of Patients	Patient Population	Location	Median Time at Assessment	Methodology	Key Findings	Other Findings
Moreno-Perez et al. [46]	277	Adult	Spain	77 days after recovery/discharge	In-person evaluation and questionnaire	Dyspnea (34.4%), cough (21.3%), headache (17.8%)	
Taboada et al. [47]	242	Adult; discharged from hospital	Spain	6 months after discharge	Structured interview	Decreased functional status (47.5%), dyspnea (10.4%)	
Petersen et al. [48]	180	Children + Adult	Faroe Islands	125 days after symptom onset	Patient questionnaire	At least one symptom (53%)	Fatigue, loss of smell and taste, arthralgia, headache, myalgia, dyspnea, etc.
Townsend et al. [49]	153	Adult	Ireland	75 days after diagnosis	Cross-sectional; Chalder Fatigue Scale, etc.	Fatigue (47%)	Decreased performance on six-minute-walk test (6MWT)
Weerahandi et al. [50]	152	Adult; discharged from hospital	U.S.	37 days after discharge	Prospective cohort; PROMIS dyspnea characteristics instrument, etc.	Dyspnea (74.3%)	Worsened mental health
Carfi et al. [22]	143	Adult; discharged from hospital	Italy	60.3 days after symptom onset	Questionnaire	Fatigue (53.1%), dyspnea (43.4%)	Joint pain, chest pain, etc.
Townsend et al. [51]	128	Adult	Ireland	72 days after symptom onset	Chalder fatigue scale	Fatigue (52.3%)	
Halpin et al. [52]	100	Adult; discharged from hospital	U.K.	48 days after discharge	Cross-sectional; telephone questionnaire	Fatigue (64%), breathlessness (50%), PTSD symptoms (31%)	Speech and swallowing dysfunction, continence, vocational difficulties
Wong et al. [53]	78	Adult; discharged from hospital	Canada	3 months after symptom onset	Prospective cohort; questionnaire	Dyspnea (50%), cough (23%)	Anxiety, depression
Le Bon et al. [54]	72	Adult	Belgium	37 days after symptom onset	Prospective cohort; "Sniffin' Sticks" test battery	Olfactory dysfunction (37%), gustatory dysfunction (7%)	
Woo et al. [55]	18	Adult	Germany	85 days after recovery	TICS-M, fatigue assessment scale, PHQ-9	Cognitive deficits (78%)	Fatigue, mood swings
Ortelli et al. [56]	12	Adult; in neurorehabilitation	Italy	9–13 weeks post COVID	Fatigue rating scale, Beck Depression Inventory, etc.	Neuromuscular fatigue, cognitive fatigue, apathy, executive dysfunction	
Ludvigsson [57]	5	Children	Sweden	6–8 months after COVID onset	Parental report	Fatigue, dyspnea, heart palpitations/chest pain (all 100%)	Headaches, concentration difficulties, muscle weakness, dizziness, etc.
Carroll et al. [58]	1	Adult female	U.S.	50 days after initial infection	Case report	Status epilepticus	
Novak [59]	1	Adult female	U.S.	2.5 months after positive test	Case report	Fatigue, headache	
Koumpa et al. [60]	1	Adult male	U.K.	55 days after symptom onset	Case report	Hearing loss	
Alhiyari et al. [61]	1	Adult	Qatar	4 months after treatment	Case Report	Cough	
Killion et al. [62]	1	Child	Ireland	3 months after hospital admission	Case report	Palmoplantar rash	

The long COVID symptoms described by each study were mapped onto a comparison chart between ME/CFS symptoms, matching long COVID symptoms, and unmatched long COVID symptoms, as seen in Table 2. All except four ME/CFS symptoms (motor disturbance, tinnitus/double vision, lymph node pain/tenderness, sensitivity to chemicals, foods, medications, odors) were reported by at least one selected study on long COVID symptoms. All three major criteria symptoms as specified by most ME/CFS case definitions (fatigue, reduced daily activity, post-exertional malaise) were reported by multiple selected long COVID studies, with fatigue being the most reported symptom (13 out of 21 eligible studies). All sub-categories within the minor criteria of ME/CFS (neurologic/pain, neurocognitive/psychiatric, etc.) were matched with long-COVID studies. Only three selected studies met the ≥6 months duration criteria for ME/CFS. There were a few reported long COVID symptoms that were unique from ME/CFS symptoms, including olfactory dysfunction, gustatory dysfunction, and rash.

Table 2. Comparison of compiled ME/CFS symptoms to reported long COVID symptoms.

ME/CFS Criteria	COVID Studies with Matching Symptoms	Non-ME/CFS Criteria Symptoms
Major criteria		
Duration ≥6 months	Huang et al., Ludvigsson	
Fatigue	Goertz et al., Huang et al., Mandal et al., Petersen et al., Townsend et al., Weerahandi et al., Carfi et al., Townsend et al., Halpin et al., Woo et al., Ortelli et al., Ludvigsson, Novak	
Reduced daily activity	Huang et al., Taboada et al., Weerahandi et al., Halpin et al., Ludvigsson	
Post-exertional malaise	Huang et al., Townsend et al., Ludvigsson	
Minor criteria		
Neurologic/Pain		
Myalgia	Goertz et al., Huang et al., Petersen et al., Carfi et al.	
Muscle weakness	Huang et al.	
Motor disturbance		
Generalized hyperalgesia (worsened pain, etc.)	Halpin et al.	
Joint pain	Goertz et al., Huang et al., Petersen et al., Carfi et al.	
Headaches	Goertz et al., Huang et al., Moreno-Perez et al., Petersen et al., Carfi et al., Novak	
Sleep difficulties	Huang et al., Mandal et al.	
	Goertz et al., Huang et al., Petersen et al., Carfi et al., Le Bon et al.	Olfactory dysfunction
	Goertz et al., Huang et al., Petersen et al., Carfi et al., Le Bon et al.	Gustatory dysfunction
	Koumpa et al.	Auditory dysfunction
	Carroll et al.	Seizure
	Halpin et al.	Speech difficulties

Table 2. Cont.

ME/CFS Criteria	COVID Studies with Matching Symptoms	Non-ME/CFS Criteria Symptoms
Neurocognitive/Psychiatric		
Difficulty thinking/processing (brain fog, confusion, etc.)	Moreno-Perez et al., Woo et al., Ortelli et al., Ludvigsson	
Memory difficulties	Moreno-Perez et al., Halpin et al., Woo et al.	
Attention difficulties	Halpin et al., Woo et al., Ortelli et al., Ludvigsson	
Psychiatric (depression, anxiety, PTSD, etc.)	Huang et al., Mandal et al., Weerahandi et al., Halpin et al., Wong et al., Woo et al., Ortelli et al., Ludvigsson	
Hypersensitivity to noise/light	Woo et al.	
Tinnitus, double vision		
Neuroendocrine		
Thermostatic instability	Goertz et al.	
Anorexia (loss of appetite, weight loss, etc.)	Goertz et al., Huang et al., Petersen et al., Carfi et al., Halpin et al., Ludvigsson	
Autonomic Manifestations		
Orthostatic intolerance (dizziness, etc.)	Goertz et al., Huang et al., Carfi et al.	
Cardiovascular (palpitations, chest pain, etc.)	Goertz et al., Huang et al., Carfi et al.	
Respiratory (dyspnea, etc.)	Goertz et al., Huang et al., Mandal et al., Moreno-Perez et al., Taboada et al., Petersen et al., Weerahandi et al., Carfi et al., Halpin et al., Wong et al., Ludvigsson	
Gastro-intestinal (Nausea/vomiting, diarrhea, abdominal pain)	Goertz et al., Huang et al., Petersen et al., Carfi et al., Ludvigsson	
Gastro-urinary (Incontinence, etc.)	Halpin et al.	
Immune		
Fever/Chills	Goertz et al., Petersen et al., Ludvigsson	
Flu-like symptoms (cough, etc.)	Goertz et al., Huang et al., Mandal et al., Moreno-Perez et al., Petersen et al., Carfi et al., Wong et al., Alhiyari et al.	
Susceptibility to virus		
Sore throat (swallow problems, etc.)	Goertz et al., Huang et al., Petersen et al., Carfi et al., Halpin et al.	
Lymph node pain/tenderness		
Sensitivity to chemicals, foods, medications, odors	Carfi et al.	Sicca Syndrome
Others		
	Goertz et al.	Ear pain
	Goertz et al., Moreno-Perez et al., Carfi et al.	Eye problems (red eyes, etc.)
	Goertz et al., Huang et al., Moreno-Perez et al., Petersen et al., Ludvigsson, Killion et al.	Dermatological symptoms (rash, etc.)
	Huang et al.	Hair loss

4. Discussions

To the authors' knowledge, this is the first review article to examine and compare the symptoms of ME/CFS and long COVID. While there are notable findings when the symptoms reported by the selected long COVID studies were juxtaposed with existing ME/CFS case definitions, it is first worth discussing the quality and design of the selected studies. Though COVID-19 has occupied the public consciousness since the early parts of 2020 [63–65], long COVID did not become a subject of public and academic interest until the latter half of 2020, as evidenced by the publication date of the earliest long COVID study included in our paper, July 2020 [22]. The majority of the included studies were published at the end of 2020/beginning of 2021. The research into long COVID is still in its infancy, though there have been ongoing calls for more research and funding into this potentially devastating chronic medical condition [66–68].

For the purpose of this systemic review, the implications are such that there is no uniform long COVID case definition, terminologies, and study methods, which leads to a heterogeneity in the study data that precludes quantitative analysis. For one, there is a huge disparity in terms of the timeline of studies, with the time of assessment ranging from a month to 6 months after symptom onset. The studies also vary greatly in assessment methodologies; while some studies utilized patient questionnaires (Goertz et al. [44], Petersen et al. [48], etc.), others utilized in-person evaluations and assessment tools (Townsend et al. [49], Ortelli et al. [56], etc.). Within individual studies, as the authors of one of the studies pointed out, external validity of the studies may be limited due to biases (Goertz et al. [44]). Yet, it is important to keep in mind that the presented studies in this article represent some of the earliest research into symptoms of long COVID, and thus they are hugely valuable in their research into long COVID symptomatology, as well as their insight into future study designs and research protocol into long COVID.

In this systemic review study, the reported symptoms of long COVID from 21 selected studies were compared to a compilation of ME/CFS symptoms from multiple case definitions [43], including Institute of Medicine [69], Fukuda et al. [70], International Consensus Criteria [71], and Canadian Consensus Criteria [72]. The results suggest a high degree of similarities between long COVID and ME/CFS. Out of 29 listed ME/CFS symptoms, all but 4 were reported by at least one long COVID study. It is particularly notable that all three major criteria symptoms, namely fatigue, reduced daily activity, and post-exertional malaise, were reported by multiple studies. Furthermore, fatigue was specifically noted in 12 of the 21 selected studies, which likely suggests fatigue as a predominant symptom of patients suffering from long COVID.

Despite the findings from this comparison, it may be too early to establish a direct causal relationship between long COVID and the development of ME/CFS. Specifically, many of the patients described do not meet the criteria for ME/CFS due to limitations of the studies in regard to duration of symptoms. The diagnosis of ME/CFS requires that the symptoms have been present for at least 6 months. Only three of the selected studies involved the assessment of patients more than 6 months after the onset of their COVID symptoms (Huang et al. [45], Taboada et al. [47], Ludvigsson [57]). The rest of the selected studies range from 37 days to 4 months. It is worthwhile pointing out that within these three studies, 63% of patients from one study reported fatigue (Huang et al. [45]) and 47.5% of patients from another reported decreased functional status (Taboada et al. [47]). In other words, a significant number of patients continue to suffer from long COVID symptoms after 6 months, seemingly at levels comparable to data from studies involving shorter time courses. While the heterogeneity in the study populations and assessment methods preclude meta-analysis of the patient data, it may be suggested that the long COVID symptoms reported by patients in other shorter-duration studies may not resolve completely by 6 months. It has previously been suggested that, even using conservative methodologies, an estimated 10% of patients with COVID-19 may develop chronic illness meeting the definition of ME/CFS [28]. With over 100 million cumulative COVID-19 cases worldwide as of March 2021 [2], the disease burden of this ME/CFS-like chronic illness will likely be devastating.

Aside from similarities in clinical features, long COVID and ME/CFS appear to have certain commonalities in their pathophysiology. As noted in the introduction, the pathogenesis of ME/CFS has been linked to multiple underlying processes including immune system dysregulation, hyperinflammatory state, oxidative stress, and autoimmunity [73]. A particular phenotype of ME/CFS has been termed post-infectious fatigue syndrome, and it has been linked to acute viral infections such as Epstein–Barr virus (EBV) and human parvovirus (HPV)-B19 [74,75]. While the etiology of long COVID is likely multifaceted and the research is still ongoing, it has been similarly linked to inflammatory state and dysregulated immune response [76,77], further underlying the resemblance between long COVID and ME/CFS [78].

Some of the included studies in this review also attempted to characterize the underlying pathophysiology of the long COVID symptoms, and the findings have been mixed. Ortelli et al. [56] noted that their study patients exhibited markedly elevated serum interleukin-6 (IL-6) levels, suggesting the role of hyperinflammation in the pathogenesis of long COVID. However, Townsend et al. [51] did not find any correlation between the patients' fatigue severity and their serum level of inflammatory markers. Alhiyari et al. [61] noted that the patient in their case report experienced a cough for at least 4 months, and this is likely attributable to the development of pulmonary fibrosis post-COVID. Townsend et al. [49], on the other hand, noted that only a small percentage of their study patients developed pulmonary fibrosis and that this does not appear to be linked with their symptom severity. Further research into the pathogenesis of long COVID and the correlation between acute illness severity and subsequent long COVID symptoms is needed.

With the early research and studies suggesting, at least on certain levels, similarities between the clinical presentation and etiologies of long COVID and ME/CFS, it would be important to consider the implication in the treatment paradigms for both conditions. It would appear that long COVID has so far avoided the earlier obscure fate of ME/CFS, with an outpouring of public and expert acknowledgement for its status as a medical illness and its significant long-term health impact [79–82]. Many have attested to the importance of providing patient support and monitoring patients' chronic symptoms post-COVID, as well as the need for further research into long COVID [83–85]. Though there is no established treatment protocol for patients with long COVID symptoms, many have acknowledged and suggested the need and benefits of rehabilitation [86,87]. With the consideration that long COVID and ME/CFS may share certain underlying pathological processes, some have suggested that ME/CFS treatment modalities, such as antioxidant therapies, may be beneficial for COVID symptoms [78,88]. In addition, as in the cases with patients with ME/CFS, patients with long COVID may also benefit from developing an energy management plan with a team of interdisciplinary physicians [89]. This may include understanding the patients' activity threshold and managing daily energy expenditure in order to maintain a healthy active lifestyle while reducing symptom flare-ups. Looking ahead to the future, it may be suggested that the research into long COVID and the ongoing research into ME/CFS may have a symbiotic relationship, with advances made in each medical illness being able to benefit patients suffering from long COVID and ME/CFS.

Limitations and Future Directions

The results of this review suggest many potential avenues for further exploration and research. While this review provides a qualitative analysis of the similarities and differences between symptoms of long COVID and ME/CFS, a quantitative analysis further delineating the characteristics of both conditions would be warranted. Such an analysis would require further research into the clinical presentation of long COVID, with studies involving standardized methodologies. Investigations into the various contributing factors to long COVID symptoms, including severity of acute disease, history of medical illness, and patient demographics would be beneficial for a future review of ME/CFS and long COVID.

5. Conclusions

This review represents the first investigation of its kind into the similarities between symptoms of ME/CFS and long COVID. Based on data from early research into patients suffering from long COVID, this review study suggests many overlaps in the clinical presentation of long COVID and ME/CFS. Further studies into the pathogenesis and symptomatology of long COVID are warranted. With the ever-increasing cumulative cases of COVID-19 worldwide, and the tremendous number of patients who are currently suffering from, or will eventually develop symptoms of long COVID, similar research into long COVID and ME/CFS will be of paramount importance for years to come.

Author Contributions: Conceptualization, T.L.W. and D.J.W.; literature search and data analysis, T.L.W.; writing—original draft preparation, T.L.W. and D.J.W.; writing—review and editing, T.L.W. and D.J.W. All authors have read and agreed to the published version of the manuscript.

Funding: This research received no external funding.

Institutional Review Board Statement: Not applicable.

Informed Consent Statement: Not applicable.

Data Availability Statement: Data available upon request.

Acknowledgments: The authors wish to acknowledge and thank the Open Medicine Foundation for supporting the cost of publishing this article.

Conflicts of Interest: The authors declare no conflict of interest.

References

1. Pollard, C.A.; Morran, M.P.; Nestor-Kalinoski, A.L. The COVID-19 pandemic: A global health crisis. *Physiol. Genom.* **2020**, *52*, 549–557. [CrossRef]
2. WHO. Weekly Epidemiological Update-9 March 2021 (Retrieved 17 March 2021). Available online: https://apps.who.int/iris/bitstream/handle/10665/340087/nCoV-weekly-sitrep9Mar21-eng.pdf?sequence=1 (accessed on 17 March 2021).
3. CDC. COVID Data Tracker (Retrieved 17 March 2021). Available online: https://covid.cdc.gov/covid-data-tracker/#cases_casesper100klast7days (accessed on 17 March 2021).
4. Zhou, F.; Yu, T.; Du, R.; Fan, G.; Liu, Y.; Liu, Z.; Xiang, J.; Wang, Y.; Song, B.; Gu, X.; et al. Clinical course and risk factors for mortality of adult inpatients with COVID-19 in Wuhan, China: A retrospective cohort study. *Lancet* **2020**, *395*, 1054–1062. [CrossRef]
5. Yuki, K.; Fujiogi, M.; Koutsogiannaki, S. COVID-19 pathophysiology: A review. *Clin. Immunol.* **2020**, *215*, 108427. [CrossRef]
6. Tian, S.; Chang, Z.; Wang, Y.; Wu, M.; Zhang, W.; Zhou, G.; Zou, X.; Tian, H.; Xiao, T.; Xing, J.; et al. Clinical Characteristics and Reasons for Differences in Duration From Symptom Onset to Release From Quarantine Among Patients With COVID-19 in Liaocheng, China. *Front. Med.* **2020**, *7*, 210. [CrossRef] [PubMed]
7. Li, J.; Huang, D.Q.; Zou, B.; Yang, H.; Hui, W.Z.; Rui, F.; Yee, N.; Liu, C.; Nerurkar, S.N.; Kai, J.; et al. Epidemiology of COVID-19: A systematic review and meta-analysis of clinical characteristics, risk factors, and outcomes. *J. Med. Virol.* **2021**, *93*, 1449–1458. [CrossRef] [PubMed]
8. Di Gennaro, F.; Pizzol, D.; Marotta, C.; Antunes, M.; Racalbuto, V.; Veronese, N.; Smith, L. Coronavirus Diseases (COVID-19) Current Status and Future Perspectives: A Narrative Review. *Int. J. Environ. Res. Public Health* **2020**, *17*, 2690. [CrossRef]
9. Somani, S.; Agnihotri, S.P. Emerging Neurology of COVID-19. *Neurohospitalist* **2020**, *10*, 281–286. [CrossRef] [PubMed]
10. Mao, R.; Qiu, Y.; He, J.S.; Tan, J.Y.; Li, X.H.; Liang, J.; Shen, J.; Zhu, L.R.; Chen, Y.; Iacucci, M.; et al. Manifestations and prognosis of gastrointestinal and liver involvement in patients with COVID-19: A systematic review and meta-analysis. *Lancet Gastroenterol. Hepatol.* **2020**, *5*, 667–678. [CrossRef]
11. Belluck, P. Many 'Long Covid' Patients had No Symptoms from Their Initial Infection (Retrieved 17 March 2021). Available online: https://www.nytimes.com/2021/03/08/health/long-covid-asymptomatic.html (accessed on 17 March 2021).
12. NIH Launches New Initiative to Study "Long COVID" (Retrieved 17 March 2021). Available online: https://www.nih.gov/about-nih/who-we-are/nih-director/statements/nih-launches-new-initiative-study-long-covid (accessed on 17 March 2021).
13. Sudre, C.H.; Murray, B.; Varsavsky, T.; Graham, M.S.; Penfold, R.S.; Bowyer, R.C.; Pujol, J.C.; Klaser, K.; Antonelli, M.; Canas, L.S.; et al. Attributes and predictors of long COVID. *Nat. Med.* **2021**, *27*, 626–631. [CrossRef]
14. Nabavi, N. Long covid: How to define it and how to manage it. *BMJ* **2020**, *370*, m3489. [CrossRef]

15. Aucott, J.N.; Rebman, A.W. Long-haul COVID: Heed the lessons from other infection-triggered illnesses. *Lancet* **2021**, *397*, 967–968. [CrossRef]
16. Nath, A. Long-Haul COVID. *Neurology* **2020**, *95*, 559–560. [CrossRef]
17. Garg, P.; Arora, U.; Kumar, A.; Wig, N. The "post-COVID" syndrome: How deep is the damage? *J. Med. Virol.* **2021**, *93*, 673–674. [CrossRef] [PubMed]
18. Baig, A.M. Deleterious Outcomes in Long-Hauler COVID-19: The Effects of SARS-CoV-2 on the CNS in Chronic COVID Syndrome. *ACS Chem. Neurosci.* **2020**, *11*, 4017–4020. [CrossRef] [PubMed]
19. Kalter, L.; WebMD Health News. Fauci Introduces New Acronym for Long COVID (Retrieved 17 March 2021). Available online: https://www.medscape.com/viewarticle/946419 (accessed on 17 March 2021).
20. Soriano, V.; Ganado-Pinilla, P.; Sánchez-Santos, M.; Barreiro, P. Unveiling Long COVID-19 Disease. *AIDS Rev.* **2020**, *22*, 227–228. [CrossRef] [PubMed]
21. Raveendran, A.V. Long COVID-19: Challenges in the diagnosis and proposed diagnostic criteria. *Diabetes Metab. Syndr.* **2021**, *15*, 145–146. [CrossRef]
22. Carfi, A.; Bernabei, R.; Landi, F.; Gemelli Against COVID-19 Post-Acute Care Study Group. Persistent Symptoms in Patients After Acute COVID-19. *JAMA* **2020**, *324*, 603–605. [CrossRef]
23. Mandal, S.; Barnett, J.; Brill, S.E.; Brown, J.S.; Denneny, E.K.; Hare, S.S.; Heightman, M.; Hillman, T.E.; Jacob, J.; Jarvis, H.C.; et al. 'Long-COVID': A cross-sectional study of persisting symptoms, biomarker and imaging abnormalities following hospitalisation for COVID-19. *Thorax* **2020**, *10*. [CrossRef]
24. Altmann, D.M.; Boyton, R.J. Decoding the unknowns in long covid. *BMJ* **2021**, *372*, n132. [CrossRef] [PubMed]
25. Bektas, A.; Schurman, S.H.; Franceschi, C.; Ferrucci, L. A public health perspective of aging: Do hyper-inflammatory syndromes such as COVID-19, SARS, ARDS, cytokine storm syndrome, and post-ICU syndrome accelerate short- and long-term inflammaging? *Immun. Ageing I A* **2020**, *17*, 23. [CrossRef]
26. Datta, S.D.; Talwar, A.; Lee, J.T. A Proposed Framework and Timeline of the Spectrum of Disease Due to SARS-CoV-2 Infection: Illness Beyond Acute Infection and Public Health Implications. *JAMA* **2020**, *324*, 2251–2252. [CrossRef]
27. #MEAction. Dr. Fauci Says POST-COVID Syndrome "Is Highly Suggestive of" Myalgic Encephalomyelitis (Retrieved 17 March 2021). Available online: https://www.meaction.net/2020/07/10/dr-anthony-fauci-says-that-post-covid-syndrome-is-highly-suggestive-of-myalgic-encephalomyelitis/ (accessed on 17 March 2021).
28. Komaroff, A.L.; Bateman, L. Will COVID-19 Lead to Myalgic Encephalomyelitis/Chronic Fatigue Syndrome? *Front. Med.* **2021**, *7*, 606824. [CrossRef]
29. Friedman, K.J.; Murovska, M.; Pheby, D.; Zalewski, P. Our Evolving Understanding of ME/CFS. *Medicina* **2021**, *57*, 200. [CrossRef]
30. Pendergrast, T.; Brown, A.; Sunnquist, M.; Jantke, R.; Newton, J.L.; Strand, E.B.; Jason, L.A. Housebound versus nonhousebound patients with myalgic encephalomyelitis and chronic fatigue syndrome. *Chronic Illn.* **2016**, *12*, 292–307. [CrossRef]
31. Bhui, K.S.; Dinos, S.; Ashby, D.; Nazroo, J.; Wessely, S.; White, P.D. Chronic fatigue syndrome in an ethnically diverse population: The influence of psychosocial adversity and physical inactivity. *BMC Med.* **2011**, *9*, 26. [CrossRef]
32. Chu, L.; Valencia, I.J.; Garvert, D.W.; Montoya, J.G. Onset Patterns and Course of Myalgic Encephalomyelitis/Chronic Fatigue Syndrome. *Front. Pediatr.* **2019**, *7*, 12. [CrossRef] [PubMed]
33. Tomas, C.; Newton, J.; Watson, S. A review of hypothalamic-pituitary-adrenal axis function in chronic fatigue syndrome. *ISRN Neurosci.* **2013**, *2013*, 784520. [CrossRef] [PubMed]
34. Kerr, J.R. Epstein-Barr Virus Induced Gene-2 Upregulation Identifies a Particular Subtype of Chronic Fatigue Syndrome/Myalgic Encephalomyelitis. *Front. Pediatr.* **2019**, *7*, 59. [CrossRef] [PubMed]
35. Chia, J.K.; Chia, A.Y. Chronic fatigue syndrome is associated with chronic enterovirus infection of the stomach. *J. Clin. Pathol.* **2008**, *61*, 43–48. [CrossRef]
36. Brenu, E.W.; Hardcastle, S.L.; Atkinson, G.M.; van Driel, M.L.; Kreijkamp-Kaspers, S.; Ashton, K.J.; Staines, D.R.; Marshall-Gradisnik, S.M. Natural killer cells in patients with severe chronic fatigue syndrome. *Auto Immun. Highlights* **2013**, *4*, 69–80. [CrossRef]
37. Landay, A.L.; Jessop, C.; Lennette, E.T.; Levy, J.A. Chronic fatigue syndrome: Clinical condition associated with immune activation. *Lancet* **1991**, *338*, 707–712. [CrossRef]
38. Naviaux, R.K.; Naviaux, J.C.; Li, K.; Bright, A.T.; Alaynick, W.A.; Wang, L.; Baxter, A.; Nathan, N.; Anderson, W.; Gordon, E. Metabolic features of chronic fatigue syndrome. *Proc. Natl. Acad. Sci. USA* **2016**, *113*, E5472–E5480. [CrossRef]
39. Liberati, A.; Altman, D.G.; Tetzlaff, J.; Mulrow, C.; Gøtzsche, P.C.; Ioannidis, J.P.; Clarke, M.; Devereaux, P.J.; Kleijnen, J.; Moher, D. The PRISMA statement for reporting systematic reviews and meta-analyses of studies that evaluate healthcare interventions: Explanation and elaboration. *BMJ* **2009**, *339*, b2700. [CrossRef] [PubMed]
40. Butland, R.J.; Pang, J.; Gross, E.R.; Woodcock, A.A.; Geddes, D.M. Two-, six-, and 12-minute walking tests in respiratory disease. *Br. Med. J.* **1982**, *284*, 1607–1608. [CrossRef] [PubMed]
41. Broadbent, S.; Coetzee, S.; Beavers, R. Effects of a short-term aquatic exercise intervention on symptoms and exercise capacity in individuals with chronic fatigue syndrome/myalgic encephalomyelitis: A pilot study. *Eur. J. Appl. Physiol.* **2018**, *118*, 1801–1810. [CrossRef] [PubMed]
42. Vink, M.; Vink-Niese, A. Graded exercise therapy for myalgic encephalomyelitis/chronic fatigue syndrome is not effective and unsafe. Re-analysis of a Cochrane review. *Health Psychol. Open* **2018**, *5*, 2055102918805187. [CrossRef]

43. Lim, E.J.; Son, C.G. Review of case definitions for myalgic encephalomyelitis/chronic fatigue syndrome (ME/CFS). *J. Transl. Med.* **2020**, *18*, 289. [CrossRef]
44. Goërtz, Y.; Van Herck, M.; Delbressine, J.M.; Vaes, A.W.; Meys, R.; Machado, F.; Houben-Wilke, S.; Burtin, C.; Posthuma, R.; Franssen, F.; et al. Persistent symptoms 3 months after a SARS-CoV-2 infection: The post-COVID-19 syndrome? *ERJ Open Res.* **2020**, *6*, 00542–02020. [CrossRef] [PubMed]
45. Huang, C.; Huang, L.; Wang, Y.; Li, X.; Ren, L.; Gu, X.; Kang, L.; Guo, L.; Liu, M.; Zhou, X.; et al. 6-month consequences of COVID-19 in patients discharged from hospital: A cohort study. *Lancet* **2021**, *397*, 220–232. [CrossRef]
46. Moreno-Pérez, O.; Merino, E.; Leon-Ramirez, J.M.; Andres, M.; Ramos, J.M.; Arenas-Jiménez, J.; Asensio, S.; Sanchez, R.; Ruiz-Torregrosa, P.; Galan, I.; et al. Post-acute COVID-19 syndrome. Incidence and risk factors: A Mediterranean cohort study. *J. Infect.* **2021**, *82*, 378–383. [CrossRef]
47. Taboada, M.; Cariñena, A.; Moreno, E.; Rodríguez, N.; Domínguez, M.J.; Casal, A.; Riveiro, V.; Diaz-Vieito, M.; Valdés, L.; Álvarez, J. Post-COVID-19 functional status six-months after hospitalization. *J. Infect.* **2021**, *82*, e31–e33. [CrossRef]
48. Petersen, M.S.; Kristiansen, M.F.; Hanusson, K.D.; Danielsen, M.E.; Steig, B.Á.; Gaini, S.; Strøm, M.; Weihe, P. Long COVID in the Faroe Islands—a longitudinal study among non-hospitalized patients. *Clin. Infect. Dis.* **2020**, ciaa1792. [CrossRef]
49. Townsend, L.; Dowds, J.; O'Brien, K.; Sheill, G.; Dyer, A.H.; O'Kelly, B.; Hynes, J.P.; Mooney, A.; Dunne, J.; Cheallaigh, C.N.; et al. Persistent Poor Health Post-COVID-19 Is Not Associated with Respiratory Complications or Initial Disease Severity. *Ann. Am. Thorac. Soc.* **2021**. [CrossRef]
50. Weerahandi, H.; Hochman, K.A.; Simon, E.; Blaum, C.; Chodosh, J.; Duan, E.; Garry, K.; Kahan, T.; Karmen-Tuohy, S.L.; Karpel, H.C.; et al. Post-Discharge Health Status and Symptoms in Patients with Severe COVID-19. *J. Gen. Intern. Med.* **2021**, *36*, 738–745. [CrossRef] [PubMed]
51. Townsend, L.; Dyer, A.H.; Jones, K.; Dunne, J.; Mooney, A.; Gaffney, F.; O'Connor, L.; Leavy, D.; O'Brien, K.; Dowds, J.; et al. Persistent fatigue following SARS-CoV-2 infection is common and independent of severity of initial infection. *PLoS ONE* **2020**, *15*, e0240784. [CrossRef] [PubMed]
52. Halpin, S.J.; McIvor, C.; Whyatt, G.; Adams, A.; Harvey, O.; McLean, L.; Walshaw, C.; Kemp, S.; Corrado, J.; Singh, R.; et al. Postdischarge symptoms and rehabilitation needs in survivors of COVID-19 infection: A cross-sectional evaluation. *J. Med. Virol.* **2021**, *93*, 1013–1022. [CrossRef] [PubMed]
53. Wong, A.W.; Shah, A.S.; Johnston, J.C.; Carlsten, C.; Ryerson, C.J. Patient-reported outcome measures after COVID-19: A prospective cohort study. *Eur. Respir. J.* **2020**, *56*, 2003276. [CrossRef] [PubMed]
54. Le Bon, S.D.; Pisarski, N.; Verbeke, J.; Prunier, L.; Cavelier, G.; Thill, M.P.; Rodriguez, A.; Dequanter, D.; Lechien, J.R.; Le Bon, O.; et al. Psychophysical evaluation of chemosensory functions 5 weeks after olfactory loss due to COVID-19: A prospective cohort study on 72 patients. *Eur. Arch. Otorhinolaryngol.* **2021**, *278*, 101–108. [CrossRef]
55. Woo, M.S.; Malsy, J.; Pöttgen, J.; Zai, S.S.; Ufer, F.; Hadjilaou, A.; Schmiedel, S.; Addo, M.M.; Gerloff, C.; Heesen, C.; et al. Frequent neurocognitive deficits after recovery from mild COVID-19. *Brain Commun.* **2020**, *2*, fcaa205. [CrossRef]
56. Ortelli, P.; Ferrazzoli, D.; Sebastianelli, L.; Engl, M.; Romanello, R.; Nardone, R.; Bonini, I.; Koch, G.; Saltuari, L.; Quartarone, A.; et al. Neuropsychological and neurophysiological correlates of fatigue in post-acute patients with neurological manifestations of COVID-19: Insights into a challenging symptom. *J. Neurol. Sci.* **2021**, *420*, 117271. [CrossRef]
57. Ludvigsson, J.F. Case report and systematic review suggest that children may experience similar long-term effects to adults after clinical COVID-19. *Acta Paediatr.* **2021**, *110*, 914–921. [CrossRef] [PubMed]
58. Carroll, E.; Neumann, H.; Aguero-Rosenfeld, M.E.; Lighter, J.; Czeisler, B.M.; Melmed, K.; Lewis, A. Post-COVID-19 inflammatory syndrome manifesting as refractory status epilepticus. *Epilepsia* **2020**, *61*, e135–e139. [CrossRef] [PubMed]
59. Novak, P. Post COVID-19 syndrome associated with orthostatic cerebral hypoperfusion syndrome, small fiber neuropathy and benefit of immunotherapy: A case report. *Eneurologicalsci* **2020**, *21*, 100276. [CrossRef]
60. Koumpa, F.S.; Forde, C.T.; Manjaly, J.G. Sudden irreversible hearing loss post COVID-19. *BMJ Case Rep.* **2020**, *13*, e238419. [CrossRef] [PubMed]
61. Alhiyari, M.A.; Ata, F.; Alghizzawi, M.I.; Bilal, A.B.I.; Abdulhadi, A.S.; Yousaf, Z. Post COVID-19 fibrosis, an emerging complicationof SARS-CoV-2 infection. *IDCases* **2020**, *23*, e01041. [CrossRef]
62. Killion, L.; Beatty, P.E.; Salim, A. Rare cutaneous manifestation of COVID-19. *BMJ Case Rep.* **2021**, *14*, e240863. [CrossRef]
63. Dyer, J.; Kolic, B. Public risk perception and emotion on Twitter during the Covid-19 pandemic. *Appl. Netw. Sci.* **2020**, *5*, 99. [CrossRef] [PubMed]
64. Parikh, P.A.; Shah, B.V.; Phatak, A.G.; Vadnerkar, A.C.; Uttekar, S.; Thacker, N.; Nimbalkar, S.M. COVID-19 Pandemic: Knowledge and Perceptions of the Public and Healthcare Professionals. *Cureus* **2020**, *12*, e8144. [CrossRef]
65. Bhagavathula, A.S.; Aldhaleei, W.A.; Rahmani, J.; Mahabadi, M.A.; Bandari, D.K. Knowledge and Perceptions of COVID-19 Among Health Care Workers: Cross-Sectional Study. *JMIR Public Health Surveill.* **2020**, *6*, e19160. [CrossRef]
66. Yelin, D.; Wirtheim, E.; Vetter, P.; Kalil, A.C.; Bruchfeld, J.; Runold, M.; Guaraldi, G.; Mussini, C.; Gudiol, C.; Pujol, M.; et al. Long-term consequences of COVID-19: Research needs. *Lancet Infect. Dis.* **2020**, *20*, 1115–1117. [CrossRef]
67. Cortinovis, M.; Perico, N.; Remuzzi, G. Long-term follow-up of recovered patients with COVID-19. *Lancet* **2021**, *397*, 173–175. [CrossRef]
68. Subbaraman, N. US Health Agency Will Invest $1 Billion to Investigate 'Long COVID' (Retrieved 17 March 2021). Available online: https://www.nature.com/articles/d41586-021-00586-y (accessed on 17 March 2021).

69. Committee on the Diagnostic Criteria for Myalgic Encephalomyelitis/Chronic Fatigue Syndrome; Board on the Health of Select Populations; Institute of Medicine. *Beyond Myalgic Encephalomyelitis/Chronic Fatigue Syndrome: Redefining an Illness*; National Academies Press (US): Washington, DC, USA, 2015.
70. Fukuda, K.; Straus, S.E.; Hickie, I.; Sharpe, M.C.; Dobbins, J.G.; Komaroff, A. The chronic fatigue syndrome: A comprehensive approach to its definition and study. International Chronic Fatigue Syndrome Study Group. *Ann. Intern. Med.* **1994**, *121*, 953–959. [CrossRef]
71. Carruthers, B.M.; van de Sande, M.I.; De Meirleir, K.L.; Klimas, N.G.; Broderick, G.; Mitchell, T.; Staines, D.; Powles, A.C.; Speight, N.; Vallings, R.; et al. Myalgic encephalomyelitis: International Consensus Criteria. *J. Intern. Med.* **2011**, *270*, 327–338. [CrossRef]
72. Myalgic Encephalomyelitis/Chronic Fatigue Syndrome (Retrieved 17 March 2021). Available online: https://www.tandfonline.com/doi/abs/10.1300/J092v11n01_02 (accessed on 17 March 2021).
73. Rivera, M.C.; Mastronardi, C.; Silva-Aldana, C.T.; Arcos-Burgos, M.; Lidbury, B.A. Myalgic Encephalomyelitis/Chronic Fatigue Syndrome: A Comprehensive Review. *Diagnostics* **2019**, *9*, 91. [CrossRef] [PubMed]
74. Ortega-Hernandez, O.D.; Shoenfeld, Y. Infection, vaccination, and autoantibodies in chronic fatigue syndrome, cause or coincidence? *Ann. N. Y. Acad. Sci.* **2009**, *1173*, 600–609. [CrossRef] [PubMed]
75. Arnett, S.V.; Alleva, L.M.; Korossy-Horwood, R.; Clark, I.A. Chronic fatigue syndrome—A neuroimmunological model. *Med. Hypotheses* **2011**, *77*, 77–83. [CrossRef] [PubMed]
76. Oronsky, B.; Larson, C.; Hammond, T.C.; Oronsky, A.; Kesari, S.; Lybeck, M.; Reid, T.R. A Review of Persistent Post-COVID Syndrome (PPCS). *Clin. Rev. Allergy Immunol.* **2021**, 1–9. [CrossRef]
77. Doykov, I.; Hällqvist, J.; Gilmour, K.C.; Grandjean, L.; Mills, K.; Heywood, W.E. 'The long tail of Covid-19'—The detection of a prolonged inflammatory response after a SARS-CoV-2 infection in asymptomatic and mildly affected patients. *F1000Research* **2020**, *9*, 1349. [CrossRef]
78. Wood, E.; Hall, K.H.; Tate, W. Role of mitochondria, oxidative stress and the response to antioxidants in myalgic encephalomyelitis/chronic fatigue syndrome: A possible approach to SARS-CoV-2 'long-haulers'? *Chronic Dis. Transl. Med.* **2021**, *7*, 14–26. [CrossRef]
79. Gupta, D. Almost A Third of People with 'Mild' COVID-19 Still Battle Symptoms Months Later, Study Finds (Retrieved 17 March 2021). Available online: https://www.cnn.com/2021/02/19/health/post-covid-syndrome-long-haulers-gupta-wellness/index.html (accessed on 17 March 2021).
80. COVID Long-Haulers Plagued by Symptoms as Experts Seek Answers (Retrieved 17 March 2021). Available online: https://www.usnews.com/news/health-news/articles/2021-03-16/covid-long-haulers-plagued-by-symptoms-as-experts-seek-answers (accessed on 17 March 2021).
81. Waldrop, T. Clinics Are Springing up around the Country for What Some Call a Potential Second Pandemic: Long Covid (Retrieved 17 March 2021). Available online: https://www.cnn.com/2021/02/22/health/long-covid-clinics/index.html (accessed on 17 March 2021).
82. Ballering, A.; Hartman, T.O.; Rosmalen, J. Long COVID-19, persistent somatic symptoms and social stigmatisation. *J. Epidemiol. Community Health* **2021**. [CrossRef]
83. Ladds, E.; Rushforth, A.; Wieringa, S.; Taylor, S.; Rayner, C.; Husain, L.; Greenhalgh, T. Developing services for long COVID: Lessons from a study of wounded healers. *Clin. Med.* **2021**, *21*, 59–65. [CrossRef]
84. Greenhalgh, T.; Knight, M. Long COVID: A Primer for Family Physicians. *Am. Fam. Physician* **2020**, *102*, 716–717.
85. The Lancet. Facing up to long COVID. *Lancet* **2020**, *396*, 1861. [CrossRef]
86. Iqbal, A.; Iqbal, K.; Ali, S.A.; Azim, D.; Farid, E.; Baig, M.D.; Arif, T.B.; Raza, M. The COVID-19 Sequelae: A Cross-Sectional Evaluation of Post-recovery Symptoms and the Need for Rehabilitation of COVID-19 Survivors. *Cureus* **2021**, *13*, e13080. [CrossRef] [PubMed]
87. Wise, J. Long covid: WHO calls on countries to offer patients more rehabilitation. *BMJ* **2021**, *372*, n405. [CrossRef] [PubMed]
88. Ouyang, L.; Gong, J. Mitochondrial-targeted ubiquinone: A potential treatment for COVID-19. *Med. Hypotheses* **2020**, *144*, 110161. [CrossRef] [PubMed]
89. O'Connor, K.; Sunnquist, M.; Nicholson, L.; Jason, L.A.; Newton, J.L.; Strand, E.B. Energy envelope maintenance among patients with myalgic encephalomyelitis and chronic fatigue syndrome: Implications of limited energy reserves. *Chronic Illn.* **2019**, *15*, 51–60. [CrossRef] [PubMed]

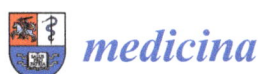

Opinion

Our Evolving Understanding of ME/CFS

Kenneth J. Friedman [1,*,†], Modra Murovska [2], Derek F. H. Pheby [3] and Paweł Zalewski [4]

1. Department of Pharmacology and Physiology, New Jersey Medical School, Newark, NJ 07103, USA
2. Institute of Microbiology and Virology, Riga Stradiņš University, LV-1067 Riga, Latvia; modra@latnet.lv
3. Society and Health, Buckinghamshire New University, High Wycombe HP11 2JZ, UK; derekpheby@btinternet.com
4. Department of Hygiene, Epidemiology, Ergonomy and Postgraduate Education, Ludwik Rydygier Collegium Medicum in Bydgoszcz Nicolaus Copernicus University in Torun, M. Skłodowskiej-Curie 9, 85-094 Bydgoszcz, Poland; p.zalewski@cm.umk.pl
* Correspondence: kenneth.j.friedman@gmail.com
† Retired.

Citation: Friedman, K.J.; Murovska, M.; Pheby, D.F.H.; Zalewski, P. Our Evolving Understanding of ME/CFS. *Medicina* **2021**, *57*, 200. https://doi.org/10.3390/medicina57030200

Academic Editor: Edgaras Stankevičius

Received: 27 January 2021
Accepted: 18 February 2021
Published: 26 February 2021

Publisher's Note: MDPI stays neutral with regard to jurisdictional claims in published maps and institutional affiliations.

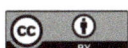

Copyright: © 2021 by the authors. Licensee MDPI, Basel, Switzerland. This article is an open access article distributed under the terms and conditions of the Creative Commons Attribution (CC BY) license (https://creativecommons.org/licenses/by/4.0/).

Abstract: The potential benefits of the scientific insights gleaned from years of treating ME/CFS for the emerging symptoms of COVID-19, and in particular Longhaul- or Longhauler-COVID-19 are discussed in this opinion article. Longhaul COVID-19 is the current name being given to the long-term sequelae (symptoms lasting beyond 6 weeks) of SARS-CoV-2 infection. Multiple case definitions for ME/CFS exist, but post-exertional malaise (PEM) is currently emerging as the 'hallmark' symptom. The inability to identify a unique trigger of ME/CFS, as well as the inability to identify a specific, diagnostic laboratory test, led many physicians to conclude that the illness was psychosomatic or non-existent. However, recent research in the US and the UK, championed by patient organizations and their use of the internet and social media, suggest underlying pathophysiologies, e.g., oxidative stress and mitochondrial dysfunction. The similarity and overlap of ME/CFS and Longhaul COVID-19 symptoms suggest to us similar pathological processes. We put forward a unifying hypothesis that explains the precipitating events such as viral triggers and other documented exposures: For their overlap in symptoms, ME/CFS and Longhaul COVID-19 should be described as Post Active Phase of Infection Syndromes (PAPIS). We further propose that the underlying biochemical pathways and pathophysiological processes of similar symptoms are similar regardless of the initiating trigger. Exploration of the biochemical pathways and pathophysiological processes should yield effective therapies for these conditions and others that may exhibit these symptoms. ME/CFS patients have suffered far too long. Longhaul COVD-19 patients should not be subject to a similar fate. We caution that failure to meet the now combined challenges of ME/CFS and Longhaul COVID-19 will impose serious socioeconomic as well as clinical consequences for patients, the families of patients, and society as a whole.

Keywords: ME/CFS; Longhaul COVID-19; pathophysiology

The development of the COVID-19 pandemic in 2020, caused by a high rate of human infection to the severe acute respiratory syndrome coronavirus 2 (SARS-CoV-2), and the unanticipated, subsequent, long-duration symptoms currently known as Longhaul COVID-19, challenges our past and present conceptualizations of ME/CFS: tens of millions of people have been infected with a specific, heretofore unknown virus [1], which has left thousands of patients chronically ill [2] with a set of symptoms remarkably similar to ME/CFS [3]. It is anticipated and estimated that approximately 10 percent of COVID-19 patients will develop Longhaul COVID-19 symptoms [4]. The occurrence of these symptoms subsequent to the acute phase of infection leaves little doubt as to the causation or that these symptoms represent a physiological abnormality.

Those of us who have been studying and researching post-viral syndromes for decades have no doubt that, as with post-viral syndromes following other viral infections, Longhaul

Covid-19 displays the constellation of symptoms that come within the scope of myalgic encephalomyelitis/chronic fatigue syndrome (ME/CFS). ME/CFS has been a cause of considerable morbidity for a large number of patients for many years, but many have suffered from disbelief and lack of understanding on the part of doctors, and those doctors and researchers who appreciated the reality of the condition have often faced an uphill struggle to advance knowledge in this area. However, the scientific knowledge that has been acquired as a result of these endeavors can now serve the interests of the wider world community, which is experiencing at first hand the trauma of a post-viral syndrome. Moreover, intensive investigation of the causation and effective treatment of these symptoms now will result in improved understanding and treatment of these symptoms regardless of triggering illness.

Arriving at a case definition and understanding of ME/CFS has been, and continues to be, difficult. For decades, attempts to define and name the disease have transpired in parallel in the United States (US) and the United Kingdom (UK) [5]. In the UK, patients suffering acute illness, both in cluster outbreaks and sporadic occurrences, developed a pattern of chronic symptoms suggestive of myalgic encephalomyelitis. In the US, several cluster outbreaks of acute disease progressing to chronic disease with a similar portfolio of symptoms were identified. The majority of cases identified were sporadic (or isolated) cases leading to confusion as to the cause of the symptoms. This led to several descriptive characterizations: Yuppie Flu, Chronic Epstein Barr, Chronic Fatigue Syndrome (CFS), and Chronic Fatigue Immune Deficiency Syndrome (CFIDS) (e.g., [6,7]).

What is clear is that the set of symptoms, although variable in presentation and expressed with different severity in differing patients, is remarkably similar. One symptom seems particularly unique to the disease; post-exertional malaise (PEM) is now considered the "hallmark" symptom [8].

Based upon the belief that this unique set of symptoms should be attributable to a single, unique organism or trigger, considerable effort—spanning at least 40 years—has been spent attempting to identify this causative agent or trigger [9]. The failure to identify a unique, causative agent, coupled with the failure to find any abnormal, routine, clinical laboratory test result, has led many healthcare professionals to conclude that the disease lacks a pathophysiological basis and, therefore, has a psychosomatic etiology. The belief in a psychosomatic origin was applied to both cluster outbreaks and sporadic occurrences of the disease. A retrospective look at one cluster outbreak, which in fact was the occurrence of several cluster outbreaks at several locations of the Royal Free Hospital in London, led to the hypothesis of the disease being mass hysteria [10]. More recently, the mass hysteria hypothesis was challenged and discredited [11].

Latterly, with the advent of social media, patients have been able to self-identify, organize into groups, and advocate for more research and an increase in the number and effectiveness of symptom relief protocols. Their awareness of diseases on both sides of the Atlantic, with almost identical sets of symptoms, has led to the realization that the ME described in the UK and the CFS described in the US are sufficiently concordant in presentation and time-course to be considered overlapping conditions. In 2011, the US National Institutes of Health concluded its CFS State of Knowledge Workshop by announcing the amalgamation of the two names into CFS/ME [12]. This was also the formulation adopted by the Chief Medical Officer's Working Group in the UK in 2002, when it concluded that the illness was a genuine clinical entity [13]. Afterwards, patient advocates lobbied for the more pathological-sounding name to be placed first. The name ME/CFS was created. The name ME/CFS is currently used despite the 2015 recommendation of the US IOM (Institute of Medicine subsequently renamed the National Academy of Medicine) to have the disease characterized by its cardinal feature and be called Systemic Exertion Intolerance Disease (SEID) [5].

The IOM report of 2015 also declared ME/CFS a disease, as opposed to its classification of being a syndrome [14], based upon the severity of the illness and its unique set of symptoms [5]. Nevertheless, and important for the hypothesis put forward here, ME/CFS remains technically a syndrome: a collection of symptoms of unknown etiology. Much work directed towards identifying the underlying pathology has been undertaken across the world, in many locations including North America and Europe, where the European ME/CFS Research Network (EUROMENE), established in 2006, has, with funding from the European Union's COST (Cooperation in Science and Technology) program, helped to address this issue (COST project CA15111) [15].

The theme of this issue of Medicina was conceived before the onset of the COVID-19 pandemic. It focuses on the causes of ME/CFS, its clinical features, and its diagnosis, but we cannot ignore the reality that we are at a moment where a pandemic virus is compelling a new understanding of the etiology of ME/CFS: The symptoms manifested by Longhaul COVID-19 patients conform closely to those manifested by ME/CFS patients, and there is some evidence that similar pathological processes, including oxidative stress and mitochondrial dysfunction, are involved in both [16]. This strongly argues against ME/CFS being caused by an unknown trigger. More likely, SARS-CoV-2 will replace the Epstein-Barr virus as being the most frequent precipitating event for ME/CFS or Longhaul COVID-19. While Epstein-Barr virus may have previously been the most frequent precipitant of ME/CFS, other viruses have been reported [17,18]. Little attention has been paid to these reports in an effort to identify a unique causation organism for ME/CFS. However, if science and discipline are to prevail, the explanation of the etiology of ME/CFS must include all identified precipitating events. Such an explanation, inclusive of all viral triggers, has not been put forward up to this time, and other triggers could not be excluded (e.g., Ehlers Danlos Syndrome, cervical spine compression, post-traumatic injury, toxic exposure, or a metabolic defect) [19]. We now put forward such a unifying hypothesis.

In consideration of the appearance of ME/CFS subsequent to the acute infection or to the reactivation of chronic/persistent infection of multiple viral species, coupled with the undeniable appearance of similar symptoms subsequent to the acute phase of SARS-CoV-2, we suggest that the set of symptoms known as ME/CFS and Longhaul COVID-19 should be described as the Post Active Phase of Infection Syndromes (PAPIS). The reason why some viruses are capable of producing PAPIS and capable of doing so more severely than others is unknown. Why some patients acquire PAPIS while others do not is also unknown. However, knowing that PAPIS exists and that the number of patients exhibiting its symptoms will dramatically increase during and subsequent to the COVID-19 pandemic, we need to explore the pathophysiological mechanisms underlying PAPIS. The similarities of symptoms between PAPIS triggered by different viral infections suggest that many of the underlying biochemical pathways and pathophysiological mechanisms will be similar, and perhaps the same. Elucidating these pathways should suggest more effective treatments, if not cures, for these symptoms. ME/CFS patients have suffered far too long. Longhaul COVID-19 patients should not experience a similar fate, and will be far too numerous to be ignored or relegated to the unemployable disabled.

Although presently unknown, the pathophysiological basis of ME/CFS and Longhaul COVID-19 symptoms should no longer be denied. Within EUROMENE, expert consensus has been developed on the diagnosis, service provision, and care of people with ME/CFS in Europe [20]. This is by no means overdue, as, without such consensus, the socioeconomic impact on the whole of the rest of society will, in the aftermath of the COVID-19 pandemic, be immense [21]. Researchers and clinicians need to admit: (1) It is not possible to find what does not exist, (2) Treatments will fail when they do not correct the underlying pathophysiology, and (3) Careful observation and correlation will yield clues to the biochemical and pathophysiological mechanisms underlying these chronic symptoms. For many of its symptoms, Longhaul COVID-19 is not like ME/CFS; it is ME/CFS. While many Longhaul COVID-19 patients will satisfy one or more of the case definitions of ME/CFS, it must be recognized that Longhaul COVID-19, for many, contains symptoms that are other than ME/CFS. Thus, while there is an overlap of the two syndromes, they cannot be considered synonymous. Nevertheless, a focus on PAPIS research is likely to lead to therapies that will make both ME/CFS and Longhaul COVID-19 patients well again.

Author Contributions: Initial conceptualization, and original draft preparation, K.J.F.; additional writing contributions, review and editing, M.M., D.F.H.P., and P.Z. All authors have read and agreed to the published version of the manuscript.

Funding: This research received no external funding.

Data Availability Statement: Not applicable.

Conflicts of Interest: The authors declare no conflict of interest.

References

1. Covid Cases Worldwide—Google. Available online: https://www.google.com/search?sxsrf=ALeKk03kiO7HPNGZZRteBNAvtHl-B1T6DFA%3A1604177564360&source=hp&ei=nM6dX8DrE8-r5wLHiJ6QBA&q=covid+cases+worldwide&oq=covid+cases+world&gs_lcp=CgZwc3ktYWIQARgAMgsIABCxAxCDARDJAzIICAAQsQMQgwEyBQgAELEDMgIIADICCAAyAggAMgIIADI-CCAAyAggAMgIIADoEC-CMQJzoFCAAQkQI6CwguELEDEMcBEKMCOgoIABCxAxAUEIcCOgcIABAUEIcCOggIABCxAxDJA-zoFCAAQkgNQ3ghYnyxgx1VoAHAAeACAAWqIAZMJkgEEMTUuMpgBAKABAaoBB2d3cy13aXXo&sclient=psy-ab (accessed on 31 October 2020).
2. Tenforde, M.W.; Kim, S.S.; Lindsell, C.J.; Rose, E.B.; Shapiro, N.I.; Files, D.C.; Gibbs, K.W.; Erickson, H.L.; Steingrub, J.S.; Smithline, H.A.; et al. Symptom Duration and Risk Factors for Delayed Return to Usual Health Among Outpatients with COVID-19 in a Multistate Health Care Systems Network—USA, March–June 2020. *MMWR. Morb. Mortal. Wkly. Rep.* **2020**, *69*, 993–998. [CrossRef] [PubMed]
3. Org Covid 19 Longhaulers: Meanings, Symptoms, Support Groups. Available online: https://covid.us.org/2020/07/12/covid-19-long-haulers-meaning-symptoms-support-groups/ (accessed on 31 October 2020).
4. Greenhalgh, T.; Knight, M.; A'Court, C.; Buxton, M.; Husain, L. Management of post-acute covid-19 in primary care. *BMJ* **2020**, *370*, m3026. [CrossRef] [PubMed]
5. Committee on the Diagnostic Criteria for Myalgic Encephalomyelitis/Chronic Fatigue Syndrome; Board on the Health of Select Populations; Institute of Medicine. *Beyond Myalgic Encephalomyelitis/Chronic Fatigue Syndrome: Redefining an Illness*; National Academies Press: Washington, DC, USA, 10 February 2015; Background. Available online: https://www.ncbi.nlm.nih.gov/books/NBK284897/ (accessed on 31 October 2020).
6. Fernandez-Sola, J. What is Chronic Fatigue Syndrome. Portal Clinic, Clinic Barcelona, 2018. Available online: https://www.clinicbarcelona.org/en/assistance/diseases/chronic-fatigue-syndrome/definition (accessed on 31 October 2020).
7. Tuller, D. Chronic Fatigue No Longer Seen As 'Yuppie Flu'. *The New York Times*. 17 July 2007. Available online: https://www.nytimes.com/2007/07/17/science/17fatigue.html (accessed on 31 October 2020).
8. Holtzman, C.S.; Bhatia, S.; Cotler, J.; Jason, L.A. Assessment of Post-Exertional Malaise (PEM) in Patients with Myalgic Encephalomyelitis (ME) and Chronic Fatigue Syndrome (CFS): A Patient-Driven Survey. *Diagnostics* **2019**, *9*, 26. [CrossRef] [PubMed]
9. Lim, E.-J.; Son, C.-G. Review of case definitions for myalgic encephalomyelitis/chronic fatigue syndrome (ME/CFS). *J. Transl. Med.* **2020**, *18*, 1–10. [CrossRef] [PubMed]
10. McEvedy, C.P.; Beard, A.W. Concept of Benign Myalgic Encephalomyelitis. *BMJ* **1970**, *1*, 11–15. [CrossRef] [PubMed]
11. Epidemic myalgic encephalomyelitis. *Br. Med. J.* **1978**, *1*, 1436–1437. Available online: https://www.bmj.com/content/1/6125/1436.2 (accessed on 29 December 2020). [CrossRef]
12. The Office of Research on Women's Health, NIH, DHHS, State of Knowledge Workshop. 7–8 April 2011. Available online: https://meassociation.org.uk/wp-content/uploads/2011/08/SoK-Workshop-Report-508-compliant-8-5-11.pdf (accessed on 31 October 2020).
13. *Chief Medical Officer's Working Group on CFS/ME*; Report; Department of Health: London, UK, 2002
14. The Free Dictionary—Medical Dictionary: Syndrome. Available online: https://medical-dictionary.thefreedictionary.com/syndrome (accessed on 30 October 2020).
15. Scheibenbogen, C.; Freitag, H.; Blanco, J.; Capelli, E.; Lacerda, E.; Authier, J.; Meeus, M.; Marrero, J.C.; Nora-Krukle, Z.; Oltra, E.; et al. The European ME/CFS Biomarker Landscape project: An initiative of the European network EUROMENE. *J. Transl. Med.* **2017**, *15*, 162. [CrossRef] [PubMed]
16. Wood, E.; Hall, K.H.; Tate, W. Role of mitochondria, oxidative stress and the response to antioxidants in myalgic encephalomyelitis/chronic fatigue syndrome: A possible approach to SARS-CoV-2 'long-haulers'? *Chronic Dis. Transl. Med.* **2020**. [CrossRef]
17. Centers for Disease Control. Myalgic Encephalomyelitis/Chronic Fatigue Syndrome Possible Causes. 2018. Available online: https://www.cdc.gov/me-cfs/about/possible-causes.html (accessed on 30 October 2020).
18. Rasa, S.; Nora-Krukle, Z.; Henning, N.; Eliassen, E.; Shikova, E.; Harrer, T.; Scheibenbogen, C.; Murovska, M.; Prusty, B.K. Chronic viral infections in myalgic encephalomyelitis/chronic fatigue syndrome (ME/CFS). European Network on ME/CFS (EUROMENE). *J. Transl. Med.* **2018**, *16*, 1–25. [CrossRef] [PubMed]
19. EUROMENE: Deliverables. Available online: http://www.euromene.eu/workinggroups/deliverables/Deliverable%20No%2013.pdf (accessed on 9 December 2020).

20. Nacul, L.; Authier, F.J.; Scheibenbogen, C.; Lorusso, L.; Helland, I.; Alegre Martin, J.; Sirbu, C.A.; Mengshoel, A.M.; Polo, O.; Behrends, U.; et al. European ME Network (EUROMENE) Expert Consensus on the Diagnosis, Service Provision and Care of People with ME/CFS in Europe. *Preprints* **2020**, 2020090688. Available online: https://www.preprints.org/manuscript/202009.0688/v2) (accessed on 25 February 2021).
21. Pheby, D.F.; Araja, D.; Berkis, U.; Brenna, E.; Cullinan, J.; De Korwin, J.-D.; Gitto, L.; A Hughes, D.; Hunter, R.M.; Trepel, D.; et al. The Development of a Consistent Europe-Wide Approach to Investigating the Economic Impact of Myalgic Encephalomyelitis (ME/CFS): A Report from the European Network on ME/CFS (EUROMENE). *Healthcare* **2020**, *8*, 88. [CrossRef] [PubMed]

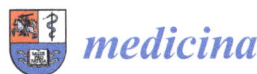 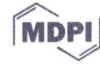

Article

Myalgic Encephalomyelitis/Chronic Fatigue Syndrome (ME/CFS): Major Impact on Lives of Both Patients and Family Members

Esme Brittain [1], Nina Muirhead [2], Andrew Y. Finlay [1] and Jui Vyas [1,*]

1. School of Medicine, Cardiff University, Cardiff CF14 4XN, UK; BrittainEL@cardiff.ac.uk (E.B.); FinlayAY@cardiff.ac.uk (A.Y.F.)
2. Buckinghamshire Healthcare NHS Trust, Amersham Hospital, Amersham HP7 0JD, UK; nina.muirhead@btinternet.com
* Correspondence: VyasJJ@cardiff.ac.uk

Abstract: *Background and objectives:* To explore the impacts that Myalgic Encephalomyelitis/Chronic Fatigue Syndrome (ME/CFS) has on the patient and their family members using the WHOQOL-BREF (Abbreviated World Health Organisation Quality of Life questionnaire) and FROM-16 (Family Reported Outcome Measure-16) quality of life assessments. *Materials and Methods:* A quantitative research study using postal questionnaires was conducted. A total of 39 adult volunteers expressed an interest in participating in the study: 24 returned appropriately completed questionnaires. Patients with ME/CFS completed the WHOQOL-BREF and up to four of their family members completed the FROM-16 questionnaire. *Results:* ME/CFS negatively affects the quality of life of the patient (median scores WHOQOL-BREF: Physical health = 19, Psychological = 44, Social relationships = 37.5, Environment = 56, n = 24) and their family members' quality of life (FROM-16: Emotional = 9.5, Personal and social = 11.5, Overall = 20.5, n = 42). There was a significant correlation between the patient's reported quality of life scores and their family members' mean FROM-16 total scores. *Conclusions:* This study identifies the major impact that having an adult family member with ME/CFS has on the lives of partners and of other family members. Quality of life of ME/CFS patients was reduced most by physical health compared to the other domains. Quality of life of family members was particularly impacted by worry, family activities, frustration and sadness. This highlights the importance of measuring the impact on the lives of family members using tools such as the FROM-16 in the ME/CFS clinical encounter and ensuring appropriate support is widely available to family members.

Keywords: ME/CFS; QoL; family impact; FROM-16; WHOQOL-BREF

Citation: Brittain, E.; Muirhead, N.; Finlay, A.Y.; Vyas, J. Myalgic Encephalomyelitis/Chronic Fatigue Syndrome (ME/CFS): Major Impact on Lives of Both Patients and Family Members. *Medicina* 2021, 57, 43. https://doi.org/10.3390/medicina57010043

Received: 3 December 2020
Accepted: 30 December 2020
Published: 7 January 2021

Publisher's Note: MDPI stays neutral with regard to jurisdictional claims in published maps and institutional affiliations.

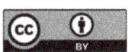

Copyright: © 2021 by the authors. Licensee MDPI, Basel, Switzerland. This article is an open access article distributed under the terms and conditions of the Creative Commons Attribution (CC BY) license (https://creativecommons.org/licenses/by/4.0/).

1. Introduction

Myalgic Encephalomyelitis/Chronic Fatigue Syndrome (ME/CFS) has profound impacts on the lives of those affected, but little is known about the impact experienced by partners and other family members. This hidden family burden is often ignored or unrecognised by health care workers.

ME/CFS is a complex, multisystem disease involving neurological, immunological, autonomic, and energy metabolism impairments [1]. Symptoms include post-exertional malaise (PEM), orthostatic intolerance, cognitive difficulties and unremitting fatigue [2]. ME/CFS is diagnosed based on clinical criteria, due to the absence of a known biomarker. The aetiology is unclear and there is no definitive pharmacological treatment; current treatment options target symptoms, rather than an underlying cause [2]. This lack of knowledge and evidence concerning diagnosis, aetiology and therapy add an additional burden to the practical issues experienced by those living with someone with ME/CFS.

Health-related quality of life (QoL) in patients with ME/CFS is significantly lower than in healthy controls and patients with other chronic illnesses [3]. Some studies have explored ME/CFS in paediatric patients and the impact on their mothers [4] and siblings [5]. However, there are no studies to date which have explored the impact of ME/CFS on both adult patients' QoL and their family members' QoL using validated questionnaires.

It is important to identify the extent to which the QoL of partners and family members of adults with ME/CFS is affected. Such knowledge may appropriately influence management decisions and also highlight areas of support that are required for both the patient and the family members. Measurement of QoL may thereby have the potential to enhance the quality of care of patients and their families.

The aim of the study was to measure the impact of ME/CFS on the patient and family using the WHOQOL-BREF (Abbreviated World Health Organisation Quality of Life questionnaire) and FROM-16 (Family Reported Outcome Measure-16) questionnaires. In families where patients reported a poorer QoL, we hypothesised that there would be a significant impact on the family member's QoL.

2. Materials and Methods

Ethical approval was granted by the Cardiff University School of Medicine Research Ethics Committee on 1 March 2019 (reference number 19/29).

Information regarding the study was posted on the Welsh Association of ME & CFS Support charity website and social media pages, through which patients made contact. Patient volunteers who expressed an interest in participating were sent packs in the post containing: research information leaflets, consent forms, one WHOQOL-BREF questionnaire for the patient and four FROM-16 questionnaires for up to four of their family members. Participants were excluded if the patient did not have a formal diagnosis of ME/CFS, if questionnaires were incomplete, or if the patient or family member were under the age of 18 years. All included patients and family members consented to participating in the study.

Participant information and questionnaire responses were recorded on separate password-protected Excel spreadsheets on a Cardiff University computer. WHOQOL-BREF questionnaires included a two-digit code number and letter A (e.g., 01 A). Each FROM-16 questionnaire included a three-digit code and letter B (e.g., 01.1 B). Each family received a different number. This coding ensured responses remained anonymous but still grouped when interpreting the data.

The WHOQOL-BREF is a 26-item questionnaire, which measures the impact of an illness on a patient's QoL [6] and is suitable for measuring the impact of ME/CFS [7]. Patients are assessed across four domains: Physical Health, Psychological, Social Relationships and Environment. A lower score in the WHOQOL-BREF indicates a poorer QoL. This questionnaire includes two additional questions regarding the patient's overall perception of their QoL and their health satisfaction. Each question has a five-point Likert interval scale where patients rate their response from 'Not at all' (1 point) to 'An extreme amount' (5 points). Patients were also asked to self-time how long it took to answer the WHOQOL-BREF.

The FROM-16 is a 16-item questionnaire designed to assess the impact of a disease on the patient's partner and family members [8]. The maximum score is out of 32, with a higher score indicating a greater impact on the family member's QoL. The questionnaire consists of two domains: Emotional (Part 1) and Personal and Social Life (Part 2). Each answer is graded on a three-point scale consisting of 'Not at all', 'A little' and 'A lot'. Statistical averages (mean, median, range, standard deviation) were used to assess the data collected by the questionnaires. Spearman's rank correlation coefficient was used to measure the strength of the correlation between different aspects of the WHOQOL-BREF and the mean FROM-16 total scores.

3. Results

Of 39 questionnaires posted in response to expression of interest, 29 were returned, giving a response rate of 74%. Five were excluded from analysis due to incomplete questionnaires and a self-reported diagnosis, resulting in 24 questionnaire packs available for analysis (24 WHOQOL-BREF questionnaires and 42 FROM-16 questionnaires).

The mean number of family members that participated within each family was 1.75 (mode = 1, median = 1) (Figure 1). The range was 1–4.

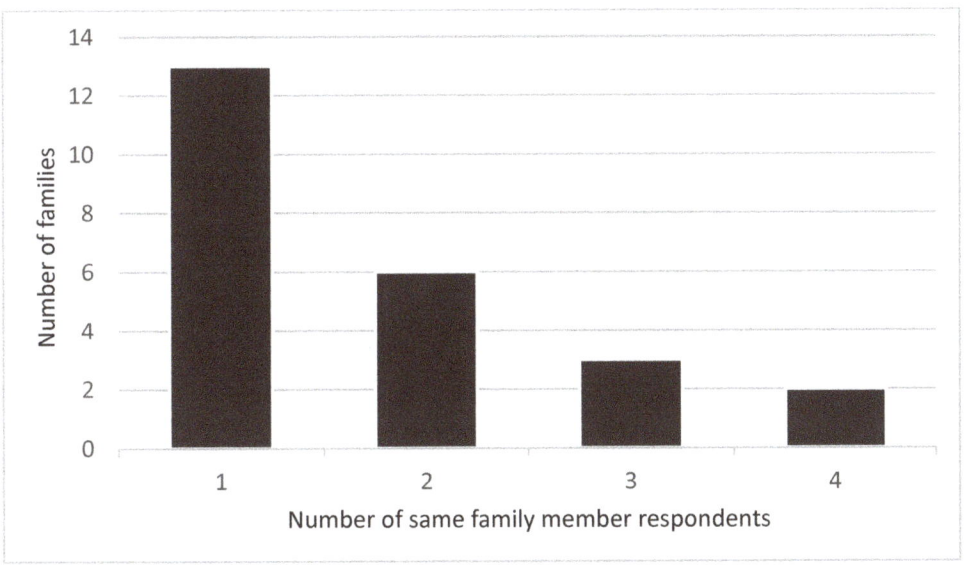

Figure 1. Bar Graph to illustrate the number of family members who completed the FROM-16 (Family Reported Outcome Measure-16) questionnaires within each family (n = 42).

Table 1 shows participant demographics. One family member did not answer the demographic questions at the start of the FROM-16 questionnaire, so the information represents 24 patients and 41 family members. The patients' mean age was 45 years (range: 18–71) and the family members mean age was 50 years (range: 18–94).

The median time it took patients to complete the WHOQOL-BREF questionnaire was 5–10 min (range from two minutes to one week). One patient did not provide this information and so was excluded from this analysis. Five of the 23 patients (21.7%) required assistance with completing their questionnaire.

One patient did not answer one of the WHOQOL-BREF questions in the Environment domain. We calculated the mean Environment score based on the other participants' answers in this domain, and then used this score to complete the question.

All patients rated their QoL as either 'Very poor', 'Poor', or 'Neither poor nor good' in Question 1 of the WHOQOL-BREF. Similarly, they were either 'Very dissatisfied' 'Dissatisfied', or 'Neither satisfied nor dissatisfied' with their health, measured using Question 2. The responses to both questions had a Spearman's rank correlation coefficient (r_s) of 0.50 [p(2-tailed) = 0.03], showing a statistically significant, strong correlation between patient QoL and health satisfaction.

The mean scores of parents, children and partners and spouses (Table 2) are very similar (range 18.0–20.1). Of the other respondents, only five siblings and grandparents responded, with a mean score of 27.0.

Table 1. Patient and family member demographics.

	Patient Demographics (n = 24)	
	Frequency	Percentage (%)
Gender:		
Female	18	75
Male	6	25
Marital Status:		
Single	6	25
Married	13	54
Living as married	3	13
Separated	1	4
Divorced	1	4
Widowed	0	0
None at all	0	0
Primary School	0	0
Secondary School	6	25
Tertiary	18	75
	Family Member Demographics (n = 41)	
	Frequency	Percentage (%)
Gender		
Female	18	43.9
Male	23	56.1
Relationship to Patient:		
Mother	11	26.8
Father	4	9.8
Spouse	12	29.3
Partner	4	9.8
Son	3	7.3
Daughter	2	4.9
Brother	2	4.9
Sister	1	2.4
Grandmother	1	2.4
Grandfather	1	2.4

Table 2. Mean FROM-16 (Family Reported Outcome Measure-16) scores of family members.

	Respondents	Number of Replies	Mean FROM-16
1	Parents	15	20.1
2	Children	5	18.0
3	Partners and Spouses	16	19.1
4	Siblings and grandparents	5	27.0

Family members, on average, scored 8.8 (max = 12) in the FROM-16 emotional domain, and 11.1 (max = 20) in the personal and social life domain (Table 3). The average overall FROM-16 score was 19.9 (n = 42). Family members are greatly affected by the ME/CFS, with no floor effect in either of the FROM-16 domains.

Table 3 shows the mean and median score for each of the 16 FROM-16 questions, and the rank of each question, based on mean scores. The median score was 2 for 6 questions: these were (given in descending order of score magnitude): questions 1 (worried), 10 (family activities), 4 (frustrated), 3 (sad), 11 (holidays), 15 (expenses). The median score for the other 10 questions was 1.

Table 3. The rank of each question based on the mean score and the median score of each question.

Rank	1	2	3	4	5	6	7	7	9	10	10	12	13	13	15	16
Question No.	1	10	4	3	11	15	5	6	2	7	14	13	12	16	8	9
Mean FROM-16 Score	1.80	1.76	1.70	1.60	1.51	1.34	1.29	1.29	1.10	1.07	1.07	0.96	0.86	0.86	0.83	0.76
Median FROM-16 Score	2	2	2	2	2	2	1	1	1	1	1	1	1	1	1	1

For patients, the average score for the physical health domain (21.8) in the WHOQOL-BREF was significantly lower compared to each of the other domains (psychological = 40.9, social relationships = 40.8, environment = 54.7, n = 24) (Table 4).

Table 4. Average results from both the FROM-16 (Family Reported Outcome Measure-16) and WHOQOL-BREF (Abbreviated World Health Organisation Quality of Life) questionnaires.

Questionnaire	Domain	Mean	Sample Standard Deviation	Median	Range	Floor Effect (%)	Ceiling Effect (%)
FROM-16 (n = 42)	Emotional (max 12)	8.8	2.7	9.5	2–12	-**	16.7
	Personal and social life (max 20)	11.1	5.2	11.5	1–20	-	2.4
	Overall score (max 32)	19.9	7.2	20.5	3–31	-	-
WHOQOL-BREF (n = 24)	Physical health *	21.8	12.5	19	0–56	4.2	-
	Psychological *	40.9	14.7	44	13–69	-	-
	Social relationships *	40.8	24.5	37.5	0–100	4.2	4.2
	Environment *	54.7	14.1	56	19–94	-	-

* Transformed score (max 100)]. The maximum FROM-16 total score is 32. The emotional and personal and social score are out of 12 and 20 respectively. ** Floor effect – all family members recorded some impact on quality of life

A statistically significant correlation [p(2-tailed) = 0.05] was found between the QoL of the patient and that of the family members, calculated from Question 1 of the WHOQOL-BREF and the mean FROM-16 total scores ($r_s = -0.41$) (Table 5). There was a negative correlation due to the different scoring directions of the two questionnaires.

Statistically significant, negative correlations were found between Physical Health (domain 1) of the WHOQOL-BREF and the mean FROM-16 total score and between the Environment (domain 4) and mean FROM-16 total score. Table 5 shows the Spearman's rank correlation coefficients for the domains with the 2-tailed probability level.

Table 5. Spearman's rank correlation coefficient and probability level of correlation between the mean FROM-16 total scores and each of the WHOQOL-BREF domains.

WHOQOL-BREF Domain Correlated with the Mean FROM-16 Total Score.	Spearman's Rank Correlation Coefficient (r_s)	p(2-Tailed) Test
Domain 1: Physical Health	−0.510	0.01
Domain 2: Psychological	−0.092	0.67
Domain 3: Social Relationships	−0.323	0.12
Domain 4: Environment	−0.453	0.03

4. Discussion

Our results confirm ME/CFS has a major negative impact on both the patient and their family members' QoL. There was no floor effect in any of the FROM-16 responses, exemplifying some degree of impact on every single family member who participated.

With a mean total FROM-16 score of 19.9, the negative impact on family members' QoL was significantly higher (mean = 19.9 SD = 7.2 n = 42) compared to previous FROM-16 scores of family members of patients with 25 other diseases (mean = 12.3, SD = 7.5, n = 120, $p < 0.001$) [8].

The statistically significant correlation between Question 1 of the WHOQOL-BREF and the mean FROM-16 total scores, confirms our hypothesis that in ME/CFS patients, a poorer QoL impacts greatly on their family members' QoL. Patient's family members' QoL is an important concept and has shown to be adversely affected in a wide range of medical specialities, from dermatology [9] to oncology [10] whereas in certain conditions such as urinary stones, there has been a negligible impact on family members [11].

From this low number of respondents, there appears to be no obvious signal suggesting that there might be differences in QoL impact experienced by relatives of different relationship with the affected person. However, the few siblings and grandparents scored more highly. Mothers and female partners/spouses scored marginally higher than fathers and male partners/spouses. The minimal clinically important score difference (MCID) for FROM-16 has not yet been determined, but the MCID of a measure is usually in the order of 10–15% of the maximum score for that measure, i.e., a score change here of three to five. If that is the case, the differences between mean scores of parents, children and partners and spouses would not have reached the MCID level. However, the mean scores for the individual FROM-16 questions reveal which aspects of family member's lives were most affected by having a family member with ME/CFS: these were worry, family activities, frustration and sadness. This emphasises the importance of providing appropriate psychological support and practical advice, including financial advice, to family members.

The finding that, for patients, the average score for the physical health domain was significantly lower compared to each of the other domains has also been shown within other ME/CFS research studies using the Medical Outcomes Study Short Form-36 Health Survey. All scores regarding physical function were significantly lower when compared to healthy controls and other illness groups [12,13]. A strong correlation was found between the WHOQOL-BREF 'Physical Health' domain and the mean FROM-16 total scores.

Also highlighted in our results, was a correlation between the WHOQOL-BREF 'Environment' domain and the mean FROM-16 total scores. Weak correlations with the other WHOQOL-BREF domains (Psychological and Social Relationships) and the mean FROM-16 total scores were expected as these aspects of QoL are not fully addressed in the FROM-16 questionnaire.

Limitations of this study include that questionnaires were not anonymous within each family—patients could see what their family members had answered and vice versa. Consequently, some participants may have over- or understated some of their responses. Self-reported questionnaires also carry their own risk of bias, for example, answering questions with socially-desirable answers. Some families had more than one family member with ME/CFS. This could confound the results. Different domains were measured between the questionnaires, therefore some of the domains were not expected to significantly correlate with the FROM-16 scores. The recruitment method used creates several biases that must be taken into account when interpreting the data. Respondents had to be motivated to be a member of a patient support group and were also part of an online environment. It is possible that these biases may have resulted in those patients and family members who were more highly educated, resourceful and dissatisfied as well as more severely affected were over-represented. This was a limitation noted by Hvidberg et al. who received questionnaire responses from 105 participants on a health related QoL (HRQoL) via the national ME/CFS patient association [3].

The median time of 5–10 min for patients to complete the WHOQOL-BREF questionnaire demonstrates that this could be a useful tool in a clinical or outpatient setting.

Positive aspects of the study included that this was the first attempt to measure the impact of adult ME/CFS on the QoL of family members using validated questionnaires. If indeed more severely affected patients are over-represented in this study, this would be an important advantage, as such patients are often poorly represented in studies, and the burden of ME/CFS may therefore be significantly underestimated [14].

5. Conclusions

To the best of our knowledge, this is the first study to measure the QoL in family members and adult patients with ME/CFS using validated questionnaires. There is a significant correlation between patient's QoL and their family members' QoL. This was a small exploratory study but provides sufficient evidence to support larger scale research to provide more robust evidence.

At present there is very little support available to family members of patients with ME/CFS. This study provides evidence of the major impact that this condition has on the QoL of family members. This lays down a challenge to the health care services to address these issues and to identify ways in which the secondary impact of ME/CFS may be alleviated.

Author Contributions: Conceptualization, N.M., A.Y.F. and J.V.; methodology, N.M., A.Y.F. and J.V.; formal analysis, E.B., N.M., A.Y.F. and J.V.; investigation, E.B.; data curation, E.B.; writing—original draft preparation, E.B.; writing—review and editing, E.B., N.M., A.Y.F. and J.V.; supervision, N.M., A.Y.F. and J.V.; project administration, J.V.; no external funding. All authors have read and agreed to the published version of the manuscript.

Funding: This research received no external funding.

Institutional Review Board Statement: The study was conducted according to the guidelines of the Declaration of Helsinki, and approved by the Cardiff University School of Medicine Research Ethics Committee on 1 March 2019 (reference number 19/29).

Informed Consent Statement: Informed consent was obtained from all subjects involved in the study.

Data Availability Statement: The data presented in this study are available on request from the corresponding author. The data are not publicly available, patients have given consent for use of their anonymous data in this study.

Acknowledgments: The authors would like to thank Jan Russell at the Welsh Association of ME & CFS Support and the ME/CFS patients and their families for volunteering to participate in this research.

Conflicts of Interest: A.Y.F. is joint copyright holder of the FROM-16. N.M. has given testimony to NICE and Ono Pharmaceutical, N.M. is also Chair of the Education Working Group of the CFS/ME Research Collaborative (CMRC) and is a member of Forward ME. J.V. has been on a paid advisory board for Amgen and has received honoraria from L'Oréal outside of this submission. E.B. has no conflicts of interest to declare.

References

1. US ME/CFS Clinician Coalition. Available online: https://www.omf.ngo/2019/09/01/new-guidelines-for-diagnosing-and-treating-me-cfs/ (accessed on 26 November 2020).
2. Baker, R.; Shaw, E. Diagnosis and management of chronic fatigue syndrome or myalgic encephalomyelitis (or encephalopathy): Summary of NICE guidance. *BMJ* **2007**, *335*, 446–448. [CrossRef] [PubMed]
3. Hvidberg, M.F.; Brinth, L.S.; Olesen, A.V.; Petersen, K.D.; Ehlers, L. The health-related quality of life for patients with myalgic encephalomyelitis/chronic fatigue syndrome (ME/CFS). *PLoS ONE* **2015**, *10*, e0132421. [CrossRef] [PubMed]
4. Missen, A.; Hollingworth, W.; Eaton, N.; Crawley, E. The financial and psychological impacts on mothers of children with chronic fatigue syndrome (CFS/ME). *Child Care Heatlh Dev.* **2012**, *38*, 505–512. [CrossRef] [PubMed]
5. Velleman, S.; Collin, S.M.; Beasant, L.; Crawley, E. Psychological wellbeing and quality-of-life among siblings of paediatric CFS/ME patients: A mixed-methods study. *Clin. Child Psychol. Psychiatry* **2016**, *21*, 618–633. [CrossRef] [PubMed]
6. Harper, A.; Power, M. Development of the World Health Organization WHOQOL-BREF quality of life assessment. *Psychol. Med.* **1998**, *28*, 551–558.
7. Roberts, D. Chronic fatigue syndrome and quality of life. *Patient Relat. Outcome Meas.* **2018**, *9*, 253–262. [CrossRef] [PubMed]
8. Golics, C.J.; Basra, M.K.A.; Finlay, A.Y.; Salek, S. The development and validation of the Family Reported Outcome Measure (FROM-16)© to assess the impact of disease on the partner or family member. *Qual. Life Res.* **2014**, *23*, 317–326. [CrossRef] [PubMed]
9. Basra, M.; Finlay, A.Y. The family impact of skin diseases: The Greater Patient concept. *Br. J. Dermatol.* **2007**, *156*, 929–937. [CrossRef] [PubMed]
10. Lee, H.J.; Park, E.C.; Seung Ju, K.; Lee, S.G. Quality of life of family members living with cancer patients. *Asian Pac. J Cancer Prev.* **2015**, *16*, 6913–6917. [CrossRef] [PubMed]
11. Raja, A.; Wood, F.; Joshi, H.B. The impact of urinary stone disease and their treatment on patients' quality of life: A qualitative study. *Urolithiasis* **2020**, *48*, 227–234. [CrossRef] [PubMed]
12. Lowry, T.J.; Pakenham, K.I. Health-related quality of life in chronic fatigue syndrome: Predictors of physical functioning and psychological distress. *Psychol. Health Med.* **2008**, *13*, 222–238. [CrossRef] [PubMed]

13. Nacul, L.C.; Lacerda, E.M.; Campion, P.; Pheby, D.; de LDrachler, M.; Leite, J.C.; Poland, F.; Howe, A.; Fayyaz, S.; Molokhia, M. The functional status and well being of people with myalgic encephalomyelitis/chronic fatigue syndrome and their carers. *BMC Public Health* **2011**, *11*, 402. [CrossRef] [PubMed]
14. Davenport, T.E.; Stevens, S.R.; Van Ness, J.M.; Stevens, J.; Snell, C.R. Checking our blind spots: Current status of research evidence summaries in ME/CFS. *Br. J. Sports Med.* **2019**, *53*, 1198. [CrossRef] [PubMed]

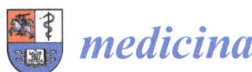

Article

Comparative Survey of People with ME/CFS in Italy, Latvia, and the UK: A Report on Behalf of the Socioeconomics Working Group of the European ME/CFS Research Network (EUROMENE)

Elenka Brenna [1,*], Diana Araja [2] and Derek F. H. Pheby [3]

1 Department of Economics and Finance, Università Cattolica del Sacro Cuore, Largo Agostino Gemelli 1, 20123 Milan, Italy
2 Department of Dosage Form Technology, Faculty of Pharmacy, Institute of Microbiology and Virology, Riga Stradins University, Dzirciema Street 16, LV-1007 Riga, Latvia; diana.araja@rsu.lv
3 Society and Health, Buckinghamshire New University (retired), High Wycombe HP11 2JZ, UK; derekpheby@btinternet.com
* Correspondence: elenka.brenna@unicatt.it

Abstract: *Background and Objectives*: A comparative survey of Myalgic Encephalomyelitis/Chronic Fatigue Syndrome (ME/CFS) patients was carried out in three countries, with the aim of identifying appropriate policy measures designed to alleviate the burden of disease both on patients and their families, and also on public institutions. The survey addressed demographic features, the economic impact of the disease on household incomes, patterns of medical and social care, specific therapies, social relationships, and the impact of the illness on quality of life. *Materials and Methods*: Parallel surveys were undertaken in Italy, Latvia, and the UK. There were 88 completed responses from Italy, 75 from Latvia, and 448 from the UK. To facilitate comparisons, 95% confidence intervals were calculated in respect of responses to questions from all three countries. To explore to what extent general practitioners (GPs) manage ME/CFS disease, a separate questionnaire for GPs, with questions about the criteria for granting a diagnosis, laboratory examinations, the involvement of specialists, and methods of treatment, was undertaken in Latvia, and there were 91 completed responses from GPs. *Results*: The results are presented in respect of sociodemographic information, household income, disease progression and management, perceived effectiveness of treatment, responsibility for medical care, personal care, difficulty explaining the illness, and quality of life. Demographic details were similar in all three countries, and the impact of illness on net household incomes and quality of life. There were significant differences between the three countries in illness progression and management, which may reflect differences in patterns of health care and in societal attitudes. Graded exercise therapy, practiced in the UK, was found to be universally ineffective. *Conclusions*: There were similarities between respondents in all three countries in terms of demographic features, the impact of the illness on household incomes and on quality of life, and on difficulties experienced by respondents in discussing their illness with doctors, but also differences in patterns of medical care, availability of social care, and societal attitudes to ME/CFS.

Keywords: Myalgic Encephalomyelitis; chronic fatigue syndrome; ME/CFS; economic impact; medical care; social care; quality of life

1. Introduction

Myalgic Encephalomyelitis/Chronic Fatigue Syndrome (ME/CFS) is a complex, multi-system disorder, with severe, profound incapacitating fatigue not alleviated by rest, and post-exertional malaise. Other symptoms include cognitive dysfunction, sleep disturbance, and muscle pain. As a result, marked reductions in functional activity and quality of life are encountered [1]. Cases vary markedly in the symptoms they manifest, in severity, and

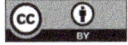

in disease progression. ME/CFS most frequently occurs between ages 20 and 50 but can affect all ages. The majority of patients are female [2]. UK experience suggests that there may be two million patients throughout Europe [3]. Much work has been carried out over several decades to investigate the nature of the syndrome, but marked uncertainty remains over its definition, diagnosis, treatment, and economic impact [4].

The problem of determining the economic impact of ME/CFS in Europe was considered by the socioeconomics working group of EUROMENE (*vide infra*). The economic burden is significant, with productivity losses appearing to be the largest cost element, while effective prevention and treatment give scope for substantial cost reductions. There are problems of economic evaluation because of the arbitrariness of case definitions, and doctors who are unable to diagnose the condition, for reasons including disbelief and lack of understanding, so there is a lack of accurate incidence and prevalence data. Recommendations of the working group include the use of the Fukuda (CDC-1994) case definition and Canadian Consensus Criteria (CCC), a pan-European common symptom checklist, implementation of prevalence-based cost-of-illness studies in different countries using an agreed data list, the use of purchasing power parities (PPP) to facilitate international comparisons, and the use of EuroQol-5D to measure health status [5].

The European Network on ME/CFS (EUROMENE) is a collaborative, Europe-wide, consortium aiming to address serious gaps in knowledge of ME/CFS. In 2016, EUROMENE received funding from the European Union through the COST programme, and was formally constituted as COST Action 15111. This action aims to "promote further research on ME/CFS with high economic impact" [6]. Working Group 3, on socioeconomics, has endeavored to appraise the economic implications of the disease, its specific objectives including surveying data from European countries on the economic losses due to ME/CFS and developing ways to calculate the direct and indirect economic burdens due to ME/CFS [7].

In pursuit of these objectives, a comparative questionnaire study of ME/CFS patients was carried out in three countries, Italy, Latvia, and the UK, with the aim of identifying appropriate policy measures designed to alleviate the burden of disease both on patients and their families, and on governments. In particular, reducing diagnostic delays should limit progression to severe, prolonged disease, with consequent reductions in its economic impact, including direct and indirect costs, and, most importantly, productivity costs.

2. Methods

Parallel surveys were undertaken in Italy, Latvia, and the UK. In Italy, a questionnaire (Supplementary Material) was distributed to 104 adult patients living in the north of the country, with the support of the Association of Patients CFS Onlus, which has an important role in assisting and supporting medical research and in disseminating knowledge of the disease [8]. The questionnaire had several sections. The first section sought general information (age, gender, education, place of residence, etc.), the second section addressed clinical history, and the third focused on the socio-economic consequences of the disease, including restrictions on daily life, sources of assistance, and understanding and awareness of the disease. The final section sought information on health status, reliance on physicians, the possible causes of illness, and future expectations. Quality of life was assessed using the instrument EuroQol-5D [9–11]. The patients were also asked to rate their quality of life in a scale from 0 to 100, where 100 represents the best imaginable QoL and 0 the worst, for the year before onset of illness, and for the year immediately preceding completion of the survey.

In Latvia, the patients' questionnaire (Supplementary Material) has been designed in accordance with the questionnaire prepared by the Italian team of Working Group 3 (socioeconomic), employed in the European program COST Action 15111 EUROMENE, in order to get a comparable data. The sample has included 75 valid observations, performed by 62 women and 13 men. Simultaneously, a questionnaire for GPs was distributed with support of the Latvian Association of Rural Family Doctors, taking into account that this association represents GPs working in urban and rural areas. The survey had included 20 questions, mostly on the criteria for granting a diagnosis, laboratory examinations, the involvement of specialists, and the methods of treatment. There were 91 completed responses from GPs.

To obtain comparison data from the UK, an internet survey was set up using the facility 'Smartsurvey'. A link to the questionnaire was circulated on 19 October 2020 via the internet group 'LocalME', with a request for UK residents with medically diagnosed ME/CFS to respond by 31 October. 448 questionnaires were completed by the deadline. The survey was structured in order to replicate as much as possible the Italian original questionnaire, though some variations were inevitable because of differences in the ways in which healthcare services are delivered. For the international comparison report we have calculated 95% confidence intervals for most of the parameters examined.

3. Results

In Italy, 88 questionnaires were correctly completed, and in Latvia, there were 75 valid responses from patients and 91 completed responses from GPs. There were 448 completed responses to the UK survey. Comparative results are presented below under the following headings—sociodemographic information, household income, disease progression and management, perceived effectiveness of treatment, responsibility for medical care, personal care, difficulty explaining the illness, and quality of life. The results of the additional GP survey in Latvia on the management of ME/CFS are provided in the concluding section.

3.1. Sociodemographic Information

The respondents ranged in age from 17 to 81, with an average of 50 years, and there was no significant difference between the three countries in terms of average age. In addition, there was no significant difference between the three countries in the gender distribution of respondents; in all three, a large majority of respondents were female. A very much higher proportion of UK respondents had post-school educational qualifications than in Latvia or Italy, but there was no significant difference between the latter two countries in that respect. Around half of all respondents in the three countries were married. In Latvia, a third of respondents lived alone. The proportions in Italy and the UK were lower, but these differences were not statistically significant. The results are detailed in Table 1.

Table 1. Sociodemographic data.

Item	Country	No. Respondents	Mean	Standard Deviation (SD)	No. Responding 'Yes'	%	95% Confidence Interval (%)
Age (years)	Italy	88	47.0	13.9			44.1–49.4
	Latvia	75	50.0	14.7			46.6–53.3
	UK	447	42.1	14.0			40.9–43.5
Gender (No. females)	Italy	88			68	77.3	67.1–87.4
	Latvia	75			62	82.7	73.1–92.3
	UK	385			332	86.3	82.5–90.0
Education (No. with post-school qualifications)	Italy	88			34	38.7	21.9–55.3
	Latvia	74			32	43.2	25.7–60.8
	UK	374			314	83.9	79.8–88.1
Marital status (No. married)	Italy	88			39	44.3	28.4–60.2
	Latvia	75			45	60.0	45.4–74.6
	UK	446			205	46.0	39.0–52.9
No. living alone	Italy	88			17	19.4	0.2–38.5
	Latvia	74			25	33.8	14.9–52.7
	UK	447			107	23.9	15.7–32.2

3.2. Household Income

According to literature, the disease significantly impacts on the personal income, because patients are frequently unable to work. International comparisons are very difficult due to the heterogeneity of average income in UE countries. Looking at Eurostat [12], the mean equivalized net income in 2018 was respectively €19,208 (Italy), €25,642 (UK), and €8740 (Latvia). However, in Italy and the UK, only 44.1% and 54.6% respondents respectively declared an income higher than €15,000, which supports the hypothesis of an impact of the disease on individual productivity. In Latvia, no patients declared an income higher than €15,000, but this is due to the fact that income is relatively lower in this country. This international comparison is summarized in Table 2.

Table 2. Household incomes.

Item	Country	No. Respondents	No. Responding 'Yes'	%	95% Confidence Interval (%)
Household income (No. with > €15,000 p.a.)	Italy	85	38	44.1	28.6–60.8
Household income, per member (No. with > €15,000 p.a.)	Latvia	65	0	0.0	-
	UK	443	242	54.6	48.2–61.0

3.3. Disease Progression and Management

There were significant differences between the three countries in the proportions of respondents reporting having had more than ten investigations, having experienced more than ten symptoms, or having had more than five treatments. Italian respondents reported the most investigations and treatments and the most symptoms, which may be associated with a lack of appropriates guidelines for diagnosing ME/CFS, and the Latvians least, with the UK respondents occupying an intermediate position. UK respondents were significantly more likely than others to report that their symptoms fluctuated in severity (Table 3).

3.4. Perceived Effectiveness of Treatment

As regards the use of non-pharmacological treatments, in all three countries there were free text responses concerning the treatments followed during the last five years, in particular physiotherapy, cognitive behaviour therapy (CBT) and graded exercise therapy (GET). For all countries, physiotherapy is the most widespread treatment, with 41.7% Italian patients receiving it (or having received it in the last five years), 30.8% Latvian patients and fewer UK patients (14.3%). CBT was also reported by 23.5% Italians, 33.3% Latvians, and 7.0% UK participants.

A specific question asked if patients considered non-pharmacological treatments effective. Whilst in Italy only 8% patients answered positively, this percentage rises at 52% for Latvia and 57.7% for UK.

With regards to this item, it seems that Italian patients are not satisfied with the therapies received. A specific response regarding GET was obtained only from the UK, and it is noteworthy that only one respondent found it effective. These findings are detailed in Table 4.

3.5. Responsibility for Medical Care

GPs were significantly more likely to have primary responsibility for medical care in Latvia than in either Italy or the UK. This probably reflects the situation that there is not a specific patients' organization for ME/CFS in Latvia, and the GP is a 'gate-keeper' for patients in diagnostic and treatment process. In Italy, the search for a correct diagnosis and the absence of appropriate guidelines for the disease identification pushes patients to ask for specialist consultations, as well as many diagnostic tests being performed before a final diagnosis is arrived at.

Table 3. Disease progression and management.

Item	Country	No. Respondents	Mean	SD	No. Responding 'Yes'	%	95% Confidence Interval (%)
No. symptoms	Italy	88	11.0	3.0			10.4–11.6
	Latvia	75	7.5	2.5			6.9–8.1
	UK	445	8.0	4.1			7.6–8.4
Treatments:							
- All	Italy	88	0.5	0.2			0.33–0.67
	Latvia	75	2.5	1.2			2.2–2.8
	UK	425	3.0	3.0			2.7–3.3
- Drug treatment	Italy	88	0.5	0.2			0.33–0.67
	Latvia	75	2.3	1.3			2.0–2.6
	UK	425	1.3	4.0			0.9–1.7
- Non-drug treatment	Italy	-	-	-			-
	Latvia	75	1.2	1.0			1.0–1.4
	UK	425	1.7	2.1			1.5–1.9
No. investigations	Italy	88	10.4	2.4			9.9–10.9
	Latvia	75	5.7	3.2			5.0–6.4
	UK	178	12.8	29.0			8.5–17.0
No. respondents reporting:							
>10 investigations	Italy	88			65	73.9	63.0–84.8
	Latvia	75			3	4.0	0.0–26.6
	UK	178			86	48.3	37.5–59.1
>10 symptoms	Italy	88			64	72.7	
	Latvia	75			7	9.3	4.6–18.0
	UK	445			86	19.3	1.8–27.8
>5 treatments	Italy	88			29	32.9	24.0–43.3
	Latvia	75			0	0.0	-
	UK	425			63	14.8	5.9–23.8
Variability of symptoms	Italy	86			48	55.8	41.5–70.1
	Latvia	75			53	70.7	58.2–83.2
	UK	446			410	91.9	89.2–94.6

On the contrary, specialists had little involvement in the care of the UK patients. Other healthcare professionals were involved in the care of a higher proportion of UK respondents than was found in either Italy or Latvia. In the latter case, there was very little involvement of other professionals (see Table 5).

3.6. Personal Care

Significantly fewer Latvian respondents had family assistance with personal care than was found in either Italy or the UK. Other (non-family) sources of personal care assistance were reported by Italian or Latvian patients while nearly a fifth of UK respondents were cared for by non-family members. No external help with personal care was reported by nearly one in five of Italian respondents and a smaller proportion of UK ones. No response from Latvian patients. A large proportion of Italian and Latvian respondents reported that they had capacity for self-care, as well as a significantly smaller proportion, but still a majority, of UK respondents (Table 6).

Table 4. Perceived effectiveness of treatment.

Item	Country	No. Respondents	No. Responding 'Yes'	%	95% Confidence Interval (%)
Treatments practiced in the last five years					
Physiotherapy	Italy	84	35	41.7	31.7–52.9
	Latvia	39	12	30.8	18.6–46.4
	UK	28	4	14.3	0.0–49.3
Cognitive behaviour therapy (CBT)	Italy	85	20	23.5	15.8–34.2
	Latvia	39	13	33.3	20.3 = 49.0
	UK	115	8	7.0	0.0–24.9
Graded exercise therapy (GET)	Italy	-	-	-	-
	Latvia	-	-	-	-
	UK	70	1	1.4	0.0–25.2
Perceived effectiveness of non-pharmacological treatments (No. finding treatment effective):	Italy	88	7	8.0	0.0–28.4
	Latvia	75	39	52.0	36.0–68.0
	UK	356	204	57.3	50.4–64.2

Table 5. Responsibility for medical care.

Item	Country	No. Respondents	No. Responding 'Yes'	%	95% Confidence Interval (%)
Responsibility for medical care:					
- GPs	Italy	85	41	48.2	32.6–63.8
	Latvia	75	57	76.0	64.7–87.3
	UK	446	189	42.4	35.2–49.6
- Specialists	Italy	85	67	78.8	68.8–88.8
	Latvia	75	44	58.7	43.8–75.5
	UK	446	35	7.9	0.0–16.9
- Other	Italy	84	18	21.4	2.1–40.8
	Latvia	75	5	6.7	0.0–29.0
	UK	446	62	35.9	5.1–22.7

Table 6. Personal care.

Item	Country	No. Respondents	No. Responding 'Yes'	%	95% Confidence Interval (%)
Assistance with Personal Care:					
- family	Italy	85	70	82.3	73.2–91.5
	Latvia	72	17	23.6	11.0–24.9
	UK	413	293	70.9	65.6–76.2
- others	Italy	85	1	1.2	0.0–22.7
	Latvia	72	0	0.0	-
	UK	413	76	18.4	9.5–27.3
- No-one	Italy	85	16	18.8	0.0–38.4
	Latvia	72	0	0.0	-
	UK	413	31	7.5	0.0–17.0
Capacity for self-care (number responding 'Yes')	Italy	84	73	86.9	79.0–94.8
	Latvia	72	58	77.3	70.2–90.9
	UK	443	253	57.1	50.9–63.3

3.7. Difficulty Explaining the Illness

One of the major difficulties for CFS/ME patients consists in explaining the symptoms. In Italy and the UK, around three-quarters of all respondents reported difficulty explaining their illnesses to physicians, but in Latvia only a quarter of respondents had this problem. This difference was statistically significant. When it came to explaining the illness to the family, though, nearly three-quarters of Italian respondents had trouble, while for Latvia and UK this figure decreases to less than 50%. Again, this difference was statistically significant. A quarter of Latvian respondents expressed difficulty explaining their illnesses to friends, compared with about two-thirds of British respondents and more than four-fifths of Italian ones. All these differences were statistically significant. The Latvians least frequently had difficulty explaining their illnesses to employers, compared with more than half of UK respondents and nearly two-thirds of Italians. However, these differences were not statistically significant (Table 7).

Table 7. Difficulty explaining the illness.

Item	Country	No. Respondents	No. Responding 'Yes'	%	95% Confidence Interval (%)
Difficulty explaining illness to:					
- Physicians	Italy	86	63	73.2	62.1–84.4
	Latvia	75	20	26.7	18.0–37.6
	UK	444	343	77.3	72.7–81.8
Family	Italy	84	60	71.4	59.8–83.1
	Latvia	75	35	46.7	35.8–57.9
	UK	446	222	49.8	43.1–56.5
Friends	Italy	83	68	81.9	72.6–91.3
	Latvia	75	20	26.7	18.0–37.6
	UK	444	290	65.3	59.7–70.9
Employers	Italy	76	49	64.5	50.8–78.1
	Latvia	75	30	40.0	29.7–51.3
	UK	407	233	57.2	50.8–63.7

3.8. Quality of Life

In all three countries, a marked diminution in quality of life (scored 0 to 100) between the year before illness and the most recent year was reported. All these changes were statistically significant. The reported quality of life prior to illness was significantly higher in Italy than in the other countries and was lowest in Latvia. The diminution in perceived life quality as a result of illness was lowest in Latvia, where the mean quality of life score during illness was significantly higher than in either Italy or the UK. Indeed, it was in Italy where the greatest decline in average quality of life as a result of illness occurred (Table 8). To this extent, a study was carried out in Italy aimed at demonstrating the impact of selected variables on the probability of experiencing a decrease higher than 50 points in self-reported quality of life. It turned out, for example, that having more than 10 symptoms and being treated with more than 5 treatments was associated with this large reduction in quality of life [13].

Table 8. Quality of life.

Item	Country	No. Respondents	Mean	SD	95% Confidence Interval (%)
Quality of life:					
- before illness	Italy	84	90.3	9.7	88.2–92.4
	Latvia	74	74.6	24.0	69.0–80.2
	UK	439	80.9	23.0	78.7–82.7
- in past year	Italy	84	34.6	20.8	30.1–39.1
	Latvia	74	57.3	16.3	53.5–61.1
	UK	440	31.5	19.8	29.6–33.1

3.9. Results of the Additional GP Survey in Latvia on the Management of CFS

In Latvia, there were 91 valid responses to the GP survey, which included questions on the criteria for making a diagnosis, laboratory examinations, referral to specialists and methods of treatment. For making the diagnosis, the results showed that 13 responders (14%) used the Fukuda case definition. 61 responders (67%) used the ICD-10 code R53 (malaise and fatigue), while 18 (20%) used code G93.3 (post viral fatigue syndrome). 5 respondents (5.5%) used ICD-10 code B94.8 (sequelae of other specified infectious and parasitic diseases). The multiplicity of codes used to record diagnoses of ME/CFS contributes to the problem of determining numbers of patients. Moreover, 70% of GPs reported that patients had difficulty in describing their symptoms. All the participating GPs used laboratory tests in the diagnostic process, some more than others, with 35 respondents (38%) using more than ten different tests. 65 GP respondents (71%) referred patients for specialist care and diagnostic support. Specialists referred to included neurologists (62%), psychiatrists or psychotherapists (30%), and infectious disease or other specialists (13%). 70% of GP respondents indicated the presence of comorbidities in their ME/CFS patients. GP management included medication, referral to physiotherapy, psychotherapy, osteopathy, homeopathy and lifestyle adjustment, but 59% of respondents regarded the disease as incurable. Improvements to the care of ME/CFS patients suggested by GP respondents included the development of a specialists' consortium, better information for patients, public funding for psychotherapy consultations, additional training, and more time for conversation with patients.

4. Discussion

In the UK, treating physicians were not identified and therefore could not be interviewed. Similarly, in Italy recruitment was via a patients' organization and did not involve treating physicians. In Latvia, participant selection was based on ICD-10 diagnoses. This was following advice from the country's only secondary referral center for ME/CFS. The diversity of recruitment methods in the three countries was probably a source of strength rather than weakness, as the findings from the survey from the three countries revealed some very similar problems and concerns, suggesting that patients' experiences were universal in nature, and not confined to any one country or health care system. It is interesting that, despite differences in health care systems, diagnostic methods, recruitment methods and survey media, there was a very considerable similarity in the experiences of respondents in all three countries.

Respondents in all three countries were similar in terms of average age and had the same preponderance of females. There were no significant differences in the proportions of respondents who were married or living alone, or who had post-school educational qualifications. In Latvia, the UK, and Italy, net household incomes were lower than the national average, indicating the impact of illness on incomes in all countries. As regards illness management and progression, there were significant differences between the three countries. Italians reported more symptoms, more investigations and more treatments than respondents from the other countries, and the Latvians the least. This may be due to the absence of appropriate guidelines for the management of the disease in Italy. We did not elicit any information on the nature of the investigations carried out, because the purpose of this question was to obtain a measure of the extent to which doctors in the three countries were taking seriously their patients' illnesses and were actively working to investigate them.

Symptom fluctuation was significantly more marked among the UK respondents than among the others. It was noteworthy that graded exercise therapy, in the UK, was found to be universally ineffective, and none of the Italians reported having had this therapy. There were reported differences between the three countries in who had responsibility for providing medical care, but these may reflect differences in the management of the disease in each country. Thus, GPs more frequently had principal responsibility for medical care in Latvia than in Italy or the UK and this probably reflects the fact that in Latvia

GPs perform the gate-keeper role for patients in the diagnostic and treatment process. Healthcare professionals other than doctors were more frequently involved in clinical care in the UK than in either Latvia or Italy, which is likely to be related to the pattern of delivery of primary care in the UK via the National Health Service.

In terms of personal care also, differences in response between the three countries were more likely to reflect differences in the way in which social care is delivered in the three countries. Thus, non-family care assistance was almost entirely confined to the UK, where capacity for self-care was less prevalent that in the other countries. Similarly, variations in difficulty explaining the disease to physicians was least widespread in Latvia, but this may be attributable to the fact that physicians there were centrally involved in the identification of potential respondents. Other variations, e.g., in explaining the illness to family, friends or employers, may reflect differences in society in the three countries. Italians were most likely to have trouble in explaining the illness to families, while Latvians had the least difficulty explaining the illness to friends or employers, which suggests that there may be greater understanding of the illness in the general population than is the case in either Italy or the UK.

While there were differences between the three countries in perceived quality of life both before and during illness, the trend was similar in Italy, Latvia, and the UK, with marked diminution in quality of life being reported in all three countries as a result of illness. In Latvia, the smaller gap in quality of life as a result of illness could be explained by a greater decrease in quality of life before diagnosis, with a subsequent smaller decrease in quality of life after diagnosis and initiation of treatment. While we do not wish to overinterpret these data, it is likely that the initial differences between the three countries reported prior to illness, for example in income and educational attainments, may reflect overall socioeconomic differences between them, while there is substantial convergence between all three countries in patient experience once illness becomes established.

The strength of this study is that this is the first study of ME/CFS patients conducted on a transnational, comparative basis in Europe. It demonstrates that the basic demographic features of the illness, in terms for example of the average age of participants and the gender distribution, are very similar in the three countries studied. Where the responses from the three countries differ, this largely reflects socioeconomic differences between countries, or differences in the way in which medical services are delivered. Although there was not a single template for the recruitment of patients, we endeavored to ensure the comparability of patients through the recruitment process. Thus, in Italy, only patients with a recognized diagnosis of CFS/ME were selected. Similarly, in Latvia, from almost 300 respondents to the on-line survey on CFS symptoms, only participants with ICD-10 diagnosis codes G93.3, R53 and B94.8 were involved in data analysis for the purposes of this paper, while in the UK patients with medically confirmed diagnoses of ME/CFS were self-selected via an internet-based patient support group.

The finding that ME/CFS has a substantial impact on net household income is consistent with the previous conclusion of the socioeconomics working group of EUROMENE that the economic impact of ME/CFS is substantial [5]. The reports of household income are worrying, given average 2018 incomes of €25,642 in the UK, €19,208 in Italy, and €8740 in Latvia [12]. International comparisons are very difficult due to the heterogeneity of average incomes in European countries, In Italy, 44.1% of respondents declared an income higher than €15,000, while the comparable proportion among UK respondents was 54.6% of respondents compared with 92% of the UK general population in 2017–18 [14]. In Latvia, annual incomes among the general population are lower than in Italy and the UK. No Latvian respondents reported an annual income per household member in excess of €15,000. Despite these differences between the three countries under consideration, the pattern is consistent; in all three countries, the respondents tended to report net incomes per household member which were substantially lower than those found among the general population. This underlines the negative impact of having ME/CFS on individual productivity and capacity to work and indicates that this impact is substantial. Our findings are consistent with other research demonstrating a very substantial impact of ME/CFS on productivity costs. Thus, Reynolds et al. analyzed data from a surveillance study of ME/CFS in Wichita, Kansas, and concluded that lost productivity due to ME/CFS was substantial both in absolute terms and in comparison with other major illnesses [15], while Collin et al. analyzed data from the UK CFS/ME National Outcomes Database, and concluded that ME/CFS causes huge productivity costs amongst the small fraction of adults with ME/CFS who access specialist services [16].

The paper did not address the relationship between severity and economic impacts, the importance of which we emphasized in a previous paper [5]. It is likely, though, that productivity costs were higher among the more severely ill patients, because being housebound or bedbound, severely ill patients are generally unable to work at all. Health care system costs are more complicated, because many severely ill patients receive no support or help from the health care system at all, due to the failure of primary care physicians to diagnose the illness. Such failure is widespread, with evidence that between a third to a half of all GPs, over several decades and a variety of geographical locations, expressing disbelief or failing to recognize ME/CFS as a genuine clinical entity [17,18].

This is consistent with the finding that a large proportion of respondents, particularly in Italy and the UK, have difficulty explaining their illness to doctors, as reported by the working group's literature review of knowledge and understanding of ME/CFS among GPs [17], which established that disbelief and lack of knowledge were widespread in primary care, while our survey of perceptions of GP knowledge and understanding among EUROMENE participants suggests that this problem exists throughout Europe [18].

This study initiative aimed to identify policy measures designed to alleviate the burden of disease on patients and their families, and on governments, in particular by reducing delays in diagnosis, and has enabled certain changes in the way in which services are delivered to be identified. Thus, in Latvia, the survey was paralleled by a survey of GPs, in which a number of improvements were suggested, including establishment of a consortium of specialists, the creation and use of clinical algorithms and patient pathways, better information for patients, reimbursement from public funds of psychotherapists' consultation fees, additional training, and more time for patient consultations. Another possible improvement recommended from Latvia was the establishment of a disease register, which would facilitate disease management by GPs, the development of patient pathways, and improved disease monitoring.

5. Conclusions

This comparative survey of ME/CFS patients in Italy, Latvia, and the UK has demonstrated marked similarities between respondents in all three countries in terms of demographic features, the impact of the illness on household incomes and on quality of life, and on difficulties experienced by respondents in discussing their illness with doctors. There were differences in terms of patterns of medical care, the availability of social care, and societal attitudes to ME/CFS. There is a need for internationally shared protocols for the disease treatment and diagnosis. More empirical research is required in Europe on ME/CFS patients' needs in order to develop adequate care pathways.

Supplementary Materials: The following are available online at https://www.mdpi.com/article/10.3390/medicina57030300/s1.

Author Contributions: Conceptualization. E.B., D.A.; methodology, E.B., D.A., D.F.H.P.; validation, E.B., D.A., D.F.H.P.; formal analysis, E.B., D.A., D.F.H.P.; investigation, E.B., D.A., D.F.H.P.; resources, E.B., D.A., D.F.H.P.; writing—original draft preparation, D.F.H.P.; writing—review and editing, E.B., D.A., D.F.H.P.; visualization, E.B., D.A., D.F.H.P.; project administration, E.B., D.A. All authors have read and agreed to the published version of the manuscript.

Funding: This research received no external funding. EUROMENE receives funding for networking activities from the COST programme (COST Action 15111), via the COST Association.

Institutional Review Board Statement: This study, 'In-depth study of Chronic Fatigue Syndrome (ME/CFS) and encouraging of a common approach in international scientific cooperation' was approved by the Research Ethics Committee of the Riga Stradins University (Decision No.6-3/3, 25 October 2018, Riga).

Informed Consent Statement: In the UK, prospective participants respondents read a detailed statement, with response indicating informed consent. In Latvia, prospective respondents read a detailed statement, which was accepted by the Research Ethics Committee of the Riga Stradins University (Decision No.6-3/3, 25 October 2018, Riga), and response therefore indicates informed consent. In Italy respondents read a detailed statement and agreed to participate.

Data Availability Statement: Initial tabulations of data from the UK are available upon request from the author. Data from Italy are available on request from the author. The aggregated data of Latvia surveys are available on request from the Riga Stradins University.

Acknowledgments: This article is based upon work from COST Action CA15111—European Network on Myalgic Encephalomyelitis/Chronic Fatigue Syndrome (EUROMENE), supported by COST (European Cooperation in Science and Technology); www.cost.eu (accessed on 15 January 2021).

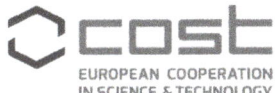
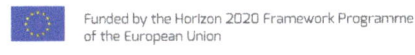

Conflicts of Interest: The authors declare no conflict of interest.

References

1. Carruthers, B.M.; Jain, A.K.; De Meirleir, K.L.; Peterson, D.L.; Klimas, N.G.; Lerner, A.M.; Bested, A.C.; Flor-Henry, P.; Joshi, P.; Powles, P.; et al. Myalgic encephalomyelitis/chronic fatigue syndrome: Clinical working case definition, diagnostic and treatment protocols. *J. Chronic Fatigue Syndr.* **2003**, *11*, 7–116. [CrossRef]
2. Pheby, D.; Lacerda, E.; Nacul, L.; Drachler, M.D.L.; Campion, P.; Howe, A.; Poland, F.; Curran, M.; Featherstone, V.; Fayyaz, S.; et al. A Disease Register for ME/CFS: Report of a Pilot Study. *BMC Res. Notes* **2011**, *4*, 139. [CrossRef] [PubMed]
3. Action for ME. Available online: https://actionforme.org.uk/what-is-me/introduction/ (accessed on 6 January 2020).
4. Brenna, E.; Gitto, L. The economic burden of Chronic Fatigue Syndrome/Myalgic Encephalomyelitis (CFS/ME): An initial summary of the existing evidence and recommendations for further research. *Eur. J. Pers. Cent. Healthc.* **2017**, *5*, 413–420. [CrossRef]
5. Pheby, D.F.; Araja, D.; Berkis, U.; Brenna, E.; Cullinan, J.; De Korwin, J.-D.; Gitto, L.; A Hughes, D.; Hunter, R.M.; Trepel, D.; et al. The Development of a Consistent Europe-Wide Approach to Investigating the Economic Impact of Myalgic Encephalomyelitis (ME/CFS): A Report from the European Network on ME/CFS (EUROMENE). *Healthcare* **2020**, *8*, 88. [CrossRef] [PubMed]
6. EUROMENE. Available online: http://www.euromene.eu (accessed on 20 October 2019).
7. Memorandum of Understanding of COST Action 15111—EUROMENE. Available online: http://www.cost.eu/actions/CA15111/#tabs/Name;overview (accessed on 18 March 2020).
8. Ardino1, R.B.; Lorusso, L. La syndrome da affaticamento cronico/encefalomielite mialgica: Le caratteristiche della malattia e il ruolo dell'Associazione malati CFS [Chronic fatigue syndrome/myalgic encephalomyelitis: The characteristics of the disease and the role of the CFS Patients Association. *Politiche Sanit.* **2018**, *19*, 91–95.
9. EuroQol Group EuroQol—A new facility for the measurement of health-related quality of life. *Health Policy* **1990**, *16*, 199–208. [CrossRef]
10. Williams, A. *The Role of EuroQol Instrument in Qaly Calculations, No 130chedp*; Working Papers; Centre for Health Economics, University of York: York, UK, 1995.
11. Dolan, P. Modeling Valuations for EuroQol Health States. *Med. Care* **1997**, *35*, 1095–1108. [CrossRef]
12. Eurostat. Available online: https://appsso.eurostat.ec.europa.eu/nui/submitViewTableAction.doc (accessed on 15 January 2021).
13. Brenna, E.; Gitto, L. Sindrome da affaticamento cronico: Una prima analisi empirica per l'Italia. *Politiche Sanit.* **2018**, *19*, 1–9. [CrossRef]
14. The Survey of Personal Incomes. Available online: https://www.gov.uk/government/statistics/percentile-points-from-1-to-99-for-total-income-before-and-after-tax (accessed on 23 November 2020).
15. Reynolds, K.J.; Vernon, S.D.; Bouchery, E.; Reeves, W.C. The economic impact of chronic fatigue syndrome. *Cost Eff. Resour. Alloc.* **2004**, *2*, 4. [CrossRef] [PubMed]
16. Collin, S.M.; Database, U.C.N.O.; Crawley, E.; May, M.T.; Sterne, J.A.; Hollingworth, W. The impact of CFS/ME on employment and productivity in the UK: A cross-sectional study based on the CFS/ME national outcomes database. *BMC Health Serv. Res.* **2011**, *11*, 217. [CrossRef] [PubMed]

17. Pheby, D.; Araja, D.; Berkis, U.; Brenna, E.; Cullinan, J.; de Korwin, J.-D.; Gitto, L.; Hughes, D.; Hunter, R.; Trepel, D.; et al. A Literature Review of GP Knowledge and Understanding of ME/CFS: A Report from the Socioeconomic Working Group of the European Network on ME/CFS (EUROMENE). *Medicina* **2020**, *57*, 7. [CrossRef] [PubMed]
18. Cullinan, J.; Pheby, D.; Araja, D.; Berkis, U.; Brenna, E.; de Korwin, J.-D.; Gitto, L.; Hughes, D.; Hunter, R.; Trepel, D.; et al. Perceptions of European ME/CFS Experts Concerning Knowledge and Understanding of ME/CFS among Primary Care Physicians in Europe: A Report from the European ME/CFS Research Network (EUROMENE). *Medicina* **2021**, *57*, 208. [CrossRef] [PubMed]

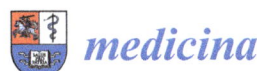

Article

Medical Care Situation of People with Myalgic Encephalomyelitis/Chronic Fatigue Syndrome in Germany

Laura Froehlich [1,*], Daniel B. R. Hattesohl [2], Leonard A. Jason [3], Carmen Scheibenbogen [4], Uta Behrends [5] and Manuel Thoma [2]

1. Research Cluster D²L², FernUniversität in Hagen, 58097 Hagen, Germany
2. German Association for ME/CFS, 20146 Hamburg, Germany; daniel.hattesohl@dg.mecfs.de (D.B.R.H.); manuel.thoma@dg.mecfs.de (M.T.)
3. Center for Community Research, DePaul University, Chicago, IL 60614, USA; ljason@depaul.edu
4. Institute of Medical Immunology, Charité University Medicine Berlin, 10117 Berlin, Germany; carmen.scheibenbogen@charite.de
5. Department of Pediatrics, School of Medicine, Technical University of Munich, 80333 München, Germany; uta.behrends@mri.tum.de
* Correspondence: laura.froehlich@fernuni-hagen.de

Abstract: *Background and Objective:* Myalgic Encephalomyelitis/Chronic Fatigue Syndrome (ME/CFS) is a severe illness with the hallmark symptom of Post-Exertional Malaise (PEM). Currently, no biomarkers or established diagnostic tests for ME/CFS exist. In Germany, it is estimated that over 300,000 people are affected by ME/CFS. Research from the United States and the UK shows that patients with ME/CFS are medically underserved, as they face barriers to medical care access and are dissatisfied with medical care. The first aim of the current research was to investigate whether patients with ME/CFS are medically underserved in Germany in terms of access to and satisfaction with medical care. Second, we aimed at providing a German-language version of the DePaul Symptom Questionnaire Short Form (DSQ-SF) as a tool for ME/CFS diagnostics and research in German-speaking countries. *Materials and Methods:* The current research conducted an online questionnaire study in Germany investigating the medical care situation of patients with ME/CFS. The questionnaire was completed by 499 participants who fulfilled the Canadian Consensus Criteria and reported PEM of 14 h or longer. *Results:* Participants frequently reported geographic and financial reasons for not using the available medical services. Furthermore, they reported low satisfaction with medical care by the physician they most frequently visited due to ME/CFS. The German version of the DSQ-SF showed good reliability, a one-factorial structure and construct validity, demonstrated by correlations with the SF-36 as a measure of functional status. *Conclusions:* Findings provide evidence that patients with ME/CFS in Germany are medically underserved. The German-language translation of the DSQ-SF provides a brief, reliable and valid instrument to assess ME/CFS symptoms to be used for research and clinical practice in German-speaking countries. Pathways to improve the medical care of patients with ME/CFS are discussed.

Keywords: Myalgic Encephalomyelitis; Chronic Fatigue Syndrome; DePaul Symptom Questionnaire; medical care

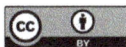

1. Introduction

The chronic illness Myalgic Encephalomyelitis or Chronic Fatigue Syndrome (we will use the acronym ME/CFS) is characterized by severe symptoms including profound exhaustion, muscle weakness and fatigability, pain, cognitive dysfunction, sleep disturbance, flu-like symptoms, and orthostatic intolerance [1–3]. The hallmark symptom of the illness is post-exertional malaise (PEM; i.e., the worsening of all symptoms after minimal exertion) [4,5]. To date, the etiology of ME/CFS is unknown, but the illness is associated with physiological abnormalities, e.g., an impaired energy metabolism [6,7], impaired cardiovascular function [8,9], as well as indicators of autoimmunity [10,11].

In the United States, it is estimated that 1.09 million adults (0.42% of the population) and 0.40 million children (0.75%) are affected by ME/CFS [12], and a meta-analysis of 46 studies conducted in 13 countries showed a pooled prevalence of 0.39% for adults [13]. A base rate of 0.4% would translate to 332,000 individuals affected by ME/CFS (including 54,000 children and adolescents) in Germany. The condition is largely unrecognized by health professionals and the public. In the United States, it is estimated that 84% of adults and 95% of children and adolescents with ME/CFS have not been diagnosed [14,15] and that ME/CFS results in annual costs between USD 35.9 and 50.9 billion in medical bills and lost incomes [12]. In the UK, an average yearly productivity loss due to employment discontinuation was estimated as GBP 22,684 per patient [16]. For the EU, an annual burden of EUROS 40 billion was estimated, although specific estimations of the cost of ME/CFS in Germany and further European countries are lacking [17]. ME/CFS is also an important health issue in children and adolescents [15], and severely affected patients in this age group often have difficulties completing their education due to ME/CFS symptoms [18].

1.1. Medical Care Situation of People with ME/CFS

Studies conducted in the United States have investigated the medical care situation of people with ME/CFS and showed that they are medically underserved [19,20] in that they lack equal access to healthcare [21]. First, people with ME/CFS report barriers to accessing medical care. These access barriers include geographical factors (e.g., low number of specialists in the area, not being able to travel large distances to see a specialist) as well as financial factors (e.g., cost for appointment not covered by insurance, travel to specialist too expensive) [20,22]. Second, people with ME/CFS report low satisfaction with the medical care they receive. The number of specialists who are knowledgeable about ME/CFS and regularly treat patients with this condition is low [23,24]. For example, Sunnquist, Nicholson, Jason, and Friedman [20] surveyed 898 US American individuals with self-reported ME/CFS; 52% of participants had never seen a specialist and only 11.5% were regularly treated by a specialist. Furthermore, 71% of participants saw four or more physicians in order to receive a diagnosis. Whereas participants who saw a specialist reported being satisfied with medical care, the satisfaction with care from non-specialists (e.g., GPs, staff of emergency departments) was reported to be low [20,24,25]. Timbol and Baraniuk [25] investigated the satisfaction with medical care in the emergency department (ED) in a sample of 282 patients with physician-diagnosed ME/CFS. Fifty-nine percent of patients reported having visited an ED in the past, predominantly due to orthostatic intolerance. Patients were dissatisfied with ED care in that they indicated that the staff were not knowledgeable about ME/CFS and half of the staff attributed patients' complaints to stress, anxiety or psychological issues [25]. Other studies also showed that patients attributed their dissatisfaction with medical care to the inadequate training of physicians in treatment of patients with their illness [20,24].

Data on the access to and satisfaction with medical care of people with ME/CFS in Germany are currently lacking. If patients with ME/CFS in Germany faced similar barriers to medical care than in other countries and reported low satisfaction with medical care, this would indicate that they are also a medically underserved community. Based on research in the United States and the UK [16,20], patients with ME/CFS being medically underserved would be associated with individual and public financial losses also in Germany. Therefore, the first objective of the current research was to assess the medical care situation (i.e., access barriers and satisfaction with medical care) of people with ME/CFS in Germany.

1.2. Assessment of ME/CFS Symptoms

A second objective of the current research was to provide researchers and medical care personnel in German-speaking countries with a concise and time-efficient German-language questionnaire to assess and diagnose ME/CFS. Research points to multi-faceted causes of ME/CFS with 72% of patients reporting an infectious illness at the onset of the disease [26]. To date, there is no diagnostic biomarker or curative treatment [27–29]. However, during the last decades the DePaul Symptom Questionnaire (DSQ) has been developed as a valid and reliable psychometric instrument to assess ME/CFS symptoms [30]. The questionnaire has been translated into multiple languages and is available in several versions, including a time-efficient short form encompassing only 14 items (DePaul Symptom Questionnaire Short Form; DSQ-SF) [30,31]. It was designed to measure the frequency and severity of symptoms from all domains of the ME/CFS Canadian Consensus Criteria: Fatigue, PEM, sleep, pain, neurocognitive, autonomic, neuroendocrine, and immune symptoms [32]. The DSQ-SF has been shown to identify a relatively similar number of patients than the longer, 99-item DSQ-1 version, and reliably distinguishes between patients with ME/CFS, adult controls, and patients with multiple sclerosis [31]. Furthermore, a brief questionnaire to assess PEM, the hallmark symptom of ME/CFS, was recently developed [33]. The DePaul Symptom Questionnaire Post-Exertional Malaise (DSQ-PEM) can be used as an efficient and reliable screening instrument to identify PEM in patients with ME/CFS. The instrument showed high sensitivity and specificity in differentiating between patients with ME/CFS and other fatiguing illnesses, namely multiple sclerosis and post-polio syndrome [33].

Thus, the second aim of the current research was to provide a translation of the DSQ-SF and the DSQ-PEM into German language. In the absence of biomarkers and established diagnostic tests, German versions of the questionnaires would provide a valuable tool for time-constrained research protocols to assess ME/CFS symptoms and for clinical practice to diagnose patients with ME/CFS in Germany and other German-speaking countries. This would be an important step towards improving patients' medical care situation.

2. Materials and Methods

2.1. Participants and Procedure

For the current project, we analyzed data collected for a superordinate research project [34], which was pre-registered at https://osf.io/spd9u/?view_only=bc79e0d225b9435caf6dd48fb6cd451b (accessed date: 22 June 2021). Participants with a self-reported diagnosis of ME/CFS were recruited via the four largest patient organizations for ME/CFS in Germany, their mailing lists, and social media. Data collection took place between May and June 2020. The online questionnaire took 30–45 min and was completed by 611 participants. We excluded participants who were under the age of 18 ($n = 7$) or did not consent to the inclusion of their data in the analyses ($n = 3$). Furthermore, we excluded participants who did not fulfil the Canadian Consensus Criteria for ME/CFS ([32]; $n = 30$; coded according to their responses to the DSQ-SF) [30]. Finally, as Cotler, Holtzman, Dudun, and Jason [33] showed that a duration of PEM longer than 14 h differentiated ME/CFS from other chronic diseases, we additionally excluded participants whose responses to the item "If you feel worse after activities, how long does this last" (item 9, DSQ-PEM) ranged between "1 h or less" and "11–13 h"; ($n = 72$). The final sample consisted of 499 participants.

After receiving information on data protection and the topic of the study, participants provided written consent in accordance with the EU General Data Protection Law, the research ethics guidelines of the American Psychological Association, as well as the Declaration of Helsinki. Then, they completed the DSQ-SF, DSQ-PEM, and SF-36, and provided information on demographics and illness history from the DSQ-2. Subsequently, they responded to items measuring their perceived barriers to medical care access and their satisfaction with medical care. For the superordinate research project, participants additionally completed measures of perceived causal attributions, perceived stigma, and satisfaction with social roles and activities (see pre-registration report, materials, and Froehlich, Hattesohl, Cotler, Jason, Scheibenbogen and Behrends [34] for a detailed description of these additional measures). Finally, participants were debriefed about the aims of the study and consented to the use of their data for analyses. The study received approval by the first author's institutional ethics commission. Scales for which no official translations were available were translated from English to German by the project team and back-translated by a professional translator. Materials, data, and analysis scripts are available on the OSF [https://osf.io/5d8vu/ (use: 22 June 2021)]. The German translations of the DSQ-SF and the DSQ-PEM are displayed in Appendix A.

2.2. Materials

ME/CFS symptoms were assessed with the De Paul Symptom Questionnaire Short Form (DSQ-SF, 14 items) [31] and the DePaul Post-Exertional Malaise Questionnaire (DSQ-PEM; eight out of 10 items assessed; due to a programming error two items identical to the DSQ-SF were not assessed) [33]. Functional status was assessed with the Short-Form Health Survey (SF-36; 36 items) [35,36]. Furthermore, to assess access to medical care, participants were asked "Did you utilize any of these services in the past 6 months in regard to your ME/CFS? Primary care physician (GP), ME/CFS-specialist, neurologist, other specialist, hospital/stationary care, ME/CFS self-help, mental health, alternative medicine" and "Are there any services that you would like to use but are not accessible to you for one or more of the following reasons? Financial/insurance reasons, lack of knowledge of service availability (who treats my disease?), ME/CFS-associated impairment prevented access to service, travel distance and lack of transportation, no ME/CFS-specialist in geographic area, ME/CFS-specialist is not covered by health insurance, ME/CFS-specialist has a full waiting-list", adapted from [20,22] to the characteristics of the German health-care system. Patient satisfaction with medical care was assessed with nine items ("Please indicate how satisfied you are with the care by your doctor that you are visiting most frequently because of ME/CFS", e.g., "Overall, I feel satisfied with my appointments", "Knowledgeable about symptoms/course of ME/CFS", 1 = strongly disagree, 4 = strongly agree) [20]. In addition, participants indicated whether the doctor is a generalized or specialized physician (further indicating the area of specialty). Finally, participants completed items on demographics and illness history from the DSQ-2 (items 3–11; 94–99; 111–115, 116; [30]; demographics adapted to the German context).

2.3. Statistical Analyses

Statistical analyses were conducted with IBM SPSS version 26 and Mplus version 7 (confirmatory factor analysis only). The level of significance was $\alpha < 0.05$, confidence intervals are displayed at the 95% level. Sample characteristics, health-related demographics and medical care access were investigated with descriptive statistics and frequency analysis. Multi-item measures (i.e., satisfaction with medical care, DSQ-SF) were aggregated to scales, as internal consistency was sufficient (Cronbach's $\alpha > 0.80$). Analyses of means was conducted with one-sample t-tests and paired-samples t-tests with bootstrapping (1000 samples). To investigate the factor structure of the DSQ-SF, we conducted the confirmatory factor analysis. Cutoffs for model fit statistics were CFI/TLI ≥ 0.90, RSMEA ≤ 0.08, and SRMR ≤ 0.05. Validity was investigated with correlational analyses, effect sizes were interpreted in accordance with Cohen (small effect: $r = 0.10$, moderate effect: $r = 0.30$, large effect: $r = 0.50$; [37]).

3. Results

3.1. Demographics

3.1.1. Sample Characteristics

Of the total sample, 372 (74.5%) participants were female, 125 (25.1%) male, and two indicated "other" as their gender (0.4%). The age ranged between 18 and 76 years ($M = 46.67$, $SD = 12.20$). The majority of participants had German nationality (97%) and indicated Germany as their country of residence (99%). Participants had various levels of education, but a substantial part of the sample had higher (university) education (no degree: $n = 5$, 1.0%, Volks-/Hauptschulabschluss (primary school/secondary school): $n = 22$, 4.4%, Realschulabschluss/Mittlere Reife (secondary school leaving certificate): $n = 118$, 23.6%, Fachabitur/Fachhochschulreife (secondary school with qualification for technical university entrance): $n = 60$, 12.0%, Abitur/Allgemeine Hochschulreife (secondary school with qualification for university entrance): $n = 80$, 16.0%, university degree: $n = 203$,

40.7%, other: $n = 10$, 2.0%, one missing). Fifty-nine percent of participants reported being on disability, whereas 17% were working part-time, 12% were unemployed, 8% retired, 6% working full-time, 6% students, and 5% homemakers (multiple answers possible).

3.1.2. Health-Related Demographics

Ninety percent of participants ($n = 450$) reported that they have been diagnosed with ME/CFS. All participants indicated that their problem with fatigue/energy lasted at least 6 months, with the majority of participants reporting a duration of 2 years or longer ("How long ago did your problem with fatigue/energy begin?", 6–12 months ($n = 8$, 1.6%), 1–2 years ($n = 16$, 3.2%), longer than 2 years ($n = 377$, 75.6%), had a problem with fatigue/energy since childhood or adolescence ($n = 98$, 19.6%)). In line with Salit [26], three quarters of the sample ($n = 378$) reported that their fatigue/energy-related illness started after they experienced an infectious illness.

3.2. Access to and Satisfaction with Medical Care

Results on service utilization ("Did you utilize any of these services in the past 6 months in regard to ME/CFS?", multiple answers possible) showed that participants predominantly visited their primary care physician, used ME/CFS self-help services, and alternative medicine. To a lesser extent, they visited specialized physicians, used mental health services or visited the hospital with regards to ME/CFS (Table 1).

Table 1. Frequencies of service utilization within the past 6 months with regards to Myalgic Encephalomyelitis/Chronic Fatigue Syndrome (ME/CFS).

Service	Frequency	Percentage
Primary care physician (GP)	344	68.9%
ME/CFS self-help (telephone hotlines for ME/CFS information, ME/CFS e-mails, ME/CFS literature, ME/CFS self-help groups)	330	66.1%
Alternative medicine (herbal medicine, self-awareness, biofeedback, acupuncture)	277	55.5%
Other specialist	200	40.1%
Neurologist	190	38.1%
Mental health (counseling, psychiatric hospitalization)	169	33.9%
Physicians specializing in the treatment of people with ME/CFS	168	33.7%
Hospital/stationary care	77	15.4%

Concerning barriers to service access ("Are there any services that you would like to use but are not accessible to you for one or more of the following reasons?"), all items except "ME/CFS specialist has a full waiting list" were affirmed by more than half of participants. The main factors participants perceived as barriers to service access were geographical reasons (i.e., lack of ME/CFS specialists in the area and lack of transportation), financial or insurance reasons, as well as lack of information about services (Table 2).

The nine items measuring patient satisfaction with medical care were averaged to a scale ($\alpha = 0.92$). On average, participants indicated that they were rather not satisfied with medical care by the doctor they most frequently visited due to ME/CFS ($M = 2.36$, 95% CI [2.29; 2.43], $SE = 0.04$) which was significantly below the scale midpoint of 2.5 ($t(469) = 4.08$, $SE = 0.03$, $p < 0.001$). Half of the sample ($n = 252$, 50.5%) indicated that they visited their GP most frequently due to ME/CFS, whereas 32.9% ($n = 164$) visited a specialized physician, and 16.2% ($n = 81$) indicated that they were currently not in treatment due to ME/CFS. The physicians' areas of specialty most frequently stated by patients were neurology/psychiatry, general medicine, internal medicine, hygiene and environmental medicine, as well as hematology and oncology (a detailed frequency table can be found on the OSF). Furthermore, 123 participants (24.6%) indicated that they were in treatment by a physician specialized in ME/CFS. These participants completed the satisfaction items again with regards to the specialist ($\alpha = 0.92$). Results showed that satisfaction with medical care by a ME/CFS specialist was higher than the scale midpoint

($M = 3.16$, 95% CI [3.05; 3.26], $SE = 0.06$; $t(122) = 11.70$, $p < 0.001$). Furthermore, participants in this subsample reported higher satisfaction with medical care by a ME/CFS specialist compared to care by a physician not specialized in ME/CFS ($M = 2.87$, 95% CI [2.74; 3.00], $SE = 0.07$, $t(121) = 4.64$, $p < 0.001$).

Table 2. Frequencies of perceived barriers to medical care access.

Barrier	Frequency	Percentage
No ME/CFS specialist in the geographic area	394	79.0%
Financial/insurance reasons	356	71.3%
Lack of knowledge of service availability (who treats my disease?)	331	66.3%
ME/CFS specialist is not covered by health insurance	287	57.5%
Travel distance and lack of transportation	278	55.7%
ME/CFS-associated impairment prevented access to service	270	54.1%
ME/CFS specialist has a full waiting list	191	38.3%

ME/CFS: Myalgic Encephalomyelitis/Chronic Fatigue Syndrome.

3.3. German Version of the DePaul Symptom Questionnaire Short Form

For the DSQ-SF, we created composite scores per item by averaging frequency and severity ratings and then multiplying them by 25 to create a scale ranging from 0 to 100 for ease of interpretation [30]. Table 3 displays descriptive statistics of the DSQ-SF items (frequency and severity displayed separately in their original metric ranging from 0 to 4).

Table 3. Descriptive statistics of German-language DePaul Symptom Questionnaire Short Form (DSQ-SF) items.

	Frequency			Severity		
Items	M [95% CI]	SE	α	M [95% CI]	SE	α
1. Fatigue/extreme tiredness	3.35 [3.28; 3.42]	0.04	0.897	3.10 [3.04; 3.17]	0.03	0.896
2. Next day soreness or fatigue after non-strenuous, everyday activities	3.22 [3.13; 3.30]	0.04	0.894	3.22 [3.14; 3.29]	0.04	0.894
3. Minimum exercise makes you physically tired	2.79 [2.68; 2.90]	0.05	0.894	2.97 [2.87; 3.06]	0.05	0.894
4. Feeling unrefreshed after you wake up in the morning	3.51 [3.45; 3.58]	0.03	0.897	3.08 [3.02; 3.14]	0.03	0.895
5. Pain or aching in your muscles	2.58 [2.48; 2.70]	0.06	0.896	2.42 [2.33; 2.51]	0.05	0.895
6. Bloating	1.90 [1.79; 2.01]	0.05	0.898	1.71 [1.62; 1.80]	0.04	0.896
7. Problems remembering things	2.00 [1.91; 2.09]	0.05	0.897	2.12 [2.03; 2.21]	0.05	0.896
8. Difficulty paying attention for a long period of time	2.90 [2.82; 2.98]	0.04	0.896	2.79 [2.72; 2.87]	0.04	0.895
9. Irritable bowel problems	2.08 [1.96; 2.19]	0.06	0.896	1.98 [1.88; 2.09]	0.05	0.894
10. Feeling unsteady on your feet, as if you might fall	1.86 [1.75; 1.97]	0.05	0.893	2.11 [2.01; 2.22]	0.06	0.893
11. Cold limbs (e.g., arms, legs, hands)	2.19 [2.08; 2.30]	0.06	0.898	1.74 [1.65; 1.83]	0.05	0.895
12. Feeling hot or cold for no reason	2.10 [2.00; 2.19]	0.05	0.894	2.02 [1.92; 2.11]	0.05	0.894
13. Flu-like symptoms	2.19 [2.10; 2.30]	0.05	0.896	2.46 [2.37; 2.55]	0.05	0.896
14. Some smells, foods, medications or chemicals make you feel sick	1.81 [1.70; 1.94]	0.06	0.894	1.80 [1.70; 1.91]	0.06	0.894

Notes. Results are displayed in the original metric before transformations. Frequency was assessed on a scale from 0 = none of the time to 4 = all of the time. Severity was assessed on a scale from 0 = symptom not present to 4 = very severe. Chronbach's αs indicate internal consistencies of the scale when the item is removed (complete scale before transformations: α = 0.899).

The confirmatory factor analysis on the composite scores (Cronbach's α = 0.83) showed that the fit of a single-factor model was acceptable ($\chi^2(73) = 222.70$, $p < 0.001$; RMSEA = 0.06, CFI = 0.92, TLI = 0.90, SRMR = 0.05) when correlated error terms of the following items were allowed: "bloating" and "irritable bowel problems", "problems remembering things" and "difficulty paying attention for a long period of time", "cold limbs" and "feeling hot or cold for no reason", as well as "unrefreshed sleep" and "muscle pain". Detailed results of the CFA can be found on the Open Science Framework.

To investigate the construct validity of the German translation of the DSQ-SF, we computed bivariate correlations of the scale with the functional status (as measured by the SF-36). Higher frequency and severity of ME/CFS symptoms was significantly associated with lower functional status on all subscales. High correlations ($r > 0.58$) were found with the subscales of physical functioning and bodily pain, whereas correlations with social functioning, general health, vitality, and mental health were moderate (0.41 > r > 0.25). Small correlations were found with role physical and role emotional (r < 0.18; Table 4).

Table 4. Bivariate correlations of the German-language DSQ-SF with the functional status.

Scales	(1)	(2)	(3)	(4)	(5)	(6)	(7)	(8)	(9)	(10)
(1) DSQ-SF	-									
(2) Physical functioning	−0.60 ***	-								
(3) Role physical	−0.18 ***	0.14 **	-							
(4) Bodily pain	−0.58 ***	0.34 ***	0.12 *	-						
(5) General health	−0.39 ***	0.23 ***	0.13 **	0.26 ***	-					
(6) Vitality	−0.32 ***	0.23 ***	0.03	0.19 ***	0.29 ***	-				
(7) Social functioning	−0.41 ***	0.40 ***	0.13 **	0.20 ***	0.25 ***	0.25 ***	-			
(8) Role emotional	−0.10 *	−0.02	0.06	0.20 ***	0.06	0.12 **	0.06	-		
(9) Mental health	−0.25 ***	0.08	0.04	0.22 ***	0.25 ***	0.29 ***	0.25 ***	0.53 ***	-	
(10) Gender	0.12 **	−0.15 ***	−0.02	−0.09	0.02	−0.04	0.00	−0.01	0.07 *	-
(11) Age	0.02	−0.01	−0.00	−0.08	0.13 **	−0.04	0.02	−0.14 **	−0.09	0.11 *

Notes. * p < 0.05, ** p < 0.01, *** p < 0.001. Gender was coded 0 = male, 1 = female. Displayed coefficients are Pearson correlations. Higher scores on the DSQ-SF represent more frequent/severe ME/CFS symptoms. Higher scores on the SF-36 subscales represent higher functioning.

4. Discussion

Myalgic Encephalomyelitis/Chronic Fatigue Syndrome (ME/CFS) is a severe and chronic illness for which currently no cure or biomarker exists. ME/CFS is associated with losses of income and economic productivity [4,16,20,38]. Based on a prevalence of 0.4% [12,13], it is estimated that 332,000 people (including 54,000 children and adolescents) in Germany are affected by ME/CFS. Evidence from the United States indicates that people with ME/CFS are medically underserved [20,24,25]. The current research shows that this is likely also the case in Germany. An online questionnaire was distributed by the four largest German ME/CFS patient organizations. The final sample consisted of 499 participants with self-reported ME/CFS who fulfilled the Canadian Consensus Criteria [32] and indicated experiencing post-exertional malaise of 14 h or longer [33]. All participants included in the final sample also fulfilled diagnostic criteria by the Institute of Medicine [4].

4.1. Patients with ME/CFS in Germany Are Medically Underserved

Results point in the direction that people with ME/CFS in Germany are severely impaired in terms of health and social, as well as economic functioning. Despite high levels of education, only less than one quarter of the sample reported working part-time or full-time, whereas more than half of the participants were on disability. This pattern shows that similar to other countries, Germany also suffers financial and economic losses due to people living with ME/CFS not being able to contribute to the labor market [12,16,20,38]. Due to the chronic nature of the illness, this is unlikely to change, as more than 95% of the sample reported having had problems with fatigue/energy for 2 years or longer.

Results on access to and satisfaction with medical care present further evidence that patients with ME/CFS are medically underserved in Germany. Most patients reported being treated by their primary care physician and only one third reported having seen a physician specialized in ME/CFS in the last 6 months. This is consistent with evidence from the United States, where the number of ME/CFS specialists was reported to be low [20,23,24]. Moreover, the majority of participants indicated using self-help and alternative medicine, but only 40% or less reported being in treatment by a neurologist or other specialized physician. This pattern might indicate that patients use alternative services in search of treatment, as they might feel that primary care and specialized physicians are not able to provide them with satisfactory medical care. This is underlined by a recent literature review and expert survey on GP knowledge and understanding of ME/CFS. Results showed that in different European countries, between one third and half of GPs did not accept ME/CFS as a genuine clinical entity and even when they did, they lacked confidence in diagnosing or managing it [39,40]. Furthermore, in line with results from Sunnquist, Nicholson, Jason, and Friedman [20] as well as Thanawala and Taylor [22], patients with ME/CFS in Germany also predominantly reported both geographical/logistic as well as financial/insurance reasons for not being able to use medical services more frequently. This pattern reflects that the number of physicians specializing in ME/CFS in Germany is too low and as a consequence, patients are required to travel long distances to visit ME/CFS specialists, which might be prevented by or even exacerbate their ME/CFS symptoms. Insurance barriers include that the current official diagnostic guidelines on fatigue in Germany [41] recommend cognitive-behavioral therapy and graded exercise therapy as treatment. Other medical care might not be covered by health insurance. Furthermore, not being able to work and suffering associated income losses might also contribute to financial barriers to service utilization.

Findings are further corroborated by results on satisfaction with medical care. Overall, satisfaction with medical care by the physician patients visited most frequently due to ME/CFS (in most cases, the primary care physician) was reported to be low. Only one third of participants reported having seen a physician specialized in ME/CFS in the last 6 months. However, this subsample was significantly more satisfied with the medical care they received from the ME/CFS specialist compared to the non-specialist care. This is in line with studies showing that the medical personnel is not knowledgeable about ME/CFS and often attributes ME/CFS symptoms to psychological causes, which leads to patients being dissatisfied with the medical care they receive [20,24,25,39,40]. To provide patients with ME/CFS in Germany with improved medical care, we conclude that a more frequent and detailed education of medical students, physicians, and other medical personnel in Germany about ME/CFS symptoms, diagnostic criteria, and treatment approaches is necessary [39].

Research has shown a link between severe viral infection and ME/CFS [42] and 75% of the current sample reported that they developed ME/CFS after an infectious illness. In light of the current COVID-19 pandemic, it is to be expected that people recovering from SARS-CoV-2 are at risk of developing ME/CFS [43,44]. For example, a recent study from Germany showed that half of the participants with chronic COVID-19 syndrome fulfilled the Canadian Consensus Criteria for ME/CFS 6 months post infection with SARS-CoV-2 [45]. The expected increase in ME/CFS cases in Germany and around the world due to the COVID-19 pandemic creates an urgency to improve the medical care situation of patients with ME/CFS by providing better care and adequate diagnostic instruments.

4.2. The German-Language DSQ-SF: A Reliable and Valid Instrument for Research and Clinical Practice

In the absence of diagnostic tests or biomarkers for ME/CFS [27,28], the DSQ has been developed based on the Canadian Consensus Criteria [32] to assess ME/CFS symptoms. The instrument is available in several versions and has been translated into a variety of languages [30]. The DSQ has demonstrated excellent psychometric properties including high reliability and validity, as well as high sensitivity and specificity to classify patients with ME/CFS [30,31]. The current research provides a German-language translation of the brief DSQ-SF, which encompasses only 14 items and is thus well-suited for time-sensitive research protocols and clinical practice to diagnose ME/CFS [31]. The German translation of the DSQ-SF showed high reliability, the expected single-factor structure, as well as construct validity. Higher scores on the frequency and severity of ME/CFS symptoms correlated negatively with all subscales of the SF-36 [35,36], an established instrument to assess the functional status. This means that stronger ME/CFS symptoms assessed by the German version of the DSQ-SF were associated with the patients' lower functional status. The pattern of interrelations of the DSQ-SF with the subscales of the SF-36 reflects the most common symptoms of ME/CFS. The strongest correlations were found with the subscales of physical functioning and bodily pain, reflecting the hallmark symptoms of post-exertional malaise, fatigability, as well as muscle weakness and pain. Moderate correlations were found with social functioning, general health, vitality and mental health, reflecting that patients with ME/CFS are severely impaired in terms of societal and social participation (see [34] for a detailed analysis on the relation of perceived stigma due to ME/CFS and lower functional status). As an indicator of discriminant validity, only small correlations of the DSQ-SF were found with the subscales of role physical and role emotional. This result reflects that due to the chronic nature of the illness, participants might have found ways to cope with the impairment they experience due to their symptoms and the associated difficulties for social relationships. Taken together, the current research provides a novel German translation of the DSQ-SF to be used for research and clinical practice in German-speaking countries.

4.3. Limitations and Future Directions

A first limitation is that the current research investigated the medical care situation of people who responded to an online questionnaire measuring only self-reported ME/CFS. This convenience sample might not be representative for the general population of patients with ME/CFS in Germany. However, we took several measures to ensure that our sample reflects the situation of patients with ME/CFS in Germany as accurately as possible. First, the questionnaire was distributed via the four largest German patient organizations, their mailing lists, and social media, increasing the likelihood of reaching patients with ME/CFS. Second, we excluded participants who did not fulfill the Canadian Consensus Criteria and did not report post-exertional malaise of at least 14 h after exertion [32,33]. Relatedly, the educational level of the sample was very high (40% reported having a university degree). It might be possible that highly educated patients with ME/CFS were particularly able or likely to participate in the online study due to higher familiarity with online questionnaires or better technical equipment/digital literacy. A combination of online recruitment and face-to-face recruitment in hospitals/doctor offices would be ideal to avoid systematic recruitment bias. However, as data were collected during the first wave of the COVID-19 pandemic (May/June 2020), such a combined recruitment approach was not possible. Future research could include a sample with a physician-confirmed diagnosis, collect data via paper-pencil questionnaires, and compare the situation of patients with ME/CFS to that of healthy controls and/or patients with other fatigue-related illnesses (e.g., multiple sclerosis).

A second limitation is that the questionnaire study was correlational and cross-sectional. Therefore, we could not investigate the medical care situation and relationships of ME/CFS symptoms with the functional status over time. Third, the current study did not include a comparison group of healthy controls or patients with other chronic illnesses to differentiate patients with ME/CFS from others. Thus, we could not investigate the Receiver Operating Characteristic analysis to set thresholds for subscores to assist with the diagnosis of ME/CFS in Germany. Future studies should include longitudinal study designs, ME/CFS screening questions in population-representative samples, studies with comparison groups, as well as cross-national surveys to shed a more encompassing light on the medical care situation of people with ME/CFS in Germany and other countries.

Finally, due to a programming error the DSQ-PEM was not fully assessed in the current research. The two items "next day soreness or fatigue after non-strenuous, everyday activities" and "minimum exercise makes you physically tired" are identical in the DSQ-SF and the DSQ-PEM, but were assessed only once in the current study. We provided the German translation for the DSQ-PEM in Appendix A, but could not investigate its psychometric properties. In our analyses, we only used one item to determine the cutoff value of >14 h of PEM duration as an inclusion criterion for our sample. Future studies should investigate the validity and reliability of the German version of the DSQ-PEM, as well as its interrelations with the DSQ-SF and functional status.

5. Conclusions

Results of the current research raise concerns about the medical care situation of people with ME/CFS in Germany, showing the need for adequate education of physicians about ME/CFS, as well as a more specialized treatment of patients with ME/CFS. Furthermore, there is a need for instruments to diagnose ME/CFS to be used in research and clinical practice. The current research provides a German version of the well-established DSQ-SF in order to provide an instrument to assess ME/CFS symptoms reliably and validly in German-speaking countries.

Author Contributions: Conceptualization, L.F., D.B.R.H., L.A.J., C.S. and U.B.; methodology, L.F., D.B.R.H. and L.A.J.; software, formal analysis, L.F. and M.T.; writing—original draft preparation, L.F., D.B.R.H. and M.T.; writing—review and editing, L.A.J., C.S. and U.B. All authors have read and agreed to the published version of the manuscript.

Funding: This research was funded by the Weidenhammer Zöbele Foundation.

Institutional Review Board Statement: The study was conducted according to the guidelines of the Declaration of Helsinki, and approved by the Institutional Review Board (or Ethics Committee) of FernUniversität in Hagen (number EA_217_2019, date of approval: 25 March 2020).

Informed Consent Statement: Informed consent was obtained from all subjects involved in the study.

Data Availability Statement: Materials, data, and analysis scripts are available on the Open Science Framework [https://osf.io/5d8vu/ (use: 22 June 2021)].

Conflicts of Interest: The authors declare no conflict of interest. The funders had no role in the design of the study; in the collection, analyses, or interpretation of data; in the writing of the manuscript, or in the decision to publish the results.

Appendix A

Table A1. German translation and original English version of the DePaul Symptom Questionnaire Short Form.

Bitte Geben Sie für jedes der folgenden Symptome die Häufigkeit und Schwere an.	For each Symptom below, Please Circle One Number for Frequency and One Number for Severity.
Häufigkeit: Innerhalb der letzten 6 Monate, wie oft hatten Sie dieses Symptom? Bitte geben Sie für jedes der untenstehenden Symptome eine Zahl an von: 0 = nie, 1 = manchmal, 2 = ca. die Hälfte der Zeit, 3 = meistens, 4 = immer	*Frequency:* Throughout the past 6 months, how often have you had this symptom? For each symptom listed below, circle a number from: 0 = none of the time, 1 = a little of the time, 2 = about half the time, 3 = most of the time, 4 = all of the time
Schwere: Innerhalb der letzten 6 Monate, wie stark hat Sie dieses Symptom Sie beeinträchtigt? Bitte geben Sie für jedes der untenstehenden Symptome eine Zahl an von: 0 = Symptom nicht vorhanden, 1 = mild, 2 = moderat, 3 = schwer, 4 = sehr schwer	*Severity:* Throughout the past 6 months, how much has this symptom bothered you? For each symptom listed below, circle a number from: 0 = symptom not present, 1 = mild, 2 = moderate, 3 = severe, 4 = very severe
Symptom	Symptom
1. Fatigue/extreme Müdigkeit	1. Fatigue/extreme tiredness
2. Am nächsten Tag Schmerzen oder Fatigue nach nicht anstrengenden, alltäglichen Aktivitäten	2. Next day soreness or fatigue after non-strenuous, everyday activities
3. Minimale Bewegung verursacht körperliche Erschöpfung	3. Minimum exercise makes you physically tired
4. Sich nicht erholt fühlen, nachdem man morgens aufwacht	4. Feeling unrefreshed after you wake up in the morning
5. Schmerzen in den Muskeln	5. Pain or aching in your muscles
6. Blähungen	6. Bloating
7. Probleme, sich an Dinge zu erinnern	7. Problems remembering things

Table A1. *Cont.*

Bitte Geben Sie für jedes der folgenden Symptome die Häufigkeit und Schwere an.	For each Symptom below, Please Circle One Number for Frequency and One Number for Severity.
8. Schwierigkeiten, über einen längeren Zeitraum aufmerksam zu sein	8. Difficulty paying attention for a long period of time
9. Reizdarmprobleme	9. Irritable bowel problems
10. Sich unsicher auf den Beinen fühlen, als wenn man hinfallen könnte	10. Feeling unsteady on your feet, as if you might fall
11. kalte Gliedmaßen (z.B. Arme, Beine, Hände)	11. Cold limbs (e.g., arms, legs, hands)
12. Gefühl von Wärme oder Kälte ohne Grund	12. Feeling hot or cold for no reason
13. Grippeartige Symptome	13. Flu-like symptoms
14. Einige Gerüche, Medikamente oder Chemikalien verursachen Unwohlsein	14. Some smells, foods, medications or chemicals make you feel sick

Table A2. German translation and original English version of the DePaul Symptom Questionnaire Post-Exertional Malaise.

Bitte geben Sie für jedes der folgenden Symptome die Häufigkeit und Schwere an.	For Each Symptom below, Please Circle One Number for Frequency and One Number for Severity.
Häufigkeit: Innerhalb der <u>letzten 6 Monate</u>, wie <u>oft</u> hatten Sie dieses Symptom? Bitte geben Sie für jedes der untenstehenden Symptome eine Zahl an von: 0 = nie, 1 = manchmal, 2 = ca. die Hälfte der Zeit, 3 = meistens, 4 = immer	*Frequency:* Throughout the <u>past 6 months</u>, how <u>often</u> have you had this symptom? For each symptom listed below, circle a number from: 0 = none of the time, 1 = a little of the time, 2 = about half the time, 3 = most of the time, 4 = all of the time
Schwere: Innerhalb der <u>letzten 6 Monate</u>, wie <u>stark</u> hat Sie dieses Symptom Sie beeinträchtigt? Bitte geben Sie für jedes der untenstehenden Symptome eine Zahl an von: 0 = Symptom nicht vorhanden, 1 = mild, 2 = moderat, 3 = schwer, 4 = sehr schwer	*Severity:* Throughout the <u>past 6 months</u>, how <u>much</u> has this symptom bothered you? For each symptom listed below, circle a number from: 0 = symptom not present, 1 = mild, 2 = moderate, 3 = severe, 4 = very severe
1. Bleiernes Gefühl nach Bewegung	1. Dead, heavy feeling after starting to exercise
2. Am nächsten Tag Schmerzen oder Fatigue nach nicht anstrengenden, alltäglichen Aktivitäten	2. Next day soreness or fatigue after non-strenuous, everyday activities
3. Geistig müde nach der geringsten Anstrengung	3. Mentally tired after the slightest effort
4. Minimale Bewegung verursacht körperliche Erschöpfung	4. Minimum exercise makes you physically tired
5. Körperlich erschöpft oder krank nach leichter Aktivität	5. Physically drained or sick after mild activity
Wählen Sie für jede der folgenden Fragen die Antwort, die Ihre PEM-Symptome am besten beschreibt.	**For each question below, choose the answer which best describes your PEM symptoms.**
6. Wenn Sie nach der aktiven Teilnahme an außerschulischen Aktivitäten, Sport oder Ausflügen mit Freunden erschöpft wären, würden Sie sich innerhalb von ein oder zwei Stunden nach Beendigung der Aktivität erholen? • 1 = Nein • 2 = Ja	6. If you were to become exhausted after actively participating in extracurricular activities, sports or outings with friends, would you recover within an hour or two after the activity ended? • 1 = No • 2 = Yes

Table A2. *Cont.*

Wählen Sie für jede der folgenden Fragen die Antwort, die Ihre PEM-Symptome am besten beschreibt.	For each question below, choose the answer which best describes your PEM symptoms.
7. Erleben Sie eine Verschlechterung Ihrer Fatigue/auf Energie bezogenen Erkrankung nach minimaler körperlicher Anstrengung? • 1 = Nein • 2 = Ja	7. Do you experience a worsening of your fatigue/energy-related illness after engaging in minimal physical effort? • 1 = No • 2 = Yes
8. Erleben Sie eine Verschlechterung Ihrer Fatigue/auf Energie bezogenen Erkrankung nach geistiger Anstrengung? • 1 = Nein • 2 = Ja	8. Do you experience a worsening of your fatigue/energy-related illness after engaging in mental effort? • 1 = No • 2 = Yes
9. Wenn Sie sich nach Aktivität schlechter fühlen, wie lange dauert es an? • 1 = ≤ 1 Stunde • 2 = 2–3 Stunden • 3 = 4–10 Stunden • 4 = 11–13 Stunden • 5 = 14–23 Stunden • 6 = 1–2 Tage • 7 = 3–7 Tage • 8 = ≥ 7 Tage	9. If you feel worse after activities, how long does it last? • 1 = ≤ 1 h • 2 = 2–3 h • 3 = 4–10 h • 4 = 11–13 h • 5 = 14–23 h • 6 = 1–2 days • 7 = 3–7 days • 8 = ≥ 7 days
10. Wenn Sie sich nicht aktivieren, liegt es daran, dass Aktivität Ihre Symptome verschlimmert? • 1 = Nein • 2 = Ja	10. If you do not exercise, is it due to the fact that exercise makes your symptoms worse? • 1 = No • 2 = Yes

References

1. Carruthers, B.M.; van de Sande, M.I.; De Meirleir, K.L.; Klimas, N.G.; Broderick, G.; Mitchell, T.; Staines, D.; Powles, A.C.P.; Speight, N.; Vallings, R.; et al. Myalgic encephalomyelitis: International Consensus Criteria. *J. Intern. Med.* **2011**, *270*, 327–338. [CrossRef]
2. Fukuda, K.; Straus, S.E.; Hickie, I.; Sharpe, M.C.; Dobbins, J.G.; Komaroff, A. The chronic fatigue syndrome: A comprehensive approach to its definition and study. International Chronic Fatigue Syndrome Study Group. *Ann. Intern. Med.* **1994**, *121*, 953–959. [CrossRef] [PubMed]
3. Van Campen, C.L.M.C.; Verheugt, F.W.A.; Rowe, P.C.; Visser, F.C. Cerebral blood flow is reduced in ME/CFS during head-up tilt testing even in the absence of hypotension or tachycardia: A quantitative, controlled study using Dop-pler echography. *Clin. Neurophysiol. Pract.* **2020**, *5*, 50–58. [CrossRef]
4. Institute of Medicine. *Beyond Myalgic Encephalomyelitis/Chronic Fatigue Syndrome: Redefining an Illness*; National Academies Press: Washington, DC, USA, 2015.
5. Stussman, B.; Williams, A.; Snow, J.; Gavin, A.; Scott, R.; Nath, A.; Walitt, B. Characterization of post-exertional malaise in patients with Myalgic Encephalomyelitis/Chronic Fatigue Syndrome. *Front. Neurol.* **2020**, *11*, 1025. [CrossRef] [PubMed]
6. Naviaux, R.K.; Naviaux, J.C.; Li, K.; Bright, A.T.; Alaynick, W.A.; Wang, L.; Baxter, A.; Nathan, N.; Anderson, W.; Gordon, E. Metabolic features of chronic fatigue syndrome. *Proc. Natl. Acad. Sci. USA* **2016**, *113*, E5472–E5480. [CrossRef]
7. Fluge, Ø.; Mella, O.; Bruland, O.; Risa, K.; Dyrstad, S.E.; Alme, K.; Rekeland, I.G.; Sapkota, D.; Røsland, G.V.; Fosså, A.; et al. Metabolic profiling indicates impaired pyruvate dehydrogenase function in myalgic encephalopathy/chronic fatigue syndrome. *JCI Insight* **2016**, *1*. [CrossRef]
8. Davenport, T.E.; Lehnen, M.; Stevens, S.R.; VanNess, J.M.; Stevens, J.; Snell, C.R. Chronotropic intolerance: An overlooked determinant of symp-toms and activity limitation in Myalgic Encephalomyelitis/Chronic Fatigue Syndrome? *Front. Pediatr.* **2019**, *7*, 82. [CrossRef] [PubMed]
9. Scherbakov, N.; Szklarski, M.; Hartwig, J.; Sotzny, F.; Lorenz, S.; Meyer, A.; Grabowski, P.; Doehner, W.; Scheibenbogen, C. Peripheral endothelial dysfunction in Myalgic Encephalomyelitis/Chronic Fatigue Syndrome. *ESC Heart Fail.* **2020**, *7*, 1064–1071. [CrossRef]

10. Wirth, K.; Scheibenbogen, C. A unifying hypothesis of the pathophysiology of Myalgic Encephalomyeli-tis/Chronic Fatigue Syndrome (ME/CFS): Recognitions from the finding of autoantibodies against ß2-adrenergic re-ceptors. *Autoimmun. Rev.* 2020, *19*, 102527. [CrossRef]
11. Fujii, H.; Sato, W.; Kimura, Y.; Matsuda, H.; Ota, M.; Maikusa, N.; Suzuki, F.; Amano, K.; Shin, I.; Yamamura, T.; et al. Altered structural brain networks related to adrenergic/muscarinic receptor autoantibodies in Chronic Fatigue Syndrome. *J. Neuroimaging* 2020, *30*, 822–827. [CrossRef] [PubMed]
12. Jason, L.A.; Mirin, A.A. Updating the National Academy of Medicine ME/CFS prevalence and economic impact figures to account for population growth and inflation. *Fatigue Biomed. Health Behav.* 2021, 9–13. [CrossRef]
13. Lim, E.J.; Ahn, Y.C.; Jang, E.S.; Lee, S.W.; Lee, S.H.; Son, C.G. Systematic review and meta-analysis of the prevalence of Chronic Fatigue Syndrome/Myalgic Encephalomyelitis (CFS/ME). *J. Transl. Med.* 2020, *18*, 100. [CrossRef]
14. Solomon, L.; Reeves, W.C. Factors influencing the diagnosis of Chronic Fatigue Syndrome. *Arch. Intern. Med.* 2004, *164*, 2241–2245. [CrossRef] [PubMed]
15. Jason, L.A.; Katz, B.Z.; Sunnquist, M.; Torres, C.; Cotler, J.; Bhatia, S. The prevalence of pediatric Myalgic Encephalomyeli-tis/Chronic Fa-tigue Syndrome in a community-based sample. *Child Youth Care Forum* 2020, *49*, 563–579. [CrossRef] [PubMed]
16. Collin, S.M.; Crawley, E.; May, M.T.; Sterne, J.A.C.; Hollingworth, W. The impact of CFS/ME on employment and productivity in the UK: A cross-sectional study based on the CFS/ME national outcomes database. *BMC Health Serv. Res.* 2011, *11*, 217. [CrossRef] [PubMed]
17. Pheby, D.F.H.; Araja, D.; Berkis, U.; Brenna, E.; Cullinan, J.; de Korwin, J.D.; Gitto, L.; Hughes, D.A.; Hunter, R.M.; Trepel, D.; et al. The development of a consistent Europe-wide approach to investigating the economic impact of Myalgic Encephalomyelitis (ME/CFS): A report from the European Network on ME/CFS (EUROMENE). *Healthcare* 2020, *8*, 88. [CrossRef] [PubMed]
18. Newton, F.R. The Impact of severe ME/CFS on student learning and K-12 educational limitations. *Healthcare* 2021, *9*, 627. [CrossRef] [PubMed]
19. Friedman, K.J. Advances in ME/CFS: Past, present, and future. *Front. Pediatr.* 2019, *7*, 131. [CrossRef] [PubMed]
20. Sunnquist, M.; Nicholson, L.; Jason, L.A.; Friedman, K.J. Access to medical care for individuals with Myalgic Encephalo-myelitis and Chronic Fatigue Syndrome: A call for centers of excellence. *Mod. Clin. Med. Res.* 2017, *1*, 28–35. [CrossRef]
21. Vanderbilt, A.A.; Dail, M.D.; Jaberi, P. Reducing health disparities in underserved communities via interprofes-sional collaboration across health care professions. *J. Multidiscip. Healthc.* 2015, *8*, 205–208. [CrossRef]
22. Thanawala, S.; Taylor, R.R. Service utilization, barriers to service access, and coping in adults with Chronic Fatigue Syndrome. *J. Chronic Fatigue Syndr.* 2007, *14*, 5–21. [CrossRef]
23. Bowen, J.; Pheby, D.F.H.; Charlett, A.; McNulty, C. Chronic Fatigue Syndrome: A survey of GPs' attitudes and knowledge. *Fam. Pract.* 2005, *22*, 389–393. [CrossRef]
24. Tidmore, T.; Jason, L.A.; Chapo-Kroger, L.; So, S.; Brown, A.; Silverman, M. Lack of knowledgeable healthcare access for patients with neuro-endocrine-immune diseases. *Front. Clin. Med.* 2015, *2*, 46–54.
25. Timbol, C.R.; Baraniuk, J.N. Chronic fatigue syndrome in the emergency department. *Open Access Emerg. Med.* 2019, *11*, 15–28. [CrossRef]
26. Salit, I.E. Precipitating factors for the chronic fatigue syndrome. *J. Psychiatr. Res.* 1997, *31*, 59–65. [CrossRef]
27. Fischer, D.B.; William, A.H.; Strauss, A.C.; Unger, E.R.; Jason, L.A.; Marshall, G.D., Jr.; Dimitrakoff, J.D. Chronic Fatigue Syndrome: The current status and future poten-tials of emerging biomarkers. *Fatigue Biomed. Health Behav.* 2014, *2*, 93–109. [CrossRef] [PubMed]
28. Bested, A.C.; Marshall, L.M. Review of Myalgic Encephalomyelitis/Chronic Fatigue Syndrome: An evi-dence-based approach to diagnosis and management by clinicians. *Rev. Environ. Health* 2015, *30*, 223–249. [CrossRef] [PubMed]
29. Nacul, L.; Authier, F.J.; Scheibenbogen, C.; Lorusso, L.; Helland, I.; Martin, J.A.; Sirbu, C.A.; Mengshoel, A.M.; Polo, O.; Behrends, U.; et al. European Network on Myalgic Encephalomyelitis/Chronic Fatigue Syndrome (EUROMENE): Expert Consensus on the Diagnosis, Service Provision, and Care of People with ME/CFS in Europe. *Medicina* 2021, *57*, 510. [CrossRef]
30. Jason, L.A.; Sunnquist, M. The development of the DePaul Symptom Questionnaire: Original, expanded, brief, and pediatric versions. *Front. Pediatr.* 2018, *6*, 330. [CrossRef]
31. Sunnquist, M.; Lazarus, S.; Jason, L.A. The development of a short form of the DePaul Symptom Questionnaire. *Rehabil. Psychol.* 2019, *64*, 453–462. [CrossRef]
32. Carruthers, B.M.; Jain, A.K.; De Meirleir, K.L.; Peterson, D.L.; Klimas, N.G.; Lerner, A.M.; Bested, A.C.; Flor-Henry, P.; Joshi, P.; Powles, A.P.; et al. Myalgic Encephalomyelitis/Chronic Fatigue Syndrome: Clinical working case definition, diagnostic and treatment protocols. *J. Chronic Fatigue Syndr.* 2003, *11*, 7–115. [CrossRef]
33. Cotler, J.; Holtzman, C.; Dudun, C.; Jason, L.A. A brief questionnaire to assess post-exertional malaise. *Diagnostics* 2018, *8*, 66. [CrossRef] [PubMed]
34. Froehlich, L.; Hattesohl, D.B.R.; Cotler, J.; Jason, L.A.; Scheibenbogen, C.; Behrends, U. Causal Attributions and Perceived Stigma for Myalgic Encephalomyelitis/Chronic Fatigue Syndrome. *J. Health Psychol.* 2021, in press.
35. Ware, J.E.; Sherbourne, C.D. The MOS 36-item short-form health survey (SF-36). I. Conceptual framework and item selection. *Med. Care* 1992, *30*, 473–483. [CrossRef] [PubMed]
36. Morfeld, M.; Kirchberger, I.; Bullinger, M. *SF-36 Fragebogen zum Gesundheitszustand: Deutsche Version des Short Form-36 Health Survey: [German Version of the Short Form-36 Health Survey]*, 2nd ed.; Hogrefe: Wiesbaden, Germany, 2011.

37. Cohen, J. *Statistical Power Analysis for the Behavioral Sciences*, 2nd ed.; Associates, L.E., Hillsdale, N.J., Eds.; Academic Press: Cambridge, MA, USA, 1988.
38. Jason, L.A.; Benton, M.C.; Valentine, L.; Johnson, A.; Torres-Harding, S. The economic impact of ME/CFS: Individual and societal costs. *Dyn. Med.* **2008**, *7*, 6. [CrossRef] [PubMed]
39. Cullinan, J.; Pheby, D.F.H.; Araja, D.; Berkis, U.; Brenna, E.; de Korwin, J.D.; Gitto, L.; Hughes, D.A.; Hunter, R.M.; Trepel, D.; et al. Perceptions of European ME/CFS experts concerning knowledge and understanding of ME/CFS among primary care physicians in Europe: A report from the European ME/CFS Re-search Network (EUROMENE). *Medicina* **2021**, *57*, 208. [CrossRef] [PubMed]
40. Pheby, D.F.H.; Araja, D.; Berkis, U.; Brenna, E.; Cullinan, J.; de Korwin, J.D.; Gitto, L.; Hughes, D.A.; Hunter, R.M.; Trepel, D.; et al. A literature review of GP knowledge and understanding of ME/CFS: A report from the socioeconomic working group of the European Network on ME/CFS (EUROMENE). *Medicina* **2020**, *57*, 7. [CrossRef] [PubMed]
41. DEGAM Leitlinie Müdigkeit [Fatigue Guideline]. 2017. Available online: https://www.degam.de/files/Inhalte/Leitlinien-Inhalte/Dokumente/DEGAM-S3-Leitlinien/053-002_Leitlinie%20Muedigkeit/Aktuelle%20Fassung%202018/053-002l_LL_Muedigkeit_180423_online22-05-18.pdf (accessed on 21 June 2021).
42. Hickie, I.; Davenport, T.; Wakefield, D.; Vollmer-Conna, U.; Cameron, B.; Vernon, S.D.; Reeves, W.C.; Lloyd, A. Post-infective and chronic fatigue syndromes precipitated by viral and non-viral pathogens: Prospective cohort study. *Br. Med J.* **2006**, *333*, 575. [CrossRef] [PubMed]
43. Islam, M.F.; Cotler, J.; Jason, L.A. Post-viral fatigue and COVID-19: Lessons from past epidemics. *Fatigue Biomed. Health Behav.* **2020**, *8*, 61–69. [CrossRef]
44. Komaroff, A.L.; Bateman, L. Will COVID-19 lead to Myalgic Encephalomyelitis/Chronic Fatigue Syndrome? *Front. Med.* **2020**, *7*, 606824. [CrossRef]
45. Kedor, C.; Freitag, H.; Meyer-Arndt, L.; Wittke, K.; Zoller, T.; Steinbeis, F.; Haffke, M.; Rudolf, G.; Heidecker, B.; Volk, H.D.; et al. Chronic COVID-19 Syndrome and Chronic Fatigue Syndrome (ME/CFS) following the first pandemic wave in Germany—A first analysis of a prospective observational study. *medRxiv* **2021**. medRxiv:2021.02.06.21249256. [CrossRef]

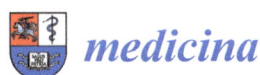

Article

Clinical Profile and Aspects of Differential Diagnosis in Patients with ME/CFS from Latvia

Angelika Krumina [1,*], Katrine Vecvagare [2], Simons Svirskis [2], Sabine Gravelsina [2], Zaiga Nora-Krukle [2], Sandra Gintere [3] and Modra Murovska [2]

[1] Department of Infectology, Rīga Stradiņš University, 16 Dzirciema St., LV-1007 Riga, Latvia
[2] Institute of Microbiology and Virology, Rīga Stradiņš University, 5 Ratsupites St., LV-1067 Riga, Latvia; katrine.vecvagare@rsu.lv (K.V.); simons.svirskis@rsu.lv (S.S.); sabine.gravelsina@rsu.lv (S.G.); zaiga.nora@rsu.lv (Z.N.-K.); modra.murovska@rsu.lv (M.M.)
[3] Department of Family Medicine, Rīga Stradiņš University, 16 Dzirciema St., LV-1007 Riga, Latvia; sandra.gintere@rsu.lv
* Correspondence: angelika.krumina@rsu.lv; Tel.: +371-2911-3833

Citation: Krumina, A.; Vecvagare, K.; Svirskis, S.; Gravelsina, S.; Nora-Krukle, Z.; Gintere, S.; Murovska, M. Clinical Profile and Aspects of Differential Diagnosis in Patients with ME/CFS from Latvia. *Medicina* 2021, 57, 958. https://doi.org/10.3390/medicina57090958

Academic Editor: Tibor Hortobágyi

Received: 16 July 2021
Accepted: 6 September 2021
Published: 11 September 2021

Publisher's Note: MDPI stays neutral with regard to jurisdictional claims in published maps and institutional affiliations.

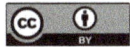

Copyright: © 2021 by the authors. Licensee MDPI, Basel, Switzerland. This article is an open access article distributed under the terms and conditions of the Creative Commons Attribution (CC BY) license (https://creativecommons.org/licenses/by/4.0/).

Abstract: *Background and objectives*: There is still an uncertainty regarding the clinical symptomatology and the diagnostic criteria in terms of myalgic encephalomyelitis/chronic fatigue syndrome (ME/CFS), as different diagnostic criteria exist. Our aim is to identify the core symptoms of ME/CFS in the outpatient setting in Riga; to distinguish symptoms in patients with ME/CFS and those with symptoms of fatigue; and to investigate patient thoughts on the onset, symptoms, treatment and effect of ME/CFS. *Materials and methods*: Total of 65 Caucasian patients from an ambulatory care setting were included in the study. Questionnaires, specialist evaluation of the patients and visual analogue scale (VAS) measurements were used to objectify the findings. *Results*: The study showed that ME/CFS with comorbidities is associated with a more severe disease. A negative correlation was found regarding an increase in age and number of current symptoms, as well as an increase in VAS score and the duration of fatigue and age in the ME/CFS without comorbidities group. *Conclusions*: Comorbidities tend to present with a more severe course of ME/CFS. Fatigue, myalgia, arthralgia and sleep disturbances tend to be more prevalent in the ME/CFS patients compared to the non-ME/CFS patients. VAS score has a tendency to decrease with age and duration of fatigue. Nonsteroidal anti-inflammatory drugs are the most commonly used pharmacological drug class that reduces ME/CFS symptoms.

Keywords: myalgic encephalomyelitis/chronic fatigue syndrome; symptoms; diagnosis; visual analogue scale

1. Introduction

Myalgic encephalomyelitis (ME) or chronic fatigue syndrome (CFS) is post-viral or post-infectious fatigue syndrome or systemic exertional intolerance disease (SEID) that affects the functioning ability of a person and reduces the energy below the level that is considered the average. It is a complex and multifactorial disease that not only dysregulates the central nervous system, immune system and cellular energy metabolism, but also influences physical and cognitive state [1].

Nowadays there are several terms that are being used in the literature to describe ME/CFS. Historically CSF and ME were used separately, as different nosologic entities, but when Federal Health Agencies in the United States of America combined them together in 2016, ME/CFS has been used as an umbrella term to identify multi-systemic, chronic disease that causes physical, cognitive, or emotional exertion [2]. SEID is a relatively new term that has been proposed by the Institute of Medicine (IOM) in 2015 [3] and introduced based on the characteristic, central elements of the disease. No matter which diagnostic criteria are being used, the recent publications aim to declare that post-exertional malaise (PEM) is one of the key symptoms [4]. In this report the term ME/CFS will be used.

As to the statistics of ME/CFS, the numbers vary and depend on the country and research. The prevalence is from 0.42% to 2.54% worldwide [5] and there are from one million to over five million people suffering from ME/CFS in Europe [4].

Several aetiological scenarios are discussed in terms of ME/CFS, but it is still considered multifactorial spectrum of illness with controversial, complex and unknown aetiology that is triggered by different factors and happens to develop in people with predisposition. There have been investigations in terms of neurological, immunological, endocrine, genetic and infectious causes, but none of these are considered the leading one [6].

As regards the diagnostics of ME/CFS, there is no single golden standard that is accepted worldwide, but several criteria systems have been used depending on the country or healthcare centre. In general, the diagnosis is based on the patient's subjective symptoms and differential diagnostics to exclude other pathologies, because there are no biomarkers or other tests that could serve to objectify this process.

In the last 30 to 40 years approximately 20 different diagnostic criteria systems have been proposed. One of the most commonly used is the Fukuda criteria (FC) [7], more recently the Canadian Consensus Criteria (CCC) [8] have been proposed, as well as the International Consensus Criteria (ICC) [1], the Oxford criteria (OC) [9] and the criteria released by the IOM in 2015 [10], the latter having received international recognition [4]. FC (1994) commonly serves as a diagnostic tool in research purposes. As to the recent suggestion from the European Network on Myalgic Encephalomyelitis/Chronic Fatigue Syndrome (EUROMENE) expert consensus, PEM should also be included in the core symptoms of the Fukuda criteria, to decrease the risk of hyperdiagnostics [4].

To better asses ME/CFS symptoms and to objectify them, several questionnaires and functional tests are being used: "UK ME/CFS Participant Questionnaire" [11]; "DePaul Symptom Questionnaire" (DSQ) [5,12]; "The RAND-36 Item Health Survey" [13,14]. There are certain strengths for each of the questionnaires, but they all have been used in both clinical and research purposes [15]. To evaluate the functioning ability, the most commonly used scales are: "Work and Social Adjustment Scale (WSAS) [16,17], "Energy Index Point Score" [18], "The Lawton Instrument Activities of Daily Living Scale" [19], VAS [20], "SF-36" [21,22], EQ-5D [23,24] and others. To evaluate sleep disturbances: "Sleep Assessment Questionnaire" [25], "Pittsburg Sleep Quality Index" [26], "PROMIS Sleep questionnaire" [27], as well as The Epworth Sleepiness Scale to detect daytime sleepiness [4] are being used.

To decrease the risk of hyperdiagnostics, several differential diagnosis should be excluded. Besides that, there are certain diseases that usually manifest together with ME/CFS and do not rule out the diagnosis of ME/CFS. Some of the overlap syndromes are: allergies, fibromyalgia, irritable bowel syndrome, postural orthostatic tachycardia syndrome, hypotension, hypogonadism and premature menopause, sleep disorders, hypersensitivities, hypoglycaemia, mitral valve prolapse, metabolic syndrome, vitamin B12 deficiency, endometriosis and others [28].

Although ME/CFS is a disabling disease with an impact on functional status and quality of life, no specific treatment or cure for ME/CFS exist, it tends to be individualised and usually vary from case to case. Nevertheless, both - pharmacological and non-pharmacological methods, as well as alternative medicine are used to reduce the symptoms and improve the quality of life and well-being [12]. But it should be noted that results of the research have been controversial, leading to reduction of the symptoms, aggravation of the symptoms, being ineffective or causing side effects. That is why these measurements should be done under control and the choice of treatment should be based according to the national guidelines.

To conclude, it is clearly seen that ME/CFS remains a challenge for medical specialists. As this disease has unclear aetiology, symptomatic variability and there are no common grounds for unified diagnostic criteria, it is challenging to find the best treatment option. However, a wide range of research is being conducted in pharmacological, non-pharmacological, as well as alternative medicine fields, therefore new strategies and potential improvements are still to come to improve the work of the clinicians and to raise the quality of life of the patients.

2. Materials and Methods

2.1. Patient Selection and Eligibility Criteria

This prospective observational study includes a Latvian population of 65 Caucasian participants (43 females, 22 males) undergoing outpatient treatment in Rīga Stradiņš University ambulance in Riga, Latvia from April 2020 to May 2021. Age ranged from 23–78 years in females and 21–72 years in males. The average age $\pm$ SD for both genders was 47.4 ± 14.92 years (47.40 ± 14.66 in females and 47.41 ± 15.78 in males).

The inclusion criteria were as follows:

- 18 years or older;
- Patient or legally authorised representative capable to give informed consent;
- Fatigue lasting for at least six consecutive months;
- Subjective symptoms of fatigue for more than six months or previously diagnosed with ME/CFS using the Fukuda et.al diagnostic criteria;
- Meets the neurologic criteria;
- Fatigue includes PEM as a compulsory symptom.

The exclusion criteria were as follows:

- Younger than 18 years;
- Pregnancy or breast feeding;
- Inability to obtain or declined informed consent;
- Cancer, radiation, chemotherapy at the time of enrolment;
- Acute infectious or inflammatory diseases;
- Previously diagnosed depression and/or any other psychiatric disorder;
- Substance abuse and/or eating disorder within two years of the onset of ME/CFS symptoms;
- Obesity with body mass index greater than 45;
- Primary brain disorder.

Patient selection was made by a qualified physician (infectologist, neurologist or general practitioner), specialised in ME/CFS diagnostics, who determined patient's suitability depending on one's clinical expertise. The selection was based on the new-onset fatigue symptoms, previously reported fatigue symptoms registered in medical histories, as well as a previous diagnosis of ME/CFS. All patients were observed by the physician, who reported demographic, medical, occupational and additional information.

2.2. Symptom Registration

Data were collected as part of care at an ambulatory outpatient health care facility. First, the participants were informed about the research, its purposes, their participation and then an informed consent was signed. Second, if the patients agreed, we asked to fill in questionnaires in the waiting room by hand. Of the 65 patients all 65 individuals returned the questionnaire. After completion, the patients were asked to share their questions and comments with a certified specialist, they were consulted and a VAS score was measured.

All patients were interviewed with questionnaires to evaluate various categories. To examine the symptom pattern in ME/CFS patients, we used adapted semi-structured interview questions created by Minnock et.al [29]. The questions were structured in six sections: causes and triggers of fatigue; character of fatigue; current symptoms; comorbidities; solutions for fatigue; and its influence on work disability. Multiple choice answers were provided for each question.

Regarding sleep disturbances, we included a self-reported questionnaire—Athens Insomnia Scale 8 [30]—to assess insomnia symptoms, which included the evaluation in various sleep-related questions: sleep induction, awakenings during the night, final awakening, sleep quality, well-being during the day, functioning capacity during the day and sleepiness during the day. We used the cut-off value of $\geq$ six points for the confirmation of sleep disturbances.

VAS, ranging from zero to ten was also measured for all patients to assess the disease-related pain intensity.

To better evaluate the differences in terms of symptoms, first, we divided the respondents into three groups—patients without ME/CFS presenting with symptoms of fatigue (n = 10), patients diagnosed with ME/CFS according to the Fukuda et.al criteria (n = 19) and patients diagnosed with ME/CFS according to the Fukuda et.al criteria, who have at least one comorbidity, which might be affecting the symptom severity and pattern of fatigue (n = 36). In some situations, we combined the two groups with the diagnosis of ME/CFS (n = 55) to better emphasise the differences between ME/CFS and non-ME/CFS patients. Second, based on the patient's self-reported answers to the questionnaires, the answers were graded by our specialists according to the severity and a total score calculated, so that the correlation analysis and comparison regarding different patterns of fatigue could be made.

2.3. Statystical Analysis

Descriptive and advanced statistical analysis, as well as graphing were done using GraphPad Prism V.9.1 for macOS (GraphPad Software, Inc., San Diego, CA, USA). The normality of the distribution of the studied data was checked by D'Agostino and Pearson, Anderson–Darling and Shapiro–Wilk normality tests. The homogeneity of variances was tested using F-test or Brown–Forsythe and Bartlett's tests. To determine and assess the correlative associations between indicators of fatigue in predefined groups, the Spearman's rank correlation test was performed. Between-group comparisons of summarised fatigue scores expressed in percentage were done by unpaired t-test or Brown-Forsythe and Welch ANOVA tests with Dunnett's T3 multiple comparison test as post-hoc procedure.

As characteristic of central tendency, arithmetic mean with $\pm$ standard deviation (SD) was applied. A p value < 0.05 was considered statistically significant for all tests.

2.4. Ethical Consideration

All of the participants received the information regarding research ethical considerations, description of the research, including the aim, the design and potential results of the inquiry, as well as an informed consent prior to study inclusion. Confidentiality was guaranteed and research subjects were informed about withdrawing from participation without any consequences.

3. Results

3.1. Subject Characteristics in ME/CFS and Non/ME/CFS Patients

Overall, there were 55 patients diagnosed with ME/CFS—with or without comorbidities. As regards results in these two groups, most of the respondents (58%) had been having fatigue for the last year or last two years (29%), whereas the minority—for the last six months (10%). In comparison, patients not diagnosed with ME/CFS reported having fatigue for the last year (60%) or the last six months (40%).

Asked about the onset of fatigue, most patients in the ME/CFS groups considered that emotional (24%) or physical (22%) stress is a contributing factor, whereas 16% reported that it developed gradually with a progression of an underlying chronic disease and 15%—because of sleep disturbances. In the group without ME/CFS on the other hand, most of the patients (60%) reported that they could not remember or identify the onset or the reason for fatigue and none reported that it begun together with a progression of a chronic disease. Emotional stress (30%) was considered a cause for fatigue in more cases than physical stress (15%) in the non-ME/CFS group.

Most patients in both groups with ME/CFS (65%), as well as patients in the non-ME/CFS (50%) group stated that fatigue is constant and invariable throughout the day, whereas for 16% of respondents in both of the ME/CFS groups, compared to none in the non-ME/CFS group fatigue was more severe in the mornings.

Regarding the core symptoms, apart from fatigue with PEM (100%), myalgia (96%), headache (87%), arthralgia (86%) and difficulty concentrating (84%) are the five most common ones in the two groups with ME/CFS, whereas in the non-ME/CFS group those are: headache (91%), myalgia (73%), difficulty concentrating (64%), neck stiffness (64%) and fatigue (55%). All of the symptoms are listed in the Table 1. A graphical representation of the differences regarding symptoms is shown in the Figure 1. It shows that fatigue, myalgia, arthralgia and sleep disturbances are the main symptoms, which have a tendency to differ in ME/CFS patients compared to non-ME/CFS patients.

Table 1. Clinical signs of ME/CFS, ME/CFS with comorbidities and non-ME/CFS patients.

Clinical Features	ME/CFS, ME/CFS + Comorbidities Patients ($n = 55$)	95% CI
Fatigue	55 (100.0)	90.5–100.0
Myalgia	53 (96.4)	87.0–100.0
Headache	48 (87.3)	78.4–96.1
Arthralgia	47 (85.5)	76.7–94.2
Difficulty concentrating	46 (83.6)	74.9–92.3
Neck stiffness	29 (52.7)	45.8–59.7
Sleep disturbances	29 (52.7)	45.8–59.7
Tachycardia	23 (41.8)	35.7–48.0
Tender lymph nodes	21 (38.2)	32.3–44.1
Night sweats	19 (32.7)	27.3–38.2
Weight loss	18 (27.3)	22.3–32.2
Orthostatic hypotension	15 (18.2)	14.1–22.2
Fever	9 (16.4)	12.5–20.2
Abdominal pain	7 (12.7)	9.3–16.1
Chest pain	4 (7.3)	4.7–9.8
Weight gain	3 (5.5)	3.2–7.7
Rash	3 (5.5)	3.2–7.7
Clinical Features	Non-ME/CFS Patients ($n = 10$)	95% CI
Headache	10 (90.9)	81.9–100.0
Myalgia	8 (72.7)	64.6–80.8
Difficulty concentrating	7 (63.6)	56.1–71.2
Neck stiffness	7 (63.6)	56.1–71.3
Fatigue	6 (54.5)	47.5–61.5
Tender lymph nodes	5 (45.5)	39.0–51.9
Arthralgia	5 (45.5)	39.0–51.9
Tachycardia	5 (45.5)	39.0–51.9
Weight loss	4 (36.4)	30.6–42.1
Night sweats	4 (36.4)	30.6–42.1
Orthostatic hypotension	4 (36.4)	30.6–42.1
Sleep disturbances	3 (27.3)	22.3–32.2
Fever	2 (18.2)	14.1–22.2
Chest pain	2 (18.2)	14.1–22.2
Abdominal pain	0 (0.0)	0.0–0.0
Weight gain	0 (0.0)	0.0–0.0
Rash	0 (0.0)	0.0–0.0

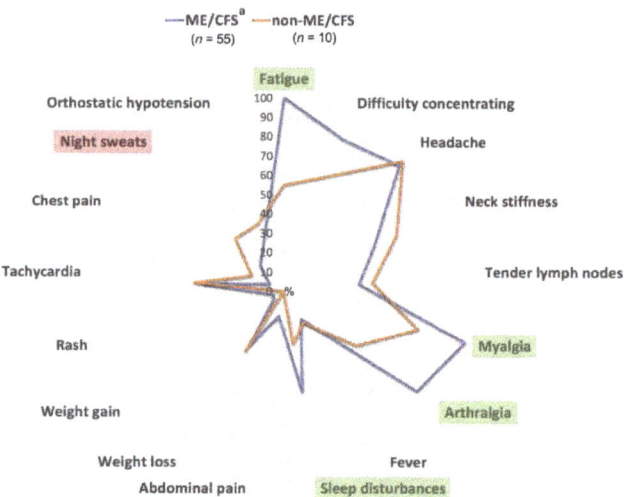

Figure 1. Comparative core symptom proportion in ME/CFS and non-ME/CFS patients using radial diagram; [a]—all ME/CFS patients including those with comorbidities; ME/CFS: myalgic encephalomyelitis/chronic fatigue.

In most cases (93%) our respondents in both of the ME/CFS groups could not identify any first-degree relatives having similar symptoms of fatigue, but if such a tendency was reported (7%), then in all of the cases the relative was mother.

Considering the effect fatigue has on the employment status, almost all respondents (82%) in both—the ME/CFS and ME/CFS with comorbidities groups had reduced their workload or become unemployed.

Regarding comorbidities presenting together with ME/CFS, the overall prevalence was 66%. Fibromyalgia, chronic hepatitis and Lyme disease occurred in 20%, 9% and 5%, respectively. EBV, enterovirus infection each occurred in 5% of cases, whereas lymphadenopathy and anaemia were registered in 4% of cases. The schematic representation of all diagnosis can be assessed in the Figure 2, where comparison of two diagnostic groups can be seen—the group with ME/CFS (*n* = 19) and the one with ME/CFS and at least one comorbidity (*n* = 36). It must be noted that all infectious or inflammatory diseases were not in their acute phase at the time of the research.

Comparing self-reported treatment methods to decrease the symptoms of fatigue, in the non-ME/CFS group almost none of the respondents (90%) had found any solutions to decrease fatigue, whereas in both groups with ME/CFS 38% reported using help-self strategies, including physical activities, sleep hygiene, physiotherapy and walking, 38% had not found any solutions and 24% reported using pharmacological drugs, the most commonly used being non-steroidal anti-inflammatory drugs (90%).

The VAS score was also calculated for each individual and the average result was seven in both—the ME/CFS and ME/CFS with comorbidities group compared to six in the non-ME/CFS group.

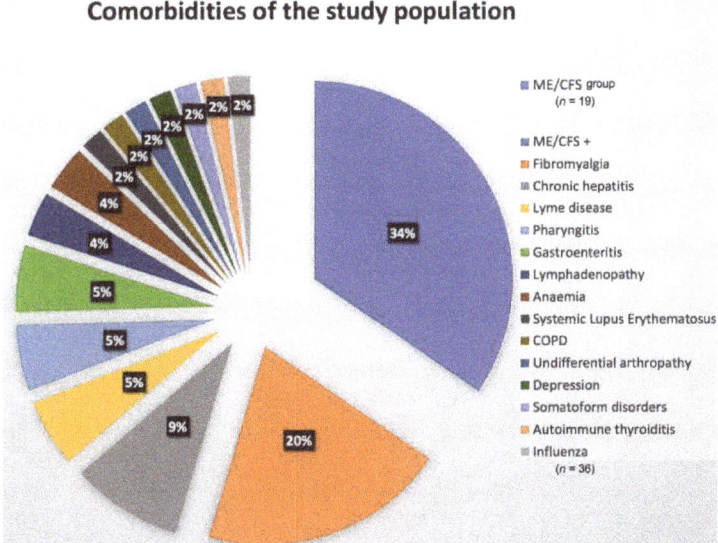

Figure 2. Representation of the proportion of ME/CFS ($n = 19$) and ME/CFS + comorbidities ($n = 36$) in the study population; COPD: Chronic obstructive pulmonary disease.

3.2. Characteristic Differences in the Three, Previously Defined Groups

As shown in the Figure 3 there is a mild but significant increase of the overall scores of the pattern of fatigue, showing the lowest mean score in the patient group with non-ME/CFS diagnosis in comparison to ME/CFS (Figure 3a), however the level of the highest individual scores was established among those patients with ME/CFS with at least one comorbidity, indicating that comorbidities might be associated with a more severe course of the disease (Figure 3b).

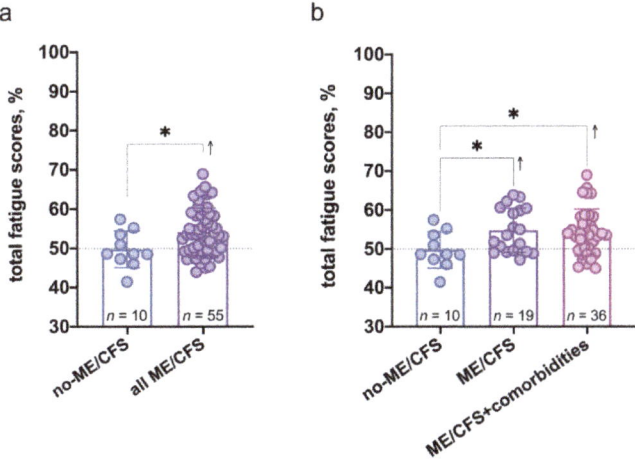

Figure 3. The overall scores of characteristics of fatigue expressed in %: (**a**)—in non-ME/CFS and all ME/CFS patients; (**b**)—in non-ME/CFS, ME/CFS and ME/CFS with at least one comorbidity patients. *—significance level $p < 0.05$ (**a**)—Unpaired *t*-test, (**b**)—Brown-Forsythe and Welch ANOVA tests with Dunnett's T3 multiple comparison test as post-hoc procedure.

Comparing the correlation coefficients in all three groups (Figure 4), those respondents in the non-ME/CFS group, who tend to identify more causes for fatigue and whose duration of fatigue was longer show an increased number of current symptoms (r = 0.59, r = 0.30, respectively). Additionally, more symptoms were identified in older patients (r = 0.30) and females (r = −0.48). In the ME/CFS group without comorbidities, on the other hand, more symptoms were identified in younger patients (r = −0.43) and in those who tend to mention less possible causes for their fatigue (r = −0.30). In both—non-ME/CFS and ME/CFS group without comorbidities more consequences of fatigue were identified by men than women (r = 30, r = 32, respectively).

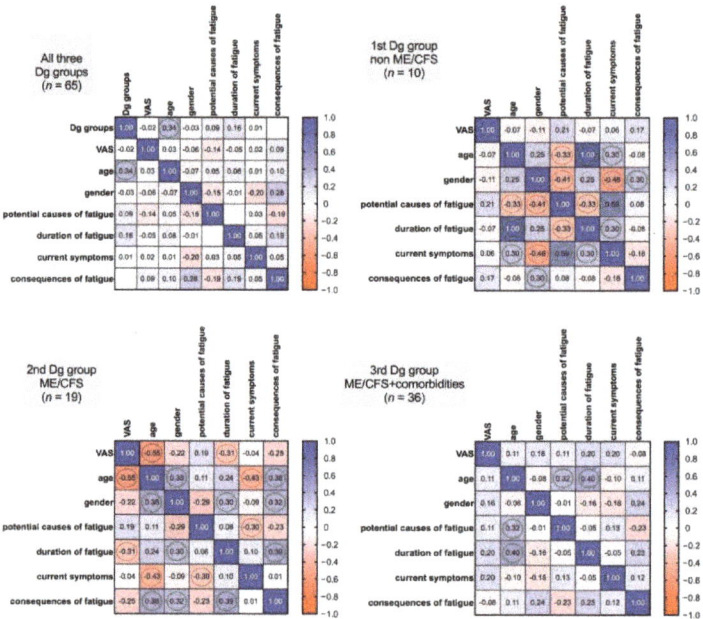

Figure 4. Presented correlograms showing the covariance of the studied variables in all three diagnostic groups—non-ME/CFS, ME/CFS and ME/CFS+comorbidities. The values in the squares represent Spearman's rank correlation coefficients, showing the strength and direction of associations and the more pronounced ones are indicated by coloured circles (red—negative association, green—positive).

Regarding VAS, there was a tendency for the VAS to be higher in younger patients (r = −0.55) and a negative correlation was found regarding an increase in VAS and the duration of fatigue in the ME/CFS group without comorbidities (r = −0.31). No correlations regarding VAS and previously mentioned parameters were found in the other two groups.

Only one correlation was found between the ME/CFS and the comorbidity group, showing that there is a tendency for the duration of fatigue to increase as the age increases (r = 0.40), as well as with an increasing age people tend to identify more possible causes for their fatigue (r = 0.32).

As to the correlation analysis in all of the groups together, only one correlation was identified, showing a tendency for the age to increase in the first (non-ME/CFS), the second (ME/CFS) and the third (ME/CFS + comorbidities) groups, respectively (r = 0.34).

4. Discussions

Comparably to the literature, where ME/CFS is said to be more commonly seen in women than men [31,32], in our study the tendency was similar (67% women, 33% men). The average age in our study was 49 years in persons diagnosed with ME/CFS (without and with comorbidities), which is more than stated in the literature, where the average age of onset is considered to be approximately 33 years [10].

According to the literature, in many cases ME/CFS follows a period of an acute infection [33–36], emotionally stressful incidents [37,38], or physical stressors. In one study the most common insidious event was considered an infection (64%) and stressful incidents (39%) [39], whereas our patients diagnosed with ME/CFS subjectively identified emotional (24%) or physical (22%) stress and to a lesser extent chronic diseases (16%)—to be possible triggers for their symptoms.

As regards the core symptoms of ME/CFS, there has been an ongoing discussion whether the diagnostic criteria identify the most prevalent symptoms and which criteria system would be the most suitable one. In our study the most prevalent symptoms apart from fatigue in the ME/CFS group were myalgia, headache, arthralgia, difficulty concentrating and neck stiffness. However, the symptoms that might be helpful in differentiating between ME/CFS and non-ME/CFS patients were fatigue, myalgia, arthralgia and sleep disturbances, which in our study were more commonly found in ME/CFS patients. Sleep disturbances were a common finding in our study (53%), which is less than in other research, where it has been found as common as in 79% of the subjects [40] showing a positive correlation regarding sleep problems and symptoms of ME/CFS [41]. As neurological and psychiatric comorbidities were excluded in our study, the identification and treatment of sleep disturbances might suggest a decrease in symptom severity. As it is stated in the literature [42], treatment of comorbidities might give promising results in attenuating the symptom severity. Although we did not make any follow-up of symptoms in this study, that would be a subject of interest in the future to evaluate the symptoms and investigate whether it is the most persistent symptom at follow-ups as stated in the literature [40] and whether treating these sleep disturbances could make any change in the current symptoms.

Some researchers have investigated the changes in the circadian rhythm in patients with fibromyalgia [43] and ME/CFS [44], showing that bright light during mornings has a tendency to improve function and pain sensitivity in fibromyalgia patients but has no effect in ME/CFS patients. In our study we concluded that ME/CFS patients report having fatigue as a rather steady symptom throughout the day (65%), but if there was a fluctuation in the severity during the day, then fatigue is more prevalent in the morning (16%), which corresponds to the information in other publications [45].

Our findings suggest that there is a rather limited association of fatigue and a positive family history. In most cases our respondents could not report any similar symptoms in their first-degree relatives in contrary to the other studies, where a positive family history showed a contribution to the predisposition of ME/CFS [46–48].

Whether the duration of the disease affects the outcome is still a debate in the literature. Some state that the duration of the illness might rather increase the ability to cope with the symptoms, in that way leading to less symptom prevalence [49], although others have found that those who have had ME/CFS for a longer period of time tend to have a more severe pattern of the disease [50,51]. Still other authors present with a finding that the duration of the illness does not predict the outcome [52]. In our study we found that there is a negative correlation regarding the age and current symptoms identified by the patients in the ME/CFS group without comorbidities, indicating that more symptoms are identified by younger patients. This caused us to think that younger patients might not yet have identified the coping mechanisms that help minimizing their symptoms. As to the effect of fatigue on work status in our study, 53% have reduced their workload or become professionally disabled, comparing to 65.1% [53] or 47% [39] in other latest studies and 40% presented in a systematic review of studies published from 1988 and 2001 [54]. In the current study those who were having the disease for 2 years or longer were more prone to change their workload and/or become professionally disabled, although follow-up surveillance would be needed to observe this tendency. Our findings regarding the effect of ME/CFS on the employment status are comparable to a study by Tiersky et al. [55], where the authors concluded that in most of the cases the patients are functionally affected and unemployed not only at the time of the diagnosis, but also on follow-ups. In our study 82% had reduced their workload or become unemployed in both of the ME/CFS groups. The authors of this study agree to the fact presented in previous research that the symptom severity decreases over time [4,39] as patients might be able to better manage their illness. It is substantiated by the fact that there was a negative correlation between the duration of fatigue, as well as age and an increase in VAS score in the ME/CFS group without comorbidities, showing no correlation in the non-ME/CFS group.

Although no treatment is found for ME/CFS, there are various strategies the patients use to decrease the severity of the symptoms. Interestingly, patients with ME/CFS were more prone to find a solution for their symptoms comparing to the non-ME/CFS group. According to the literature, the best way to decrease the symptom severity is to treat pain and sleep problems, because they might also be leading to a more severe pattern of other symptoms [4]. As it is seen in this study, nonsteroidal anti-inflammatory drugs are one of the most used pharmacological drugs and are considered effective in 90% of users in both of the ME/CFS groups. None of the patients reported taking supplements or undergoing cognitive behavioural therapy, which might be due to the fact that patients and their caregivers might not be informed about variable strategies to manage the disease.

5. Conclusions

This small-scale study provides important information on the evidence of symptom burden of ME/CFS patients from Riga, Latvia. ME/CFS with at least one comorbidity is associated with a more severe course of the disease. Fatigue, myalgia, arthralgia and sleep disturbances are the symptoms that have a tendency to be more prevalent in the ME/CFS compared to the non-ME/CFS patients. Symptoms in the ME/CFS group without comorbidities tend to decrease by increasing age, as well as more consequences of fatigue are identified by males in both—the non-ME/CFS group and the ME/CFS group without comorbidities. Younger patients and those who present with a shorter duration of the disease tend to have a higher VAS score in the ME/CFS group without comorbidities. An increase in age positively correlates with the duration of the disease, as well as potential causes identified in the ME/CFS group with at least one comorbidity. As to the treatment, the most frequently used pharmacological drug class that reduces the symptoms in patients with ME/CFS are nonsteroidal anti-inflammatory drugs.

It must be acknowledged that this paper can indicate the common patterns patients in particular region present with, although more research is needed to give access to a larger sample size and wider range of examples in order to better distinguish between ME/CFS and patients with fatigue symptoms (non-ME/CFS) in the clinical setting.

Author Contributions: Conceptualisation, A.K.; software, S.S.; validation, A.K., K.V., S.S.; investigation, A.K., K.V.; resources, A.K.; data curation, S.S.; writing—original draft preparation, K.V.; writing—review and editing, K.V., A.K., S.G. (Sabine Gravelsina), S.G. (Sandra Gintere), S.S., Z.N.-K., M.M.; visualisation, S.S.; supervision, M.M.; project administration, M.M.; funding acquisition, M.M. All authors have read and agreed to the published version of the manuscript.

Funding: This research was funded by the Latvian Science Council's Fundamental and Applied Research project, grant number LZP-2019/1-0380.

Institutional Review Board Statement: The study was conducted according to the guidelines of the Declaration of Helsinki, and approved by the Ethical Committee of Rīga Stradiņš University (Ethical code Nr.6-1/05/33 and date of approval 30.04.2020.).

Informed Consent Statement: Informed consent was obtained from all subjects involved in the study. Written informed consent has been obtained from the patients to publish this paper.

Conflicts of Interest: The authors declare no conflict of interest.

References

1. Carruthers, B.M.; van de Sande, M.I.; De Meirleir, K.L.; Klimas, N.G.; Broderick, G.; Mitchell, T.; Staines, D.; Powles, A.C.; Speight, N.; Vallings, R.; et al. Myalgic encephalomyelitis: International Consensus Criteria. *J. Intern. Med.* **2011**, *270*, 327–338. [CrossRef]
2. Valdez, A.R.; Hancock, E.E.; Adebayo, S.; Kiernicki, D.J.; Proskauer, D.; Attewell, J.R.; Bateman, L.; DeMaria, A.; Lapp, C.W.; Rowe, P.C.; et al. Estimating Prevalence, Demographics, and Costs of ME/CFS Using Large Scale Medical Claims Data and Machine Learning. *Front. Pediatrics* **2018**, *6*, 412. [CrossRef]
3. Jason, L.A.; Sunnquist, M.; Brown, A.; McManimen, S.; Furst, J. Reflections on the Institute of Medicine's systemic exertion intolerance disease. *Pol. Arch. Med. Wewn.* **2015**, *125*, 576–581. [CrossRef] [PubMed]
4. Nacul, L.; Authier, F.J.; Scheibenbogen, C.; Lorusso, L.; Helland, I.B.; Martin, J.A.; Sirbu, C.A.; Mengshoel, A.M.; Polo, O.; Behrends, U.; et al. European Network on Myalgic Encephalomyelitis/Chronic Fatigue Syndrome (EUROMENE): Expert Consensus on the Diagnosis, Service Provision, and Care of People with ME/CFS in Europe. *Medicina* **2021**, *57*, 510. [CrossRef] [PubMed]
5. Jason, L.A.; Kot, B.; Sunnquist, M.; Brown, A.; Evans, M.; Jantke, R.; Williams, Y.; Furst, J.; Vernon, S.D. Chronic fatigue syndrome and myalgic encephalomyelitis: Towards an empirical case definition. *Health Psychol. Behav. Med.* **2015**, *3*, 82–93. [CrossRef]
6. Cortes, R.M.; Mastronardi, C.; Silva-Aldana, C.T.; Arcos-Burgos, M.; Lidbury, B.A. Myalgic Encephalomyelitis/Chronic Fatigue Syndrome: A Comprehensive Review. *Diagnostics* **2019**, *9*, 91. [CrossRef]
7. Fukuda, K.; Straus, S.E.; Hickie, I.; Sharpe, M.C.; Dobbins, J.G.; Komaroff, A. The chronic fatigue syndrome: A comprehensive approach to its definition and study. *Ann. Intern. Med.* **1994**, *121*, 953–959. [CrossRef] [PubMed]
8. Strand, E.B.; Nacul, L.; Mengshoel, A.M.; Helland, I.B.; Grabowski, P.; Krumina, A.; Alegre-Martin, J.; Efrim-Budisteanu, M.; Sekulic, S.; Pheby, D. Myalgic encephalomyelitis/chronic fatigue Syndrome (ME/CFS): Investigating care practices pointed out to disparities in diagnosis and treatment across European Union. *PLoS ONE* **2019**, *14*, e0225995. [CrossRef]
9. Sharpe, M. A report–chronic fatigue syndrome: Guidelines for research. *J. R. Soc. Med.* **1991**, *84*, 118–121. [CrossRef]
10. Committee on the Diagnostic Criteria for Myalgic Encephalomyelitis/Chronic Fatigue Syndrome; Board on the Health of Select Populations; Institute of Medicine. *Beyond Myalgic Encephalomyelitis/Chronic Fatigue Syndrome: Redefining an Illness*; National Academies Press (US): Washington, DC, USA, 2015.
11. Lacerda, E.M.; Bowman, E.W.; Cliff, J.M.; Kingdon, C.C.; King, E.C.; Lee, J.-S.; Clark, T.G.; Dockrell, H.M.; Riley, E.M.; Curran, H. The UK ME/CFS biobank for biomedical research on myalgic encephalomyelitis/chronic fatigue syndrome (ME/CFS) and multiple sclerosis. *Open J. Bioresour.* **2017**, *4*. [CrossRef]
12. Jason, L.A.; McManimen, S.; Sunnquist, M.; Newton, J.L.; Strand, E.B. Clinical criteria versus a possible research case definition in chronic fatigue syndrome/myalgic encephalomyelitis. *Fatigue: Biomed. Health Behav.* **2017**, *5*, 89–102. [CrossRef] [PubMed]
13. Hays, R.D.; Sherbourne, C.D.; Mazel, R.M. The rand 36-item health survey 1.0. *Health Econ.* **1993**, *2*, 217–227. [CrossRef]
14. Varni, J.W.; Seid, M.; Kurtin, P.S. PedsQL™ 4.0: Reliability and validity of the Pediatric Quality of Life Inventory™ Version 4.0 Generic Core Scales in healthy and patient populations. *Med. Care* **2001**, *39*, 800–812. [CrossRef] [PubMed]
15. Mundt, J.C.; Marks, I.M.; Shear, M.K.; Greist, J.H. The Work and Social Adjustment Scale: A simple measure of impairment in functioning. *Br. J. Psychiatry* **2002**, *180*, 461–464. [CrossRef]
16. Cella, M.; Sharpe, M.; Chalder, T. Measuring disability in patients with chronic fatigue syndrome: Reliability and validity of the Work and Social Adjustment Scale. *J. Psychosom. Res.* **2011**, *71*, 124–128. [CrossRef] [PubMed]
17. Lerner, A.M.; Beqaj, S.H.; Fitzgerald, J.T. Validation of the energy index point score to serially measure the degree of disability in patients with chronic fatigue syndrome. *In Vivo* **2008**, *22*, 799–801. [PubMed]
18. Graf, C. The Lawton instrumental activities of daily living scale. *AJN Am. J. Nurs.* **2008**, *108*, 52–62. [CrossRef]
19. Vink, M.; Vink-Niese, A. The draft updated NICE guidance for ME/CFS highlights the unreliability of subjective outcome measures in non-blinded trials. *J. Health Psychol.* **2021**. [CrossRef]
20. Jason, L.A.; Evans, M.; Brown, M.; Porter, N.; Brown, A.; Hunnell, J.; Anderson, V.; Lerch, A. Fatigue scales and chronic fatigue syndrome: Issues of sensitivity and specificity. *Disabil. Stud. Q. DSQ* **2011**, *31*, 9–10. [CrossRef]
21. Maruish, M. *User's Manual for the SF-12v2 Health Survey*, 3rd ed.; QualityMetric Incorporated: Lincoln, RI, USA, 2012.
22. Ware Jr, J.E.; Scherbourne, C.D. The MOS 36-Item Short-Form Health Survey (SF-36): I. Conceptual Framework and Item Selection. *Med. Care* **1992**, *30*, 473–483.
23. Schrag, A.; Selai, C.; Jahanshahi, M.; Quinn, N.P. The EQ-5D—A generic quality of life measure—Is a useful instrument to measure quality of life in patients with Parkinson's disease. *J. Neurol. Neurosurg. Psychiatry* **2000**, *69*, 67–73. [CrossRef] [PubMed]
24. Devlin, N.J.; Brooks, R. EQ-5D and the EuroQol group: Past, present and future. *Appl. Health Econ. Health Policy* **2017**, *15*, 127–137. [CrossRef] [PubMed]
25. Roth, T.; Zammit, G.; Kushida, C.; Doghramji, K.; Mathias, S.D.; Wong, J.M.; Buysse, D.J. A new questionnaire to detect sleep disorders. *Sleep Med.* **2002**, *3*, 99–108. [CrossRef]
26. Josev, E.K.; Jackson, M.L.; Bei, B.; Trinder, J.; Harvey, A.; Clarke, C.; Snodgrass, K.; Scheinberg, A.; Knight, S.J. Sleep quality in adolescents with chronic fatigue syndrome/myalgic encephalomyelitis (CFS/ME). *J. Clin. Sleep Med.* **2017**, *13*, 1057–1066. [CrossRef] [PubMed]
27. Yu, L.; Buysse, D.J.; Germain, A.; Moul, D.E.; Stover, A.; Dodds, N.E.; Johnston, K.L.; Pilkonis, P.A. Development of short forms from the PROMIS™ sleep disturbance and sleep-related impairment item banks. *Behav. Sleep Med.* **2012**, *10*, 6–24. [CrossRef]

28. Lapp, C.W. Initiating Care of a Patient With Myalgic Encephalomyelitis/Chronic Fatigue Syndrome (ME/CFS). *Front. Pediatrics* **2019**, *6*, 415. [CrossRef]
29. Minnock, P.; Ringnér, A.; Bresnihan, B.; Veale, D.; FitzGerald, O.; McKee, G. Perceptions of the Cause, Impact and Management of Persistent Fatigue in Patients with Rheumatoid Arthritis Following Tumour Necrosing Factor Inhibition Therapy. *Musculoskelet. Care* **2017**, *15*, 23–35. [CrossRef]
30. Soldatos, C.R.; Dikeos, D.G.; Paparrigopoulos, T.J. Athens Insomnia Scale: Validation of an instrument based on ICD-10 criteria. *J. Psychosom. Res.* **2000**, *48*, 555–560. [CrossRef]
31. Reyes, M.; Nisenbaum, R.; Hoaglin, D.C.; Unger, E.R.; Emmons, C.; Randall, B.; Stewart, J.A.; Abbey, S.; Jones, J.F.; Gantz, N. Prevalence and incidence of chronic fatigue syndrome in Wichita, Kansas. *Arch. Intern. Med.* **2003**, *163*, 1530–1536. [CrossRef]
32. Torres-Harding, S.R.; Jason, L.A.; Taylor, R.R. Fatigue severity, attributions, medical utilization, and symptoms in persons with chronic fatigue. *J. Behav. Med.* **2002**, *25*, 99–113. [CrossRef]
33. Hickie, I.; Davenport, T.; Wakefield, D.; Vollmer-Conna, U.; Cameron, B.; Vernon, S. Prospective cohort study precipitated by viral and non-viral pathogens: Post-infective and chronic fatigue syndromes. *BMJ* **2006**, *333*, 575. [CrossRef]
34. Rasa, S.; Nora-Krukle, Z.; Henning, N.; Eliassen, E.; Shikova, E.; Harrer, T.; Scheibenbogen, C.; Murovska, M.; Prusty, B.K. Chronic viral infections in myalgic encephalomyelitis/chronic fatigue syndrome (ME/CFS). *J. Transl. Med.* **2018**, *16*, 1–25. [CrossRef]
35. Cameron, B.; Flamand, L.; Juwana, H.; Middeldorp, J.; Naing, Z.; Rawlinson, W.; Ablashi, D.; Lloyd, A. Serological and virological investigation of the role of the herpesviruses EBV, CMV and HHV-6 in post-infective fatigue syndrome. *J. Med. Virol.* **2010**, *82*, 1684–1688. [CrossRef]
36. Bested, A.; Saunders, P.; Logan, A. Chronic fatigue syndrome: Neurological findings may be related to blood–brain barrier permeability. *Med. Hypotheses* **2001**, *57*, 231–237. [CrossRef] [PubMed]
37. Heim, C.; Nater, U.M.; Maloney, E.; Boneva, R.; Jones, J.F.; Reeves, W.C. Childhood trauma and risk for chronic fatigue syndrome: Association with neuroendocrine dysfunction. *Arch. Gen. Psychiatry* **2009**, *66*, 72–80. [CrossRef]
38. Nater, U.M.; Maloney, E.; Heim, C.; Reeves, W.C. Cumulative life stress in chronic fatigue syndrome. *Psychiatry Res.* **2011**, *189*, 318–320. [CrossRef] [PubMed]
39. Chu, L.; Valencia, I.J.; Garvert, D.W.; Montoya, J.G. Onset Patterns and Course of Myalgic Encephalomyelitis/Chronic Fatigue Syndrome. *Front. Pediatrics* **2019**, *7*, 12. [CrossRef]
40. Nisenbaum, R.; Jones, J.F.; Unger, E.R.; Reyes, M.; Reeves, W.C. A population-based study of the clinical course of chronic fatigue syndrome. *Health Qual. Life Outcomes* **2003**, *1*, 1–9. [CrossRef] [PubMed]
41. Milrad, S.F.; Hall, D.L.; Jutagir, D.R.; Lattie, E.G.; Ironson, G.H.; Wohlgemuth, W.; Nunez, M.V.; Garcia, L.; Czaja, S.J.; Perdomo, D.M. Poor sleep quality is associated with greater circulating pro-inflammatory cytokines and severity and frequency of chronic fatigue syndrome/myalgic encephalomyelitis (CFS/ME) symptoms in women. *J. Neuroimmunol.* **2017**, *303*, 43–50. [CrossRef]
42. Comhaire, F.; Deslypere, J.P. News and views in myalgic encephalomyelitis/chronic fatigue syndrome (ME/CFS): The role of co-morbidity and novel treatments. *Med. Hypotheses* **2020**, *134*, 109444. [CrossRef] [PubMed]
43. Burgess, H.J.; Park, M.; Ong, J.C.; Shakoor, N.; Williams, D.A.; Burns, J. Morning versus evening bright light treatment at home to improve function and pain sensitivity for women with fibromyalgia: A pilot study. *Pain Med.* **2017**, *18*, 116–123. [CrossRef]
44. Williams, G.; Waterhouse, J.; Mugarza, J.; Minors, D.; Hayden, K. Therapy of circadian rhythm disorders in chronic fatigue syndrome: No symptomatic improvement with melatonin or phototherapy. *Eur. J. Clin. Investig.* **2002**, *32*, 831–837. [CrossRef]
45. Jones, D.; Gray, J.; Frith, J.; Newton, J. Fatigue severity remains stable over time and independently associated with orthostatic symptoms in chronic fatigue syndrome: A longitudinal study. *J. Intern. Med.* **2011**, *269*, 182–188. [CrossRef] [PubMed]
46. Whistler, T.; Jones, J.F.; Unger, E.R.; Vernon, S.D. Exercise responsive genes measured in peripheral blood of women with chronic fatigue syndrome and matched control subjects. *BMC Physiol* **2005**, *5*, 5. [CrossRef] [PubMed]
47. Walsh, C.; Zainal, N.; Middleton, S.; Paykel, E. A family history study of chronic fatigue syndrome. *Psychiatr. Genet.* **2001**, *11*, 123–128. [CrossRef] [PubMed]
48. Albright, F.; Light, K.; Light, A.; Bateman, L.; Cannon-Albright, L.A. Evidence for a heritable predisposition to Chronic Fatigue Syndrome. *BMC Neurol.* **2011**, *11*, 62. [CrossRef]
49. Jason, L.; Benton, M.; Torres-Harding, S.; Muldowney, K. The impact of energy modulation on physical functioning and fatigue severity among patients with ME/CFS. *Patient Educ. Couns.* **2009**, *77*, 237–241. [CrossRef]
50. Friedberg, F.; Dechene, L.; McKenzie, M.J., II; Fontanetta, R. Symptom patterns in long-duration chronic fatigue syndrome. *J. Psychosom Res.* **2000**, *48*, 59–68. [CrossRef]
51. Brown, M.M.; Brown, A.A.; Jason, L.A. Illness duration and coping style in chronic fatigue syndrome. *Psychol. Rep.* **2010**, *106*, 383–393. [CrossRef]
52. Twisk, F.N. Accurate diagnosis of myalgic encephalomyelitis and chronic fatigue syndrome based upon objective test methods for characteristic symptoms. *World J. Methodol.* **2015**, *5*, 68–87. [CrossRef]
53. Kidd, E.; Brown, A.; McManimen, S.; Jason, L.A.; Newton, J.L.; Strand, E.B. The Relationship between Age and Illness Duration in Chronic Fatigue Syndrome. *Diagnostics* **2016**, *6*, 16. [CrossRef] [PubMed]

54. Ross, S.D.; Levine, C.; Ganz, N.; Frame, D.; Estok, R.; Stone, L.; Ludensky, V. Systematic review of the current literature related to disability and chronic fatigue syndrome. *Evid. Rep./Technol. Assess. (Summ.)* **2002**, 1–3. [CrossRef]
55. Tiersky, L.; Deluca, J.; Hill, N.; Dhar, S.; Johnson, S.; Lange, G.; Rappolt-Schlichtmann, G.; Natelson, B. Longitudinal Assessment of Neuropsychological Functioning, Psychiatric Status, Functional Disability and Employment Status in Chronic Fatigue Syndrome. *Appl. Neuropsychol.* **2001**, *8*, 41–50. [CrossRef] [PubMed]

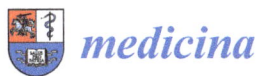 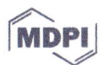

Opinion

European Network on Myalgic Encephalomyelitis/Chronic Fatigue Syndrome (EUROMENE): Expert Consensus on the Diagnosis, Service Provision, and Care of People with ME/CFS in Europe

Luis Nacul [1,2,*,†], François Jérôme Authier [3,†], Carmen Scheibenbogen [4], Lorenzo Lorusso [5], Ingrid Bergliot Helland [6], Jose Alegre Martin [7], Carmen Adella Sirbu [8], Anne Marit Mengshoel [9], Olli Polo [10], Uta Behrends [11], Henrik Nielsen [12], Patricia Grabowski [13], Slobodan Sekulic [14], Nuno Sepulveda [15], Fernando Estévez-López [16], Pawel Zalewski [17], Derek F. H. Pheby [18], Jesus Castro-Marrero [19], Giorgos K. Sakkas [20], Enrica Capelli [21], Ivan Brundsdlund [22], John Cullinan [23], Angelika Krumina [24], Jonas Bergquist [25,26], Modra Murovska [27], Ruud C. W. Vermuelen [28,‡] and Eliana M. Lacerda [29,‡]

Citation: Nacul, L.; Authier, F.J.; Scheibenbogen, C.; Lorusso, L.; Helland, I.B.; Martin, J.A.; Sirbu, C.A.; Mengshoel, A.M.; Polo, O.; Behrends, U.; et al. European Network on Myalgic Encephalomyelitis/Chronic Fatigue Syndrome (EUROMENE): Expert Consensus on the Diagnosis, Service Provision, and Care of People with ME/CFS in Europe. *Medicina* **2021**, *57*, 510. https://doi.org/10.3390/medicina57050510

Academic Editor: Tibor Hortobágyi

Received: 11 April 2021
Accepted: 13 May 2021
Published: 19 May 2021

Publisher's Note: MDPI stays neutral with regard to jurisdictional claims in published maps and institutional affiliations.

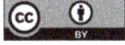

Copyright: © 2021 by the authors. Licensee MDPI, Basel, Switzerland. This article is an open access article distributed under the terms and conditions of the Creative Commons Attribution (CC BY) license (https://creativecommons.org/licenses/by/4.0/).

1. London School of Hygiene and Tropical Medicine, Faculty of Infectious and Tropical Diseases, London WC1E 7HT, UK
2. BC Women's Hospital, Vancouver, BC V6H 3N1, Canada
3. Faculty of Medicine Créteil—Paris Est, 94010 Creteil, France; fj.authier@gmail.com
4. Institute of Medical Immunology, Charité-Universitätsmedizin Berlin, 10117 Berlin, Germany; Carmen.Scheibenbogen@charite.de
5. Neurology and Stroke Unit—Neuroscience Department—A.S.S.T.—Lecco, 23900 Merate, Italy; lorusso.lorenzo@gmail.com
6. National Advisory Unit on CFS/ME, Oslo University Hospital, Rikshospitalet OUS, 0372 Oslo, Norway; ihelland@ous-hf.no
7. Chronic Fatigue Unit, Hospital Universitari Vall d'Hebron University Hospital (VHIR), Universitat Autònoma de Barcelona, E-08035 Barcelona, Spain; jalegre@vhebron.net
8. Central Military Emergency University Hospital, Titu Maiorescu University, 040441 Bucharest, Romania; sircar13@yahoo.com
9. Institute of Health and Society, Medical Faculty, University of Oslo, Box 1089 Blindern, 0317 Oslo, Norway; a.m.mengshoel@medisin.uio.no
10. Bragée ME/CFS Center, 115 26 Stockholm, Sweden; olli.polo@unesta.fi
11. Department of Pediatrics, School of Medicine, Technical University of Munich, 80333 Munich, Germany; uta.behrends@mri.tum.de
12. Privat Hospitalet Danmark, 2920 Charlottenlund, Denmark; hnreum@dadlnet.dk
13. Department of Hematology, Oncology and Tumor Immunology, Institute for Medical Immunology, Charite Medical School, 10117 Berlin, Germany; patricia.grabowski@charite.de
14. Medical Faculty Novi Sad, University of Novi Sad, 21000 Novi Sad, Serbia; slobodan.sekulic@mf.uns.ac.rs
15. Centre of Statistics and Its Applications, University of Lisbon, 1749-016 Lisbon, Portugal; Nuno.Sepulveda@lshtm.ac.uk
16. Erasmus MC University Medical Center, 3015 Rotterdam, The Netherlands; fer@estevez-lopez.com
17. Department of Hygiene, Epidemiology, Ergonomics and Postgraduate Education, Nicolaus Copernicus University in Torun, Collegium Medicum, 85-067 Bydgoszcz, Poland; p.zalewski@cm.umk.pl
18. Society and Health, Buckinghamshire New University (retired), High Wycombe HP11 2JZ, UK; derekpheby@btinternet.com
19. Division of Rheumatology, ME/CFS Research Unit (Lab 009—Box 02), Vall d'Hebron Hospital Research Institute (VHIR), Val d'Hebron Hospital Research Unit (VIHR), Passeig de la Val d'Hebron 119-129, E-08035 Barcelona, Spain; jesus.castro@vhir.org
20. Department of PE and Sports Science, University of Thessaly, 421 00 Trikala, Greece; gsakkas@med.uth.gr
21. Department of Earth and Environmental Sciences, University of Pavia, 27100 Pavia, Italy; enrica.capelli@unipv.it
22. Department of Regional Health Research, University Hospital of Southern Denmark, 5000 Odense, Denmark; Ivan.Brandslund@rsyd.dk
23. School of Business & Economics, National University of Ireland Galway, University Road, H91 TK33 Galway, Ireland; john.cullinan@nuigalway.ie
24. Department of Infectiology and Dermatology, Riga Stradins University, LV-1067 Riga, Latvia; angelika.krumina@rsu.lv
25. Department of Chemistry—Biomedical Center, Analytical Chemistry and Neuro Chemistry, Uppsala University, 751 23 Uppsala, Sweden; jonas.bergquist@kemi.uu.se

26 The Myalgic Encephalomyelitis/Chronic Fatigue Syndrome (ME/CFS) Collaborative Research Centre, Uppsala University, 751 23 Uppsala, Sweden
27 Institute of Microbiology and Virology, Riga Stradins University, LV-1067 Riga, Latvia; Modra.Murovska@rsu.lv
28 CFS/ME Medical Centre, 1078 Amsterdam, The Netherlands; rv@cvsmemc.nl
29 Department of Clinical Research, Faculty of Infectious and Tropical Diseases, London School of Hygiene and Tropical Medicine, Keppel Street, London WC1E 7HT, UK; Eliana.Lacerda@lshtm.ac.uk
* Correspondence: luis.nacul@cw.bc.ca
† Shared first authorship.
‡ Shared last authorship.

Abstract: Designed by a group of ME/CFS researchers and health professionals, the European Network on Myalgic Encephalomyelitis/Chronic Fatigue Syndrome (EUROMENE) has received funding from the European Cooperation in Science and Technology (COST)—COST action 15111— from 2016 to 2020. The main goal of the Cost Action was to assess the existing knowledge and experience on health care delivery for people with Myalgic Encephalomyelitis/Chronic Fatigue Syndrome (ME/CFS) in European countries, and to enhance coordinated research and health care provision in this field. We report our findings and make recommendations for clinical diagnosis, health services and care for people with ME/CFS in Europe, as prepared by the group of clinicians and researchers from 22 countries and 55 European health professionals and researchers, who have been informed by people with ME/CFS.

Keywords: Myalgic Encephalomyelitis/Chronic Fatigue Syndrome; diagnosis; health services; care

1. Introduction

1.1. Standardization of Clinical Procedures and Services for Myalgic Encephalomyelitis/Chronic Fatigue Syndrome (ME/CFS) in Europe: The Origins

Initially designed by a group of ME/CFS researchers and health professionals, the European Network on Myalgic Encephalomyelitis/Chronic Fatigue Syndrome (EUROMENE) has received funding from the European Cooperation in Science and Technology (COST)— COST action 15111 [1] —from 2016 to 2020. The main goal of the Cost Action was to assess the existing knowledge and experience on health care delivery for people with Myalgic Encephalomyelitis/Chronic Fatigue Syndrome (ME/CFS) in European countries and to enhance coordinated research and health care provision in this field.

One of the aims of the network was to *define a standardised clinical diagnosis for ME/CFS for clinical and research use*. With the paucity and lack of integration of clinical guidelines in European countries [1], a high need has been identified for addressing the uncertainties around diagnosis and treatment, and to support the development of health services and standard clinical practices for people with ME/CFS across the continent. We report here on the recommendations for clinical diagnosis and management of ME/CFS in Europe, as prepared by the group of clinicians and researchers from 22 countries participating in the network activities (including on Near Neighbour Country–Belarus), and 55 European researchers and health professionals, who have been informed by people with ME/CFS. The participating countries are Austria, Belarus, Belgium, Bulgaria, Denmark, Finland, France, Germany, Greece, Ireland, Italy, Latvia, Netherlands, Norway, Poland, Portugal, Romania, Serbia, Slovenia, Spain, Sweden, United Kingdom. The researchers' names and affiliations are listed in the COST Action website [1].

1.2. The Population Burden of the Disease and the Need for Better Recognition

ME/CF is characterised by intolerance to efforts expressed by profound or pathological fatigue, malaise, and other symptoms aggravated by physical or cognitive efforts at intensities previously well tolerated by the individual. Intolerance to efforts may be experienced immediately or typically be delayed for hours or a day or more after exertion and is associated with slow recovery. This marked and prolonged exacerbation of symptoms of ME/CFS, which follows physical activity and, in some cases, cognitive activity, is termed post-exertional malaise (PEM) and may last several days.

Other key symptoms include unrefreshing sleep, cognitive impairment, orthostatic intolerance, and pain, including muscle and joint pain and headaches. The symptoms are persistent or recurrent over long periods of time and lead to a significant reduction in previous levels of functioning. Diagnosis is clinical, owing to the absence of biomarkers, and based on detailed clinical history and physical examination by a competent clinician [2–5]. There is no causal treatment for the disease. With symptom-oriented support, there can be improvement with time, or patients may learn to manage their illness. There is little evidence on long term prognosis. However, full recovery is not the norm, particularly in adults [2–7], and in addition, there has been a small number of studies reviewing mortality among people with ME/CFS. These are consistent in demonstrating increases in mortality from suicide, in the UK [8] and in the US [9,10]. One American study demonstrated increased cardiovascular and cancer mortality [11], but this has not been confirmed by other studies.

Prevalence rates have been estimated as between 0.1 and 0.7%, and the incidence rate as 0.015 new cases/1000-year [12]. This could represent between 1 million and over 5 million people, probably around 3 million, in the European continent living with ME/CFS. However, there are no European-wide estimates of disease burden [13]. A much larger number of people will have chronic fatigue for other reasons, and many of them will also be significantly incapacitated. At least 2/3 of the cases are in women [12,13], with young people in their most productive phases of life being preferentially affected. However, ME/CFS has been reported in all age groups [14,15]. Quality of life of those with ME/CFS is on average lower than with other chronic or disabling diseases, such as multiple sclerosis [16], cancer, rheumatoid arthritis, depression [17], diabetes, epilepsy, or cystic fibrosis [18]. Economic costs are considerable [19–23] with repercussions for the individuals affected, their families and society, as well as to educational and occupational services.

Many will be unable to work or do so only on a part-time basis; with some in the milder spectrum of the disease able to work full time, however, often at the cost of enduring significant symptoms and sacrificing their social life and other interests due to the need to rest when not working [24,25]. In the absence of economic analysis on the costs of the disease in Europe, we estimate, based on data from the UK, ME/CFS may cost some 40 billion Euros per year to health services and society [22]. There is, however, a large degree of imprecision in these estimates, due to variation in coverage and costs of health services provision and living costs across the Continent, as well as in many cases failure to recognize or diagnose the disease, which not only contributes to this imprecision but also may result in patients being treated inappropriately through their being misdiagnosed as having a psychiatric illness.

Despite the substantial disease burden, the health needs of people with ME/CFS remain largely unmet in Europe, as in many other parts of the world. Clinical services for people with the disease are in small numbers and sparse. A large proportion of the population with the disease has very limited access to health services, including in the public, mixed, and private sectors, because of either geographical inaccessibility, disability, or unsympathetic responses from healthcare professionals. The still limited knowledge of health professionals about the disease, including those in primary care, who are often the first port of call for those with ME/CFS, means diagnosis is often missed or delayed, and not infrequently patients remain undiagnosed and do not receive appropriate care for long periods of time. While waiting for diagnosis, patients often encounter difficulties in getting help from the health and other services, and their suffering and needs are not fully recognised, not only by health professionals but also by employers and educators. On the other hand, on some occasions, patients are over-investigated, with inherent risks and unnecessary costs to individuals and society. People with ME/CFS may easily get trapped into a situation where, while unable to carry on or start meaningful work- or school-related activities, they receive very little guidance from the health sector or support from social services—where they feel disbelieved and neglected and are often failed by the welfare system [24]. Their disability contributes to social isolation, which adds to their burden, and limits their chances of recovery or re-integration in society, by restricting access to healthcare and social support.

2. Methods

2.1. Development of Recommendations

The EUROMENE network activities were organised in Working Groups (WG), including the Clinical Group, tasked to explore existing methods used for the diagnosis of cases in Europe and to develop recommendations for the diagnosis and treatment of people with ME/CFS in the continent. The recommendations for standardising the diagnostic criteria for ME/CFS to be used by European researchers are covered in a related EUROMENE document [26], which will allow comparability and better estimates.

We have not systematically reviewed the evidence in relation to diagnostic criteria and interventions, as this has been done by others. Thus, the following recommendations are pragmatic and were based on the working group member's collective and consensual assessment of key documents on clinical definitions of ME/CFS [2,4–6,27,28] and existing studies and guidelines for clinical assessments and care used in Europe and internationally [1]. The WG members met on various occasions (WG meetings) to agree on key documents and to consider them, based on the members' experiences and expertise and relevance for clinical practice in Europe. We recognise that there is still limited evidence-based research on ME/CFS; as we witness progresses in this field, we recognise the need for frequent reviews of these recommendations, in line with emerging evidence.

2.2. Considerations on ME/CFS Diagnosis for Clinical Purposes

Many diagnostic criteria have been proposed for use in clinical practice, of which those by the Institute of Medicine (currently, National Academy of Medicine), known as the IOM criteria, have received international recognition. Their relative simplicity makes them ideal for use in primary care. An editorial in the Lancet in 2015 [29] suggested that the adoption of the new name Systemic Exertion Intolerance Disease (SEID) could lead to changed attitudes and greater acceptance of the condition. However, despite the fact that the term ME/CFS implies a particular underlying pathology which has yet to be demonstrated, this remains the most widely used diagnostic term, and it is arguable also that SEID understates the severity of the condition, since exertion intolerance is by no means its only clinical feature. The term ME, an abbreviation for myalgic encephalomyelitis, in particular, is unsatisfactory as it suggests that the pathological process underlying the disease is an inflammatory process affecting the brain. There is a lack of convincing evidence for this, and the truth is undoubtedly both more arcane and more complex. The term CFS, short for chronic fatigue syndrome, is equally unsatisfactory, as it implies that fatigue is the main symptom of the illness, whereas in fact its clinical features are far more wide-ranging. The composite term ME/CFS thus carries the disadvantages and shortcomings of both contributary terms. We use it and recommend its use, on purely pragmatic grounds despite these problems, since most clinicians and researchers working in the field use the term and understand its shortcomings. It is part of the lingua franca and enables those working in the field to communicate effectively with each other and, it is to be hoped, to make progress which will enable us ultimately to establish the underlying pathology with greater precision, leading in turn to the development of more appropriate and accurate terminology.

A case of ME/CFS in an adult patient requires the presence of symptoms for at least 6 months and are typically present for at least half of the time (Box 1).

Box 1. Institute of Medicine (IOM) criteria for the diagnosis of ME/CFS.

Required symptoms
1. Substantial reduction or impairment in the ability to engage in pre-illness levels of activity (occupational, educational, social, or personal life) with profound fatigue of new onset, which is present for at least 6 months, is not explained by ongoing or unusual excessive exertion and is not substantially relieved by rest
2. Post-exertional malaise (PEM)
3. Unrefreshing sleep
At least one of the following:
1. Cognitive impairment
2. Orthostatic intolerance

For full details, see Institute of Medicine (IOM), 2015 [6].

The Canadian Consensus Criteria (CCC) are particularly suitable for diagnosis confirmation and case sub-grouping in secondary care, as well as in research (Box 2). The CDC-1994/Fukuda et al. criteria [27] may also be used as a screening tool for diagnosis in clinical practice, but we recommend that only cases with post-exertional malaise (PEM) (which is optional in that definition), are included for diagnosis (Box 3). Note that although the CDC-1994 criteria have been developed for research purposes, they have often been used for diagnosis purposes in clinical practice and are still a preferred case definition by some in Europe.

For children, the IOM [6] and Rowe et al., 2017, criteria [4] (Box 4) may be used. The latter is based on 6 cardinal paediatric symptoms and a disease duration of 6 months; a diagnosis of "postinfectious fatigue syndrome" (PFS) is made when the symptoms are present for 3 months following an acute infection. The Canadian Consensus criteria [2] may also be used in children, as proposed by Jason et al. [5,30]. However, using 3 months of symptoms is sufficient for diagnosis in children and adolescents.

Diagnosis in both adults and children can be suspected earlier, and the primary care physician should be proactive in starting diagnostic investigations. Initial management and referral may be considered when diagnosis is suspected or with 3 months of symptoms, as appropriate.

Box 2. Canadian Consensus Criteria for the diagnosis of ME/CFS.

The required symptoms, listed below, must be persistently or recurrently present for at least 6 months in adults (3 months in children and adolescents). If other conditions have the same symptoms, those conditions must be assessed and treated optimally first before a diagnosis of ME/CFS can be made. Exclusionary conditions should be ruled out by a combination of clinical history, physical examination, and complementary tests.
• Pathological fatigue
• Post-exertional malaise and worsening of symptoms
• Sleep dysfunction
• Pain
• Cognitive symptoms (at least two symptoms from a list provided)
In addition, at least one symptom from two from the following categories of symptoms are required:
• Autonomic
• Neuroendocrine
• Immune

For full details, see Carruthers et al., 2003 [2]. The structure of the CCC definition in adults and some aspects of the CDC-1994 [26] criteria were used to create a paediatric cases definition of ME/CFS [5,30].

Box 3. Modified* CDC-1994 Criteria for the diagnosis of ME/CFS.

Primary symptoms
Clinically evaluated, unexplained, persistent, or relapsing chronic fatigue that is:

- Of new or definite onset (has not been lifelong);
- Is not the result of ongoing exertion;
- Is not substantially alleviated by rest;
- Results in substantial reduction in previous levels of occupational, educational, social, or personal activities;
- Is associated with post-exertional malaise (PEM)*.

Additional symptoms
The concurrent occurrence of three or more of the following symptoms:

- Substantial impairment in short-term memory or concentration;
- Sore throat;
- Tender lymph nodes;
- Muscle pain;
- Multi-joint pain without swelling or redness;
- Headaches of a new type, pattern, or severity;
- Unrefreshing sleep.

These symptoms must have persisted or reoccurred during 6 or more consecutive months of illness and must not have started before the fatigue.
* Modified for use in clinical diagnosis of ME/CFS, to include PEM as compulsory symptom (EUROMENE recommendation). Source: Fukuda et al. 1994 [27].

Box 4. Paediatric diagnosis of ME/CFS.

A diagnosis is based on persistent symptoms as below:
Compulsory symptoms:

- Impaired function
- Post-exertional symptoms
- Fatigue

In addition, 2 of 3 groups of symptoms are required:

- Sleep problems
- Cognitive problems
- Pain

A diagnosis is made if all the criteria below apply:

- Symptoms are persistent for 6 months (or for 3 months if post-infection) and at least some occur daily and are at least of moderate severity
- Other diagnoses are excluded by history, physical examination, and medical testing, including learning disabilities
- Severity of symptoms over a pre-determined cut-off score

For full details, see Rowe et al., 2017 [4]. For research we recommend using the DePaul Symptom Questionnaire Pediatric (DSQ-Ped) [5].

3. Approach to the Diagnosis and Characterisation of Patients

3.1. Steps to Recognising ME/CFS Cases in Clinical Practice

Clinical History

History reveals the main symptoms, including extreme fatigue, fatigability, and cognitive difficulties that are worsened by physical or mental effort. Physical fatigue is often expressed as "lack of energy or stamina", profound tiredness, or general weakness (Box 5).

Mental fatigue is expressed as cognitive problems, such as slowness of response, attention, and concentration problems; they are often referred by patients as "brain-fog" and result in reduced ability to perform "mental tasks".

There is significant intolerance to efforts, both physical and mental, with post-exertional aggravation of symptoms or PEM. PEM typically has delayed onset, often noticed hours later or the following day, and lasts for variable and often extended periods of time—

e.g., from a day in milder cases to many days or weeks in moderately and severely affected individuals.

Sleep is characteristically "non-restorative" or "unrefreshing", and difficulty in initiating or maintaining sleep is common.

Orthostatic intolerance may be manifested with light-headedness and worsening of symptoms (such as fatigue, malaise, dizziness, nausea, palpitations) when assuming or persisting in the upright position for some time, usually a few minutes, but it may happen very soon after raising from the recumbent position or within up to 10 min or more, depending on severity of the dysautonomia. The most severely affected may be unable to stand for more than a few seconds.

Pain can be generalised and referred to joints, muscles, and adjacent soft tissues, with frequent headaches commonly reported. Pain may be migratory and variable in nature and is not associated with signs of inflammatory arthritis or myositis, with typical absence of joint swelling or redness.

There is considerable symptom overlap between ME/CFS and fibromyalgia [30], and a concomitant diagnosis of fibromyalgia [31,32] is often made. The latter requires pain to be generalised (present in at least 4 of 5 body regions) and is widespread and accompanied by other symptoms, such as fatigue, poor sleep, and cognitive difficulties [33].

Importantly, the symptoms of ME/CFS lead to substantial reductions in previous levels of activity and function. Some individuals will still manage full-time work or education, at least for some time. However, very often patients are unable to take up or continue full-time work or education, or any at all, with a significant minority (often quoted as corresponding to 25% of all patients) virtually home- or bedbound. Educational, social, and economic consequences take their toll, with a resulting compromise in emotional wellbeing.

3.2. Clinical Examination

- General physical examination may be entirely normal. However, some patients present with general aspect of tiredness or of being unwell. Nutritional status is usually satisfactory, though overweight or obesity may result from long-term inactivity or as a neuro-endocrine manifestation of the disease. On the other hand, signs of weight loss or low body mass index (BMI) may be present, more commonly in severely affected patients, although they may also raise suspicion of other severe morbidity; signs of neglect or poor care with basic needs, if noticed, should raise concerns about the wellbeing of the patient. Paleness and cold extremities may be noted.
- Orientation and cognition; patients are oriented, but they may show signs of slow thinking, poor attention and short memory and be lost for words; long consultations may elicit increasing cognitive and physical difficulties as the patient tires; on the other hand, some patients may show signs of anxiety and "wired-tiredness", where they are restless in spite of being very tired physically and mentally. Emotional responses may be triggered as patients go through their histories and common difficulties experienced with their symptoms and lack of validation of their diagnosis and degree of disability, which are often not obvious to the untrained observer. In general, patients are highly motivated and willing to do whatever may be needed to improve their symptoms. However, secondary anxiety and depressed mood may be observed, and lack of motivation or despondency should raise the possibility of associated low mood.
- Skin: Paleness and cold extremities may be noted, often aggravated by upright position, which may be associated with low peripheral perfusion or autonomic dysfunction. Redness of lower extremities when sitting or standing may also be noted as a consequence of venous congestion.
- Head and neck: Enlarged lymph nodes may be noted especially on the neck and might be tender; non-exudative pharyngitis might be observed, and crimson crescents in the oral pharyngeal region have often been described [34].

Box 5. Symptoms and complaints to consider when taking a clinical history.

Key symptoms
- Persistent, debilitating symptoms that include extreme fatigue or lack of energy, assessed by the impairment in the ability to work, study, or undertake domestic tasks, leisure activities, and social interactions.
- Persistent exhaustion or unusually high levels of fatigue, aggravated by low levels of exertion, still, upright position, and stress (physical or emotional, such as infections or raised anxiety levels).
- Post-exertional malaise, or post-exertional exacerbation of symptoms: any or all symptoms can get worse following physical or mental efforts and stress—this can happen immediately or more typically delayed after a period following the exertion, e.g., which may be longer than 24 h; recovery to previous levels of functioning and symptom severity may last long (typically from a day to weeks).
- Sleep dysfunction with unrefreshing sleep, i.e., waking up not feeling rested as one would expect following a good night's sleep.
- Complaints of cognitive impairment, such as poor memory, attention, and concentration, slow thinking, reasoning difficulties, sense of disorientation, or "brain fog".
- Pain: muscle and joint pains, which may affect multiple sites and be migratory, but without local signs of inflammation; headaches (tension or migraine type); existing musculoskeletal symptoms may worsen.

Additional symptoms
- Orthostatic intolerance, defined by symptoms occurring only or worsened in the upright position (particularly when not associated with movement—i.e., in the still position), and improved by lying down, e.g., palpitations, tremors, light-headedness, dizziness, weakness, nausea.
- Over-sensitivity to stresses and sensory stimuli such as light, noise, temperature changes, or touch.
- Intolerance to dietary and environmental factors, such as to alcohol, selected or multiple food intolerances and medications, new allergies.
- Infection-like immune symptoms, e.g., frequent and prolonged symptoms of upper respiratory tract infections, such as flu-like symptoms, tender cervical lymph nodes, sore throat, congested nose, shortness of breath.
- Symptoms of irritable bowel syndrome.
- Weight loss or gain.
- Sicca-symptoms (dry eyes, mouth, or the opposite: hypersalivation).
- Emotional instability, anxiety, and depression.

Symptoms' characteristics
- Symptoms may start following infectious or other insults or insidiously. These are persistent, but they may fluctuate from day to day or during the day. Some people experience temporary partial remission of symptoms, which is followed by recurrence and may occur after physical or mental exertion beyond their tolerance level.

Although *specific symptoms* vary in presentation and severity, the symptoms tend to follow a typical pattern of inter-relatedness. This means that patients may have difficulties in distinguishing whether their symptoms arise from lack of energy, pain, or sleep deprivation, for example.

Fatigue and intolerance to efforts are key symptoms which are not always easy to interpret
- *Fatigue* is a main symptom, but its description and interpretation are variable. It usually represents a feeling of intense lack of physical energy or stamina and mental tiredness (reduced mental clarity with slowness in thinking and difficulty in understanding and processing information, focusing attention and forgetfulness), which restricts the ability to undertake physical and mental activities.
- *Intolerance to efforts is a key symptom, which relates to disease severity and previous levels of functioning*. The most severely affected may be limited in simple movements in bed, speaking or engaging in conversation, eating, and activities of daily living such as going to bathroom, bathing, showering, or dressing), milder cases who were previously very active (e.g., athletes) may remain active, though much less than previously.

- Chest and cardio-vascular: Examination of the lungs and heart is usually unremarkable, except for possible changes in heart rate and blood pressure. Mild regular tachycardia may be present at rest. Postural tachycardia (standing heart rate of

>30/min above normal in patients older than 20 years and > 40/min above normal in younger patients, compared to lying down or >120 standing heart rate at any age) may happen immediately or within 10 min or more after standing up from the recumbent or sitting position; it may result from dysautonomia or relative hypovolemia and result in the diagnosis of postural tachycardia syndrome (POTS). Some patients develop hypotension upon standing, sometimes after a brief period of raised blood pressure. These signs are more common in the young and in some over-medicated patients and may be associated with postural hyperaemia or cold extremities.

- Abdomen: General standard examination is conducted to rule out other explaining diseases; mild diffuse abdominal tenderness is not uncommon.
- Musculoskeletal: Joints appearance is usually normal (no oedema or redness); tenderness of joints and soft tissues may also be present. Some patients have hypermobile joints or fulfil the clinical criteria of hypermobile Ehlers–Danlos syndrome (hEDS) [35,36], which should be recognized as a comorbidity.
- Brief neurological examination: This is usually normal, muscle fatiguability is shown by lower handgrip strength compared to healthy individuals or by a rapid fall in grip strength measures during repetitive muscle contractions, particularly in severely affected cases [37]. Sensory examination may be normal, though hyperalgesia or allodynia may be present. Cognitive difficulties and the occasional fasciculation may be noticeable [38]. Brisk symmetrical reflexes in arms and legs may be observed. Cranial nerve examination is usually normal; however, pupil reaction might be slow. Subtle gait abnormalities may be associated with a feeling of instability, although a full-blown Romberg sign at examination is atypical [39]. A brief psychiatric assessment may show signs of associated anxiety or mood disorders or the presence of an alternative diagnosis. Signs suggestive of specific neurological or psychiatric abnormalities should be investigated further.
- In the more severely affected, signs of frailty may be evident; patients may be virtually bed-bound, sit in a wheelchair, have a pale and puffy face, have cold extremities, and not be able to remain or feel very uncomfortable in the upright position for longer than a few seconds or minutes. There is a general sense of weakness and lack of stamina, and short periods of break during clinical assessment may be required as the patient becomes visibly tired and shows signs of increasing cognitive difficulty. Symmetrical reduction in limb muscle strength may be observed on formal neurological examination, and the hand grip manometer will usually show reduced power, with decreasing values on repeated measurements.

3.3. Differential Diagnosis

Since fatigue is a common complaint in daily life and in association with a range of medical problems, it is important to note that most people with ongoing fatigue do not have ME/CFS but rather have symptoms that are caused by other conditions, emotional well-being, or life-style-factors. The presence of PEM, however, raises the level of suspicion, as this is quite typical, though not specific of ME/CFS.

The list of co-morbid conditions and differential diagnoses is not exhaustive. Examples are listed in Boxes 6 and 7. Some conditions are often present concomitantly to ME/CFS (co-morbidities). Other conditions may potentially exclude a diagnosis if they fully or mainly explain the symptoms. However, such conditions may also be co-morbid when their presence does not explain most of the symptoms and signs observed. In general, when one of these conditions is present and is not well-controlled, the patient should be offered optimum treatment and stabilization, before a diagnosis of ME/CFS is considered. Severe conditions should be explored early and excluded or treated promptly. Action is prompted by clinical suspicion and red flags, such as unintentional weight loss, prolonged fever $\geq 38\,°C$, persistently elevated inflammatory markers, significant abnormalities in physical examination, or suicidal ideation. Box 8 includes suggested diagnostic sub-categories, which may change as the clinical picture and further clinical and related information arise. It should be noted also that some comorbid conditions occur largely in the presence of ME/CFS and so their presence or otherwise should be noted when considering whether the possible comorbid condition fully explains the patient's symptoms.

Box 6. Co-morbid conditions which do not exclude ME/CFS diagnosis.

- Fibromyalgia
- Restless legs syndrome, periodic limb disorder
- Postural orthostatic tachycardia syndrome (POTS)
- Neuro-mediated hypotension
- Irritable bowel syndrome
- Food intolerances and atopic conditions
- Mild anxiety
- Mild depression
- Hypermobility Ehlers–Danlos syndrome
- Myofascial pain syndrome
- Small fibre neuropathy
- Sicca symptoms
- Chronic pelvic pain, endometriosis
- Interstitial cystitis
- Hashimoto thyroiditis; hypothyroidism controlled clinically)
- Migraine
- Mast cell activation disorder, eosinophilic esophagitis

Box 7. List of diseases where fatigue may be a prominent feature, which may preclude a diagnosis of ME/CFS if the disease largely explains the symptoms. They may, however, be co-morbidities with ME/CFS if they do not fully explain symptoms characteristic of ME/CFS (including fatigue, cognitive complains, sleep dysfunction, PEM).

- Hypothyroidism
- Hyperthyroidism
- Malignancy
- Rheumatoid arthritis, systemic lupus erythematosus, polymyositis, Sjogren syndrome, psoriasis arthritis
- Crohn's disease, ulcerative colitis, coeliac disease
- Post-concussion syndrome, post-ICU syndrome, post-traumatic stress disorder
- Heart disease, such as heart failure
- Severe chronic obstructive pulmonary disease, other severe respiratory diseases
- Severe anaemia, vitamin B12 deficiency, haemochromatosis
- Renal failure
- Diabetes mellitus
- Addison's or Cushing's disease, hyperparathyroidism, and other endocrine disorders
- Bipolar disorder, schizophrenia, major depression, anorexia, bulimia, autism
- Multiple sclerosis, myasthenia gravis, other neuroimmunological diseases, paraneoplastic syndromes
- Parkinson's disease, Alzheimer's disease, stroke, other serious neurodegenerative diseases
- Sleep apnoea
- Narcolepsy
- Hepatitis, tuberculosis, HIV/AIDS, neuroborreliosis, other chronic infections
- Excessive consumption/abuse of alcohol or other substances

3.4. Detailed Clinical Characterization, Laboratory, and Other Tests

Further patient characterization may involve the use of standard questionnaires—which may be self-completed or applied by an interviewer, and physical measures, which are used to assess function and disease severity. They are useful for patient's baseline evaluation, and, when repeated subsequently, they provide indicators of disease course and evaluation of response to treatment. Core assessments shown in Box 8 include examples of tests that may be used routinely for that aim. When research studies are linked to clinical practice, these and other questionnaires and instruments may also be used [26]. Further laboratory tests and imaging studies may be needed to identify potential co-morbidities, and/or to exclude other diagnoses. These should be guided by clinical assessment and the need to exclude conditions that may explain the symptoms.

Examples of useful screening tests for initial investigations in primary care include full blood count, ferritin, liver enzymes, renal function, thyroid function, high-sensitivity C reactive protein (CRP) or erythrocyte sedimentation rate, electrolytes including sodium, potassium, calcium, inorganic phosphate, creatine phosphokinase (CK), and fasting glucose or glycated haemoglobin.

Serology screening for EBV, hepatitis B and C, HIV, Lyme, and other tick-borne diseases may be useful according to clinical and epidemiological features [40].

Other tests may be required according to availability of resources or as clinically guided. These are usually reserved for specialist centres or are done through referral to other specialties. These are usually aimed at differential diagnosis but could also be used for better characterization of pathology or for the assessment of function and disability (Box 6). Examples include anti-CCP, transglutaminase antibodies, morning cortisol, vitamin B12, NT-pro BNP, and vitamin D3 or 25(OH)D. In some cases, an extended auto-immune screening, allergy testing, serum tryptase levels, and/or lymphocyte differentiation may be required. Imaging and other specialised tests may be appropriate in some cases but are usually reserved for specialist centres, e.g., brain or spine MRI, cardiopulmonary exercise testing (CPET), cognitive testing panel, echocardiography, and tilt table or standing test.

Tests results will often be unremarkable, though subtle abnormalities may be observed [40]. Routine inflammatory markers are usually not elevated in ME/CFS. Low CK suggests severe disease or very low physical activity levels [41]. Elevated LDH and GPT/GOT are found in a subset of patients. Elevated NT-pro BNP might be found and is associated with lower cardiac volume [42]; this should be investigated further. A subset of patients has diminished IgG/A/M levels and/or IgG subclass deficiency [43]. Marked abnormalities should raise the suspicion of an alternative diagnosis.

3.5. Steps to Recognising ME/CFS in Children

None of the criteria used in adults have been validated for the diagnosis of paediatric ME/CFS. Diagnosis of ME/CFS in children is especially challenging for two main reasons: First, younger children may not report symptoms accurately and might assume fatigue as normal, when not remembering the experience of full health. Second, there are differences in how children perceive and report symptoms of ill health, and proxy reporting by parents may not always accurately reflect children's experience. To account for the latter, paediatric ME/CFS should be diagnosed if CCC are fulfilled for as little as 3 months and no other underlying disease has been identified (Box 2). Owing to differences in manifestations and their ascertainment in children, compared to adults, a paediatric case definition that uses the structure of the CCC 2003 adults' definition and some aspects of the CDC-1994 criteria was published in 2006 [30] and modified in 2018 [5]. Most recently, a group of experienced paediatricians suggested a "Clinical Diagnostic Worksheet" [4] (Box 4). This guidance refers to "impaired function" or a "substantial reduction in the child's ability to take part in personal, educational, and/or social activities" associated with fatigue and PEM as cardinal symptoms. Other symptoms including headaches, myalgia, joint pain, sore throat, painful lymph nodes, and abdominal pain are scored as "pain" [4].

Symptoms usually start acutely, often following symptoms of infection, e.g., flu-like symptoms, or gastroenteritis, but may have an insidious or episodic onset. In children, about half of the cases of ME/postinfectious fatigue syndrome manifest after typical Epstein–Barr-virus (EBV)-associated infectious mononucleosis [44–46]. Symptoms are usually fluctuating in type and severity (especially in the early stages of the disease), with patients typically reporting "good" and "bad" days. A more careful analysis of the pattern of symptoms may reveal correlation with physical or mental efforts.

Primary care professionals may suspect a diagnosis in children and adolescents presenting with persistent or recurrent moderate to severely impaired function, fatigue, and post-exertional symptoms, especially if associated with autonomic symptoms, sleep disturbance, neurocognitive problems, and pain (e.g., headaches and abdominal pain), following history, clinical examination, and routine tests that exclude other diagnoses that may explain the symptoms. We recommend paediatricians use the full criteria from Rowe et al.

(2017) [4] as part of diagnostic approach and the CCC 2003 criteria [2] if symptoms are present for 3 months.

Box 8. Core and additional assessments that may be recommended for ME/CFS secondary care services.

Domain or Specific Clinical Situations	Clinical, Laboratory, and Imaging Assessments or Measurement Instruments
CORE ASSESSMENTS	
Severity assessment	UKMEB-PQsymp; DPQ, RAND-36, Pain and fatigue analogue scales
Disability screening	RAND-36 summary scales (physical and mental component summaries)
Muscle power and general health	Hand grip measurements, dynamometer
ADDITIONAL ASSESSMENTS	
Routine tests not done recently and justified clinically	Tests as appropriate
If clinical history suggests autoimmune or immunodeficiency	ANA, ENA, TPO, AMA, APA, immunoglobulins, and others according to clinical findings
Serious neurocognitive symptoms that increase risks for patients	Neurocognitive tests—e.g., Creteil battery of tests; NIH CDE Toolbox (National Institute of Neurological Disorders and Stroke (NINDS), 2018) [43]
Neuroimaging as needed for further neurological investigations	MRI scan, CT
Obstructive sleep apnoea suspected	Sleep studies, polysomnography
Signs of small fibre neuropathy, peripheral neuropathy, marked muscle symptoms, objective peripheral findings	Nerve conduction studies, electromyography (EMG), skin (for intradermal nerve fibre density) or muscle (rarely necessary) biopsy
POTS, orthostatic intolerance	Tilt table test or repeated recumbent and standing heart rate and blood pressure (standing test)
Objective assessment of PEM or disability	2-day CPT (use with caution as can cause or aggravate PEM)
Other more recent tests which may be useful	Metabolomics, e.g., those revealed through organic acid testing and amino acid urine and serum, cytokine panels, and autoantibodies to receptors such as adrenergic receptors.
* A selection or the full range of tests may be conducted routinely or in support of disability assessment. AMA: anti-mitochondrial antibody. ANA: anti-nuclear antibodies. APA: anti-phospholipid antibodies. CPT: cardio-pulmonary testing. DPQ: DePaul Symptom Questionnaire. ENA: extractable nuclear antigens. PEM: post-exertional malaise. POTS: postural orthostatic tachycardia syndrome. TPO: thyroid peroxidase. UKMEB PQsym.: UK ME/CF Participant Questionnaire.	

3.6. Diagnostic Categories

A proposed diagnostic characterization of patients, which builds on previous disease criteria definitions, is shown in Box 9, which also suggests stratification variables that may be used for sub-grouping of cases.

Chronic fatigue-spectrum disorder (CFSd) is an encompassing term and may be used to refer to persistent profound fatigue for over 3–6 months associated with other symptoms, including the following sub-categories: (a) cases meeting diagnostic criteria for ME/CFS; (b) cases that do not fully meet diagnostic criteria (Non-ME chronic fatigue-Sd) but cannot be explained otherwise; (c) cases totally or partially explained by other diseases known to cause chronic fatigue (disease-associated CFS; or ME/CFS of combined aetiology).

Box 9. Diagnostic categories and sub-grouping.

Symptom description

Prolonged fatigue: persistent profound fatigue or lack of energy, usually (but not necessarily) accompanied by other symptoms; should be present for at least one month

Chronic fatigue (CF): persistent fatigue or lack of energy, that leads to reduced activity levels lasting over 3–6 months*. This may be explained by a condition other than ME/CFS (e.g., cancer-related fatigue) or unexplained ("idiopathic chronic fatigue"). It does not require other symptoms that are typically found in ME/CFS

Post-infectious fatigue or post-viral illness (PIF or PVI): new onset symptom complex including persistent profound fatigue with exercise intolerance following an infectious trigger and which is not otherwise explained by a diagnosed condition or lifestyle. It is usually accompanied by at least 2 further symptoms** from: post-exertional malaise, unrefreshing or poor sleep quality, cognitive or autonomic symptoms for at least 3 months (i.e., this is a subset, where the viral aetiology is clear, of patients with chronic fatigue).

Diagnostic categories

- *ME or ME/CFS:* persistent fatigue or lack of energy that leads to reduced activity levels lasting over 3–6 months, when diagnostic criteria according to IOM or Canadian Consensus criteria (CCC) are fully met for adults, and CCC or Rowe's criteria are fully met in children.
- *ME/PVFS (ME/Post-viral fatigue syndrome or post-infectious fatigue syndrome, post-infectious ME/CFS):* As for ME/CFS, when symptoms follow a presumed or confirmed infection (e.g., post-COVID-19 fatigue syndrome, post-mononucleosis fatigue syndrome, post-Lyme ME/CFS) (NB. This does not preclude there being triggers other than infections involved in the origins of the illness in other cases)
- *Non-ME chronic fatigue:* chronic fatigue cases that do not fulfil the diagnostic criteria for ME/CFS, lasting for at least 3–6 months, but are attributable to other underlying causes.
- *ME/CFS of combined aetiology:* when symptoms are attributed to a combination of ME/CFS and other known disease(s), e.g., ME/CFS and diabetes type 2 (NB. This is not in itself a diagnosis, which requires identification of the disease(s) to which the condition is attributable).

Examples of stratification categories:

- Age-group (e.g., children, adolescents, adults, elderly), gender
- Illness onset: acute or gradual; post-infection, following other triggers, e.g., environment exposure
- Presence of co-morbidities, e.g., fibromyalgia, hypermobility, mild mood disorders
- Phase of disease (or disease duration), e.g., early, established, and complicated disease (Nacul et al., 2020) [7]
- Severity (based on symptoms score or measures of function); a broad categorisation of severe/non-severe is based on being virtually house-bound or able to regularly be outside home. Very severe cases are virtually bed-bound.
- Clinical phenotype: based on predominance of symptoms by type (e.g., based on CCC symptoms sub-groups); e.g., neuro-cognitive, immune, sleep phenotypes (NB. There are distinct clinical phenotypes in ME/CFS which can be identified from gene expression data [47,48]). One study identified seven genomically derived subtypes of ME/CFS which manifested distinct phenotypes [49,50].
- Molecular phenotype: i.e., based on well-defined profiles based on results of specialised investigations, e.g., metabolic, immunological.

* CCC 2003 [2], IOM 2015 [6], and Rowe et al., 2017 [4], criteria require 6 months of symptoms; experienced clinicians should be able to diagnose adults with 3 months of symptoms. For children, CCC criteria requires 3 months [2], and Rowe et al., 2017 [4], require 3 months in post-infectious cases. ** The 2 additional symptoms criterion is not required when the fatigue symptoms can be clearly linked to the triggering infection and are not explained by other pathologies.

3.7. Recommendations for Health Care provision

Primary care professionals have an important role in the initial diagnosis, including consideration of alternative conditions leading to similar symptoms. It is important to note that many symptoms commonly reported in ME/CFS have a low disease-specificity and may occur in a number of diseases. Acute infectious onset and PEM should always prompt to consider ME/CFS. Although diagnostic confirmation may require a 3- to 6-month period, it is important to contemplate the diagnosis at earlier stages, so that disease management may start, and diagnosis and treatment of alternative diseases are not delayed (See Box 7).

Careful medical history, including social and occupational history and circumstances associated with the start of symptoms and subsequent progress will give significant clues on diagnosis. Information should be obtained on current and previous treatments, including prescribed and over the counter medicines and supplements as well as self-management strategies and alternative therapies. It is important to check for medications potentially leading to fatigue as well as autonomic-related and other symptoms. Physical examination and routine bloods tests are required to increase diagnostic accuracy and detect alternative conditions explaining the symptoms [51].

Patients with ME/CFS tend to be multi-symptomatic and often have long clinical histories, which may include various failed attempts to obtain a diagnosis and treatment. Multiple previous investigations are not uncommon; however, often, symptoms presented are discarded by clinicians as "exaggerated" or "imagined", related to excessive work or studies or as mood-related. Such a scenario is to be avoided through early recognition and diagnosis, which are reliant on better knowledge of the disease and education of doctors and other health professionals.

When a diagnosis is suspected in primary care, regular reviews are warranted, when the possibility of alternative diagnoses is explored at the same time as initial management, strategies are put in place. In such cases, it may be helpful to ask the patient to record their symptoms and other health parameters using standard instruments in advance of follow-up consultations (see Core Assessments, Box 8).

Education of patients in advance of, during, and following consultation may be useful, and reliable educational materials should be recommended, e.g., booklets, videos, or other online information materials. These should cover concepts and practical recommendations for "pacing" (pacing is a self-management tool to implement a strategy designed to help people live within their energy envelope, minimise PEM, and improve quality of life [52]) with adequate rest periods or breaks in activity, sleep hygiene, and pain management strategies. Both mental and physical activities should be taken in such a way to avoid over-exertion, which may trigger post-exertional aggravation of symptoms or "crashes", and as a key strategy to optimise chances of recovery. A main goal of educational activities is to empower the patient for self-management and to be in control of their disease and healing process.

3.8. Criteria for Referral for Specialist Services

Although with good education of primary care physicians, diagnosis and monitoring of people with ME/CFS in primary care are possible and desirable, and referral for specialist services may be indicated in some circumstances (Box 10), viz. for confirmation of diagnosis, when there is doubt; for cases who may benefit from a multi-disciplinary team with specific expertise, including drug treatments or care of those with severe or complicated disease; and for a range of service offerings, such as occupational therapy, supportive counselling, education on self-management and energy/activity management with "pacing", social services, and advice on access to community support, e.g., for educational, occupational, and social matters, such as benefits (see below on secondary services). Patients with more recent disease onset, such as those with less than 1–2 years of symptoms and the young (children, adolescents, and young adults) may also benefit from referral for initiation of multicomponent therapy, as early referral at this age might especially affect long-term prognosis. The more severely affected, including those who are house- or bedbound and severely disabled, should also be priority for referral, especially where appropriate home-visits or telemedicine are available, and, when necessary, for occupational, educational, and disability support. Note that some cases may be best served by referral to alternative services, especially where ME/CFS or Complex Chronic Diseases (CCD) Services are not well developed, such as to pain management, rehabilitation, neurology, psychiatry, and rheumatology services.

Box 10. Examples of criteria for referral to secondary services caring from people with ME/CFS.

Diagnosis confirmation
Young people
Severe cases or significant disability, especially if local support is limited
Short duration of symptoms (less than 1 or 2 years)
Rapid deterioration of symptoms
Complex diseases, where diagnosis and treatment are challenging
Inability to provide adequate care in the community or when management and treatment are only available at specialist services

3.9. The Continuing Role of Primary Care and the General Practitioner

In general, irrespective of referral to secondary care, whenever possible, the primary care team should continue to take responsibility for the long-term care and monitoring of patients with ME/CFS and their treatment, whenever possible in partnership with the specialist team. This includes facilitating the provision of emotional, social care, and occupational health support, and medical advice to teachers, employers, and caregivers, in response to the specific needs of patients. This could involve access to resources in the community, such as to physiotherapy, occupational therapy, dietician, or home visits by the primary care team (especially for the more severely affected), e.g., by district nurses. Support for self-management, education, and work activities may require further contacts with the patients and their carers/families, as well as with educators and employers. Here, online educational materials may be of value, as well as group educational activities for patients. Organization of care for people with ME/CFS and in particular the severely affected may be complex and requires communication by primary care professionals with others from various disciplines.

The primary care provider will still have major responsibilities for searching for alternative diagnoses where relevant and dictated by clinical judgement, for dealing with co-morbidities, the onset of new co-morbidities, and other diseases that may be not directly related to the diagnosis of ME/CFS, and for referring to different specialists as appropriate. Pharmacological and non-pharmacological approaches to treatment and clinical progress should be reviewed. It is important to consider that patients with ME/CFS may be more sensitive to a range of medications; this also needs to be considered when treating other conditions, having in mind also the possibility of drug interactions.

Needless to say, the strength of primary and secondary care services in particular settings will be relevant to determine roles at each care level and the best ways of cooperation between services at different levels. We appreciate limitations of access and service provision in primary care in many places, and local solutions will need to be found in line with local needs and resources. Virtual healthcare or virtual support from the specialist to the primary care team may have an important role.

4. The ME/CFS Specialist Consultation

4.1. Preparing for the Consultation and the Waiting Room

Before specialist consultation, it may be helpful to obtain relevant information, using standardised questionnaires or data/information otherwise obtained that may help with diagnostic confirmation, characterization of symptoms and their severity, and life impact. Forms may also be used as baseline clinical information for monitoring disease progress and response to management or treatment. These can be completed before consultation.

Standard questionnaires include the UKMEB Symptoms Assessment Questionnaire (SAQ) [53], to aid diagnosis and the Participant Phenotyping Questionnaire (PPQ), for severity profiling [54] or the DePaul Symptom Questionnaire, allowing diagnosis and symptom severity profiling [6]. The Impact on function and quality of life may be measured by standard instruments, such as Rand-36 [55,56], some of which have been validated in many languages. The Epworth Sleepiness Scale [57] can be used to assess excess daytime sleepiness and as a screening for obstructive sleep apnoea. Other instruments may be used to screen for mood disorders, e.g., neuroQOL [58] or HADS [59] for depression and anxiety or GAD-7 [60] for anxiety. Fatigue severity may be measured by instruments validated for ME/CFS, e.g., the fatigue severity scale [61]; visual scales such as pain and fatigue analogue scales are simple to use [62,63]. The same applies to sleep disorders (e.g., the Pittsburgh Sleep Quality Index [64]), and autonomic symptoms (e.g., Compass 31 [65]). A diagnosis of fibromyalgia may be established with a good degree of confidence by the annotation of pain symptomatology in pictorial representation of the human body [66]. The same is true for the evaluation of hypermobility syndromes, using the Beighton criteria [35].

4.2. Diagnosis Confirmation and Continued Search for Alternative Diagnoses and Co-Morbidities

The list of differential diagnoses of fatigue is exhaustive. Examples are listed in Box 7. Some conditions are often present concomitantly to ME/CFS (co-morbidities). Other conditions may potentially exclude a diagnosis if they may fully or mainly explain the symptoms. However, such conditions may also be co-morbid when their presence does not explain most of the symptoms and signs observed.

For diagnosis confirmation, we recommend the use of the CCC in both adults and children [2]. Additional tools for adults include The IOM criteria [6] and for children the paediatric "Diagnostic Work Sheet" [4] and/or the DSQ-PED [5]. Full consideration needs to be given to differential diagnosis and co-morbidities, and the need for detailed history, physical examination, and complementary tests, as appropriate, cannot be overestimated. Further tests may be recommended in secondary care settings, according to the need for supporting ME/CFS diagnosis and/or severity, and for differential diagnosis. Box 8 lists some assessments that may be considered. Those marked are suggested to be run routinely at the first assessment, and the others should be evaluated on a case-by-case basis, based on the clinical presentation. RAST tests for specific allergies, echocardiography, and serology for specific infectious diseases, as guided by clinical and epidemiological information, are other modalities that may be considered as appropriate.

Treatment for children and young people should usually be started by a paediatrician or a ME/CFS secondary care specialist centre that includes a paediatrician.

Further referral may be required when alternative diagnoses are suspected. This may include referral to a neurology or multiple sclerosis (MS) clinic and/or to specialists in ophthalmology, ENT, immunology (autoimmunity, immune dysfunction), allergology, orthopaedics, physical therapy, infectious diseases (travel-related disease), psychiatry, or gastroenterology.

4.3. Management and Treatment

In the absence of disease-specific treatment, key roles of the health professional include confirming the diagnosis, explaining to the patient the importance of avoiding overexertion and mental stress, "pacing", and symptomatic medication as needed and appropriate for the patient. Regular monitoring is important, when progress should be assessed, and the possible development of new diagnoses and co-morbidities considered, as the management plan is reviewed. "Pacing" refers to breaking up physical or mental activities with periods of rest, before a significant level of tiredness or exacerbation of symptoms is achieved or is expected following exertion, e.g., PEM, which may manifest many hours after the effort. A general rule of thumb is the recommendation to keep the activity at 2/3 of the duration and of the intensity that is expected (based on previous experience) to cause post-exertional symptoms, though flexibility should be exercised in order to reflect the particular needs and circumstances of individual patients.

The goal of the management/treatment programme is to treat the most distressing symptoms (sleep disturbance, pain, orthostatic intolerance, or others) and empower the patients to be in control of symptoms and the disease by encouraging them to trust their own experiences and enhance their awareness of the activities and environments in which they can cope without exacerbating symptoms, and "pace" themselves accordingly. The program should aim at optimizing the patient's ability to maintain function in everyday activities, being as active as possible within their boundaries and then gently extending those boundaries [2]. This may be challenging, especially in the more severely affected who may be able to tolerate only very low levels of activity; those with less severe forms of disease are likely to "overdo" and may have frequent exacerbations of symptoms ("crashes") as a consequence.

Recent studies suggest that there may be a role for cognitive behaviour therapy (CBT) in the management of ME/CFS. It may have long-term benefits in chronic fatigue [67], but there is little evidence of this, and it needs to be used with considerable care to avoid distress [68]. It should be appreciated that it is a supportive therapy and not curative [69].

Wearables can assist objective measurement of activity and sleep patterns, and in some cases heart rate variability [70]. They may be combined with a symptom diary, which will help the interpretation of symptoms and management.

4.4. Professional-Patient Partnership, Self-Management, and Support

It is important to establish a supportive and collaborative relationship with the patient suffering from ME/CFS and, as appropriate, with their caregivers. Engagement with the family may be essential, especially for children and young people, and for people with severe ME/CFS. A named healthcare specialist should be involved for coordinating care for the person with ME/CFS. Information to people at all disease stages should be according to the person's circumstances, including clinical, personal, and social factors. Information should be available in a variety of formats as appropriate (printed materials, electronic videos, and audios).

The doctor-patient partnership, informed choices and risk minimisation are essential components of care. Partnership between patient and health care providers should be based on trust, and consideration of their interactions as encounters between two experts with different, but complementary backgrounds (the patient and the healthcare provider), who recognise that knowledge about the disease and its management is incomplete. Basic management principles should apply, but often different treatments may be attempted (preferably one at a time, on a trial-and-error basis) and reassessed according to response or potential adverse effects. This is when the strength of the partnership becomes even more important, as partners engage in a journey where uncertainty is gradually replaced by increasing understanding of the disease/health process, as treatment and management strategies are regularly reviewed and adapted to suit patient characteristics and preferences. Over-investigation and over-treatment are discouraged, but a very passive approach to illness may also be counterproductive, and such discouragement should not result in patients being denied treatment or testing needed to monitor changes in their condition.

4.5. Managing Patients' Expectations

It is essential that the professional is upfront in explaining the current limits of treatment and understanding of potential pathophysiology and the approach to symptom management. This will greatly address discrepancies between patients' and doctors' expectations and set up the conditions for an open and positive patient-doctor relationship where patients are empowered to make informed choices.

There is no known pharmacological treatment or cure for ME/CFS. However, symptoms should be managed as in usual clinical practice. Physicians may consider starting symptomatic treatment at a lower than usual dose, due to frequent medication sensitivities in this population. The dose may be carefully increased. Treatment and repeat prescription may be continued in primary care, depending on the patient's preference and local circumstances.

4.6. Non-Pharmacological Treatment for Symptoms Relief and Available Support Therapies

Recommendations considered appropriate are shown in Box 11. It is important that these are provided by practitioners with experience in ME/CFS.

Box 11. Recommendations for a non-pharmacological approach to the relief of ME/CFS symptoms.

Pain
- Relaxation
- Meditation/mindfulness
- Manual methods (e.g., physiotherapy, acupuncture, and acupressure)

Sleep
- Sleep hygiene
- Relaxation strategies

Autonomic dysfunction, e.g., POTS
- Stockings
- Increase in water intake (>2 litres/day) or rehydration solutions, drinking frequently
- Increase in salt intake
- Sleep with feet in higher position (a few centimetres higher, increasing very slowly each night, up to what is tolerated)

Diet
- Healthy and balanced diet
- Anti-inflammatory diet
- Reduce ingestion of simple carbohydrates
- Adequate fluid intake
- Adequate ingestion of protein
- Increase unsaturated fatty acids and omega-3 fatty acids
- May try exclusion diets with support from dietician, especially for food with reported intolerances by the patient. It may be worth trying to avoid gluten, lactose, or fructose during a few weeks to test if there is any improvement in symptoms [71].

Support measures
- "Pacing" and activity management to work with the "energy envelope" [72]
- Supporting therapies that could help with coping and adapting to changes in life due to symptoms, within the "energy envelope", and counselling or psychotherapy
- Occupational therapy provided by professionals with experience in ME/CFS patients
- Social workers who could help with social welfare
- Educational needs: welfare and educational sectors should be involved in the planning and care for affected patients, particularly children, adolescents, and young adults

---

A professional view on symptom management and relief

"Periods of rest and "pacing" are important components of all management strategies for ME/CFS patients. Physicians should advise people with ME/CFS on the role of adequate rest, how to introduce breaks into their daily routine, and their frequency and length which may be appropriate for each patient. Excessive rest may be counterproductive, except in the initial stages of disease, in the very severe cases, or in cases of acute exacerbation; so it is important to introduce 'low level' physical and cognitive activities within the patient's capacity, according to the severity of symptoms.
Sleep management is tailored to the individual, the role and effect of disordered sleep is explained, common changes in sleep dysfunction that may exacerbate fatigue symptoms are identified; common manifestations include insomnia, hypersomnia, sleep reversal, altered sleep-awake cycle and non-refreshing sleep. The professional provides general advice on good sleep hygiene and encourages gradual changes in sleep pattern, though of course there is no implication that poor sleep hygiene is the cause of non-refreshing sleep.
Relaxation techniques appropriate for ME/CFS should be offered for the management of pain, sleep problems and comorbid stress or anxiety. Examples include guided visualisation and breathing techniques, which can be incorporated into daily routines and rest periods", while mindfulness ma be of value as a sympathetic nervous system modulator. Although exclusion diets are not generally recommended for managing ME/CFS, many people find them helpful for some symptoms, including bowel symptoms. The patient may attempt an exclusion diet or dietary manipulation under professional guidance and supervision, e.g., from a dietitian. For those with nausea, advice includes eating small portions and snacking on dry starchy food and sipping fluids. The use of anti-emetic drugs should be considered if the nausea is severe." Dr. L. Lorusso (personal communication)

4.7. Symptoms Relief and Management Using Available Pharmacological Drugs

Treatment of pain and sleep dysfunction are key, as they may have an indirect impact on other symptoms. Options for the pharmacological treatment of fatigue, including mental fatigue are more restricted. A balance between benefits and side effects, and significant individual variability in treatment response, call for individualised treatment. Costs are also a consideration, especially in settings where patients pay for medications out of pocket or where there are restrictions in prescribing medications.

Evidence of the effects of various drugs or supplements is scarce and often based on their use for related conditions or on reported use in ME/CFS and clinicians experience. It is important to observe legislations in different countries and to ensure that prescription of any drugs not specifically approved or licensed for ME/CFS is discussed with the patient and an informed choice is made. In some settings, it may be appropriate to obtain formal signed consent from the patient before introduction of a drug that has not been approved for use in ME/CFS. Regulations on supplements and over the counter medications are usually much less strict, but again, use by patients should be based on informed decision. Finally, it is important to note that many patients have already been taking a range of medications and supplements before reaching the ME/CFS specialist; again, in these cases, it is important to discuss continuation or otherwise with the patient; evidence of benefit on the individual patient, costs, potential side effects, or interactions with other medicines are important considerations. Some examples of pharmacological drugs that could be considered, where appropriate, are listed in Box 12. The use of medications that may address multiple symptoms may be considered.

4.8. Following the Consultation and Clinical Monitoring

Regular follow-ups are opportunities for education, including on self-management, assessment of usefulness of medications and other treatments and side-effects. Follow-up should include monitoring of symptoms, using similar instruments to those used at or before the initial consultation. Examples of instruments that may be used in monitoring patients include hand grip strength measurement, standing test, serum CK, severity assessment using specific instruments or scales (such as analogue scales for pain, fatigue, sleep, and other symptoms), and specific questionnaires for assessing symptom severity.

4.9. Needs of Patients with Different Severities

People who have severe ME/CFS may be unable to carry out activities of daily living and may spend a significant proportion, or all, of the day in bed. The symptoms experienced by patients with severe ME/CFS are diverse and debilitating, and these may fluctuate and change, both in type and in severity. It is therefore important that the management and care plan is flexible and reviewed regularly. People may have severe ME/CFS for years, and recovery is uncertain. Health services need to be prepared to attend to the specific needs of the severely affected, including home visits or virtual health consultations.

5. Concluding Remarks and Recommendations for Developing and Organising ME/CFS Services

The following are general recommendations for fully implemented services, but we appreciate that they are not achievable in the short term in many places, especially where knowledge and training in the field are limited or other resources are scarce. We encourage countries and regions to plan for their services, training, and educational needs according to the specific needs and characteristics of their population and patients and their organizational structures and resources. A national champion for each country or regions within countries would be highly desirable, especially in places with no or very scarce provision of services for ME/CFS.

Box 12. Examples of pharmacological approaches for relieving/managing ME/CFS symptoms*.

Pain
- Paracetamol
- NSAID (for short periods, e.g., up to 7 days)
- Gabapentin or pregabalin
- Tricyclics, such as amitriptyline
- Low dose naltrexone
- Duloxetine
- Venlafaxine

Sleep
- Tricyclics, e.g., amitriptyline
- Trazodone
- Melatonin
- Doxepin low dose
- Diphenhydramine
- Promethazine
- Benzodiazepines and Z-drugs (for short periods only)
- Gabapentin/pregabalin

Autonomic dysfunction, e.g., POTS
- Fludrocortisone
- SSRI
- Midodrine
- Ivabradine
- Pyridostigmine

Anti-allergic/anti-inflammatory
- Antihistamines, e.g., fexofenadine or famotidine
- Sodium cromoglicate

Supplements which may be tried for symptoms such as fatigue or cognitive dysfunction
- Iron (if ferritin < 50 ug/l, transferrin saturation <20%)
- Vitamin D
- L-carnitine or acetyl-carnitine
- CoQ-10 or MitoQ
- NADH
- Vitamin B12.
- α-lipoic acid
- Magnesium
- Omega-3 or omega-3/omega-6 combination
- D-Ribose
- Vitamin B1, B2, and/or B6
- Vitamin C

* Refer to local guidelines on the use of medications that are not specifically licensed for use in ME/CFS.

For fully functioning services, we recommend 2–4 ME/CFS specialist doctors/1 million population, with a supporting multi-disciplinary team, to include professionals such as nurses, nurse practitioners, occupational therapists, psychologists, dieticians, social workers, etc.; these would staff outpatient services for diagnosis and follow up. The specialist may be a doctor with expertise in ME/CFS. Internists, neurologists, immunologists, rheumatologists, infectious diseases specialists, and general practitioners are particularly suited for this role, but it may be done by doctors of any specialty, as long as they have the right expertise or training. For children, this role is to be filled by paediatricians. At the time of writing, we are not aware of any specific programme for the training of doctors to become specialists in ME/CFS, something that has often occurred informally so far. The training and provision of services in secondary care should be aligned with the training of primary care physicians to manage cases in the community. We recognize that the above target is ambitious, considering the current capacity and status of service provision in the continent. They should be seen as tentative and should not replace the assessment of patients' needs and structure and capacity of services at local and national levels.

The current reality of health services suggests that, where specialist services are not well developed, we follow a minimum standard of care for those with ME/CFS that may rely on virtual health and app-technology as well as on a strong partnership with primary care.

The minimum desirable is one ME/CFS centre providing specialist services for a 10 million population. These services should also consider the characteristics of the population, including ethnic and cultural diversity. Furthermore, we recommend that the specialist services should have the primary aim of confirming diagnosis and setting up treatment/management plans, which should be agreed upon and carried out by a multidisciplinary team. The follow-up could use multi-media approaches, such as remote consultations or telemedicine, as appropriate according to local circumstances and medical regulations. Local care for people with significant disability may need to be provided by primary care teams or local doctors with knowledge about ME/CFS, with support from the specialist services as appropriate. The option of smaller satellite clinics linked to the specialist service would provide full assistance for most and the "eyes" of a competent health professional, in support of remote consultations from the specialist for complex cases.

There is no suggestion that people with ME/CFS require more social support than people with other chronic diseases, and we are most certainly not implying that the disease is primarily psychological in nature. We are, though, very well aware that people with other chronic diseases, such as for example diabetes or multiple sclerosis, do not have the same problems of disbelief and lack of legitimisation experienced by people with ME/CFS. All people with chronic diseases need, and should be entitled to, social support, but few experience the same difficulty accessing it as people with ME/CFS.

Finally, it is important to consider that addressing the substantial needs of people with ME/CFS requires a multi-sectoral approach (Box 13), as well as ensuring that health services are organised and delivered effectively. Much of the needs of people affected by ME/CFS arise from their reduced ability to function in society and in more extreme cases on their total dependence on care for basic needs. Work, life, and education may be disrupted, with substantial economic and personal impacts on individuals and their families; lack of understanding and support, and often stigma, adding to the burden of physical suffering from symptoms. It is extremely important to prioritize research and education of health professionals and others in society, so as to address the scientific and societal poor understanding of the scale of the problem faced.

Box 13. Multi-sectoral approach to ME/CFS.

Specific societal sectors
Higher education:
• Development of training for under-graduates and post-graduates, including training for primary care staff and occupational physicians
Educational sector:
• Development of materials for teachers and education staff, as well as for pupils with ME/CFS and their parents
Work and pensions:
• Development of adequate instruments for assessing disability and flexibility in workplaces, particularly after returning to work, to minimise the risk of relapse
Health sector and public health:
• Adoption of guidelines, flexibility on the use of medications for management of symptoms
• Public health strategy for raising awareness about stigma, importance of care and education to avoid aggravation of symptoms and/or relapse
• ME/CFS services development and evaluation
Funding agencies and pharmaceutical industry:
• Research funding and support for well-designed clinical trials

Author Contributions: Conceptualisation—L.N., F.J.A., R.C.W.V. and E.M.L.; methodology—L.N., F.J.A., R.C.W.V., and E.M.L.; validation— L.N., F.J.A., C.S., L.L., I.B.H., J.A.M., C.A.S., A.M.M., O.P., U.B., H.N., P.G., S.S., N.S., F.E.-L., P.Z., D.F.H.P., J.C.-M., G.K.S., E.C., I.B., J.C., A.K., J.B., M.M., R.C.W.V. and E.M.L.; formal analysis—not applicable; investigation— L.N., F.J.A., C.S., L.L., I.B.H., J.A.M., C.A.S., A.M.M., O.P., U.B., H.N., P.G., S.S., N.S., F.E.-L., P.Z., D.F.H.P., J.C.-M., G.K.S., E.C., I.B., J.C., A.K., J.B., M.M., R.C.W.V. and E.M.L.; resources—not applicable; writing—original draft preparation— L.N., F.J.A., C.S., L.L., I.B.H., J.A.M., C.A.S., A.M.M., O.P., U.B., H.N., P.G., S.S., N.S., F.E.-L., P.Z., D.F.H.P., J.C.-M., G.K.S., E.C., I.B., J.C., A.K., J.B., M.M., R.C.W.V. and E.M.L.; writing—review and editing— L.N., F.J.A., C.S., L.L., I.B.H., J.A.M., C.A.S., A.M.M., O.P., U.B., H.N., P.G., S.S., N.S., F.E.-L., P.Z., D.F.H.P., J.C.-M., G.K.S., E.C., I.B., J.C., A.K., J.B., M.M., R.C.W.V. and E.M.L.; visualization—not applicable; project administration—L.N., F.J.A., R.C.W.V., and E.M.L. All authors have read and agreed to the published version of the manuscript.

Funding: This research received no external funding. EUROMENE receives funding for networking activities from the COST programme (COST Action 15111), via the COST Association.

Institutional Review Board Statement: Not applicable.

Informed Consent Statement: Not applicable. The manuscript does include patient-related data or samples.

Data Availability Statement: No new data were created or analysed in this study. Data sharing is not applicable to this article.

Acknowledgments: The Latvian Council of Sciences is supporting the project No lzp-2019/1-0380 "Selection of bi-omarkers in ME/CFS for patient stratification and treatment surveillance/optimisation". The Open Medicine Foundation is supporting the ME centre in Uppsala in projects to identify diagnostic and prognostic biomarkers relevant for the clinical care of ME patients (and other related diseases).

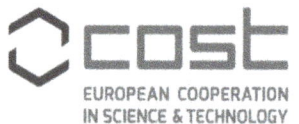
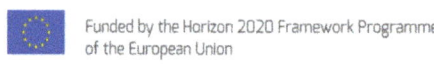

This article/publication is based upon work from the COST Action "European network on Myalgic Encephalomyelitis/Chronic Fatigue Syndrome", EUROMENE, supported by COST (European Cooperation in Science and Technology). COST (European Cooperation in Science and Technology) is a funding agency for research and innovation networks. Its actions help connect research initiatives across Europe and enable scientists to grow their ideas by sharing them with their peers. This boosts their research, careers, and innovation. www.cost.eu.

Conflicts of Interest: CS has a clinical study grant and speaker honoraria from Takeda and Fresenius and is consultant for Celltrend. RV is consultant for Alfasigma SpA Bologna Italy. JAM has collaborated with Vitae, Pharmanord, Vinas Laboratories, in research on coenzyme Q10, NADH, selenium, and melatonin and has a patent with Grifols Laboratories for the use of alpha-1-antiprypsin in CFS. LN has been a Committee Member, UK NICE guidelines on ME/CFS 2021. JC-M has received research support and honoraria from VITAE Health Innovation, PharmaNord, Viñas Laboratories on treatments of Coenzyme Q10 plus NADH, selenium, and melatonin plus zinc in people with ME/CFS from Spain. All other authors declare no conflicts of interest.

References

1. EUROMENE. Available online: https://www.cost.eu/actions/CA15111/#tabs\T1\textbar{}Name:overview (accessed on 14 May 2021).
2. Strand, E.B.; Nacul, L.; Mengshoel, A.M.; Helland, I.B.; Grabowski, P.; Krumina, A.; Alegre-Martin, J.; Efrim-Budisteanu, M.; Sekulic, S.; Pheby, D.; et al. Myalgic encephalomyelitis/chronic fatigue Syndrome (ME/CFS): Investigating care practices pointed out to disparities in diagnosis and treatment across European Union. *PLoS ONE* **2019**, *14*, e0225995. [CrossRef]
3. Carruthers, B.; Jain, A.K.; de Meirleir, K.L.; Peterson, D.L.; Klimas, N.G.; Lerner, A.M.; Bested, A.C.; Flor-Henry, P.; Joshi, P.; Powles, A.P.; et al. Myalgic encephalomyelitis/chronic fatigue syndrome: Clinical working case definition, diagnostic and treatment protocols. *J. Chronic Fatigue Syndr.* **2003**, *11*, 7–115. [CrossRef]

4. Carruthers, B.M.; van de Sande, M.I.; De Meirleir, K.L.; Klimas, N.G.; Broderick, G.; Mitchell, T.; Staines, D.; Powles, A.C.; Speight, N.; Vallings, R.; et al. Myalgic encephalomyelitis: International Consensus Criteria. *J. Intern. Med.* **2011**, *270*, 327–338. [CrossRef]
5. Rowe, P.C.; Underhill, R.A.; Friedman, K.J.; Gurwitt, A.; Medow, M.S.; Schwartz, M.S.; Speight, N.; Stewart, J.M.; Vallings, R.; Rowe, K.S. Myalgic Encephalomyelitis/Chronic Fatigue Syndrome Diagnosis and Management in Young People: A Primer. *Front. Pediatr.* **2017**, *5*, 121. [CrossRef] [PubMed]
6. Jason, L.A.; Sunnquist, M. The Development of the DePaul Symptom Questionnaire: Original, Expanded, Brief, and Pediatric Versions. *Front. Pediatr.* **2018**, *6*, 330. [CrossRef]
7. Institute of Medicine (IOM). *Beyond Myalgic Encephalomyelitis/Chronic Fatigue Syndrome: Redefining an Illness*; The National Academies Press: Washington, DC, USA, 2015.
8. Nacul, L.; O'Boyle, S.; Palla, L.; Nacul, F.E.; Mudie, K.; Kingdon, C.C.; Cliff, J.M.; Clark, T.G.; Dockrell, H.M.; Lacerda, E.M. How Myalgic Encephalomyelitis/Chronic Fatigue Syndrome (ME/CFS) Progresses: The Natural History of ME/CFS. *Front. Neurol.* **2020**, *11*, 826. [CrossRef] [PubMed]
9. Roberts, E.; Wessely, S.; Chalder, T.; Chang, C.-K.; Hotopf, M. Mortality of people with chronic fatigue syndrome: A retrospective cohort study in England and Wales from the South London and Maudsley NHS Foundation Trust Biomedical Research Centre (SLaM BRC) Clinical Record Interactive Search (CRIS) Register. *Lancet* **2016**, *387*, 1638–1643. [CrossRef]
10. Smith, W.R.; Noonan, C.; Buchwald, D. Mortality in a cohort of chronically fatigued patients. *Psychol. Med.* **2006**, *36*, 1301–1306. [CrossRef]
11. McManimen, S.L.; Devendorf, A.R.; Brown, A.A.; Moore, B.C.; Moore, J.H.; Jason, L.A. Mortality in patients with myalgic encephalomyelitis and chronic fatigue syndrome. *Fatigue Biomed. Health Behav.* **2016**, *4*, 195–207. [CrossRef] [PubMed]
12. Nacul, L.C.; Lacerda, E.M.; Pheby, D.; Campion, P.; Molokhia, M.; Fayyaz, S.; Leite, J.C.; Poland, F.; Howe, A.; Drachler, M.L. Prevalence of myalgic encephalomyelitis/chronic fatigue syndrome (ME/CFS) in three regions of England: A repeated cross-sectional study in primary care. *BMC Med.* **2011**, *9*, 91. [CrossRef] [PubMed]
13. Estevez-Lopez, F.; Castro-Marrero, J.; Wang, X.; Bakken, I.J.; Ivanovs, A.; Nacul, L.; Sepulveda, N.; Strand, E.B.; Pheby, D.; Alegre, J.; et al. Prevalence and incidence of myalgic encephalomyelitis/chronic fatigue syndrome in Europe-the Euro-epiME study from the European network EUROMENE: A protocol for a systematic review. *BMJ Open* **2018**, *8*, e020817. [CrossRef] [PubMed]
14. Valdez, A.R.; Hancock, E.E.; Adebayo, S.; Kiernicki, D.J.; Proskauer, D.; Attewell, J.R.; Bateman, L.; Demaria, A., Jr.; Lapp, C.W.; Rowe, P.C.; et al. Estimating Prevalence, Demographics, and Costs of ME/CFS Using Large Scale Medical Claims Data and Machine Learning. *Front. Pediatr.* **2019**, *6*, 412. [CrossRef] [PubMed]
15. Bakken, I.J.; Tveito, K.; Gunnes, N. Two age peaks in the incidence of chronic fatigue syndrome/myalgic encephalomyelitis: A population-based registry study from Norway 2008–2012. *BMC Med.* **2014**, *12*, 167.
16. Kingdon, C.C.; Bowman, E.W.; Curran, H.; Nacul, L.; Lacerda, E.M. Functional Status and Well-Being in People with Myalgic Encephalomyelitis/Chronic Fatigue Syndrome Compared with People with Multiple Sclerosis and Healthy Controls. *Pharm. Open* **2018**, *2*, 381–392. [CrossRef]
17. Nacul, L.C.; Lacerda, E.M.; Campion, P.; Pheby, D.; de L Drachler, M.; Leite, J.C.; Poland, F.; Howe, A.; Fayyaz, S. The functional status and well being of people with myalgic encephalomyelitis/chronic fatigue syndrome and their carers. *BMC Public Health* **2011**, *11*, 402. [CrossRef]
18. Kennedy, G.; Underwood, C.; Belch, J.J. Physical and functional impact of chronic fatigue syndrome/myalgic encephalomyelitis in childhood. *Pediatrics* **2010**, *125*, e1324–e1330. [CrossRef]
19. Jason, L.A.; Benton, M.C.; Valentine, L.; Johnson, A.; Torres-Harding, S. The economic impact of ME/CFS: Individual and societal costs. *Dyn. Med.* **2008**, *7*, 6. [CrossRef]
20. Lloyd, A.R.; Pender, H. The economic impact of chronic fatigue syndrome. *Med. J. Aust.* **1992**, *157*, 599–601. [CrossRef]
21. Hunter, R.M.; James, M.; Paxman, J. *Counting the Cost—Chronic Fatigue Syndrome/Myalgic Encephalomyelitis*; 2020health, The Optimum Health Clinic Foundation: London, UK, 2017.
22. Pheby, D.F.; Araja, D.; Berkis, U.; Brenna, E.; Cullinan, J.; De Korwin, J.D.; Gitto, L.; Hughes, D.A.; Hunter, R.M.; Trepel, D.; et al. The Development of a Consistent Europe-Wide Approach to Investigating the Economic Impact of Myalgic Encephalomyelitis (ME/CFS): A Report from the European Network on ME/CFS (EUROMENE). *Healthcare* **2020**, *8*, 88. [CrossRef]
23. Castro-Marrero, J.; Faro, M.; Zaragoza, M.C.; Aliste, L.; de Sevilla, T.F.; Alegre, J. Unemployment and work disability in individuals with chronic fatigue syndrome/myalgic encephalomyelitis: A community-based cross-sectional study from Spain. *BMC Public Health* **2019**, *19*, 840. [CrossRef]
24. Lacerda, E.M.; Mcdermott, C.; Kingdon, C.C.; Butterworth, J.; Cliff, J.M.; Nacul, L. Hope, disappointment and perseverance: Reflections of people with Myalgic encephalomyelitis/Chronic Fatigue Syndrome (ME/CFS) and Multiple Sclerosis participating in biomedical research: A qualitative focus group study. *Health Expect.* **2019**, *22*, 373–384. [CrossRef] [PubMed]
25. Bhatia, S.; Olczyk, N.; Jason, L.A.; Alegre, J.; Fuentes-Llanos, J.; Castro-Marrero, J. A Cross-National Comparison of Myalgic Encephalomyelitis and Chronic Fatigue Syndrome at Tertiary Care Settings from the US and Spain. *Am. J. Soc. Sci. Humanit.* **2019**, *5*, 104–115. [CrossRef]
26. Mudie, K.; Esteves-Lopez, F.; Sekulik, S.; Ivanovs, A.; Sepulveda, N.; Zalewsky, P.; Mengshoel, A.M.; de Korwin, J.; Hinic Capo, N.; Alegre-Martin, J.; et al. Recommendations for Epidemiological Research in ME/CFS from the EUROMENE Epidemiology Working Group. *Preprints* **2020**, 2020090744. [CrossRef]

27. Fukuda, K.; Straus, S.E.; Hickie, I.; Sharpe, M.C.; Dobbins, J.G.; Komaroff, A. The chronic fatigue syndrome: A comprehensive approach to its definition and study. International Chronic Fatigue Syndrome Study Group. *Ann. Intern. Med.* **1994**, *121*, 953–959. [CrossRef]
28. Friedberg, F.; Batemen, L.; Bested, A.C.; Davenport, T.; Friedman, K.J.; Gurwitt, A.; Jason, L.A.; Lapp, C.W.; Stevens, S.R.; Underhill, R.A.; et al. *ME/CFS: A Primer for Clinical Practitioners*; IACFS/ME: International Association for Chronic Fatigue Syndrome/Myalgic Encephalomyelitis: Chicago, IL, USA, 2012.
29. Editorial. What's in a name? Systemic exertion intolerance disease. *Lancet* **2015**, *385*, 663, (21 February 2015). Available online: www.thelancet.com (accessed on 5 May 2021). [CrossRef]
30. Jason, L.A.; Jordan, K.; Miike, T.; Bell, D.S.; Lapp, C.; Torres-Harding, S.; Rowe, K.; Gurwitt, A.; de Meirleir, K.; van Hoof, E.L.S. A Pediatric Case Definition for Myalgic Encephalomyelitis and Chronic Fatigue Syndrome. *J. Chronic Fatigue Syndr.* **2006**, *13*, 1–44. [CrossRef]
31. Faro, M.; Sáez-Francàs, N.; Castro-Marrero, J.; Aliste, L.; Collado, A.; Alegre, J. Impacto de la fibromialgia en el síndrome de fatiga crónica. *Med. Clín.* **2014**, *142*, 519–525. [CrossRef]
32. Ferrari, R.; Russell, A.S. A Questionnaire Using the Modified 2010 American College of Rheumatology Criteria for Fibromyalgia: Specificity and Sensitivity in Clinical Practice. *J. Rheumatol.* **2014**, *40*, 1590. [CrossRef] [PubMed]
33. Wolfe, F.; Clauw, D.J.; Fitzcharles, M.A.; Goldenberg, D.L.; Häuser, W.; Katz, R.L.; Mease, P.J.; Russell, A.S.; Russell, I.J.; Walitt, B. 2016 Revisions to the 2010/2011 fibromyalgia diagnostic criteria. *Semin. Arthritis Rheum.* **2016**, *46*, 319–329. [CrossRef]
34. Lapp, C.W. Initiating Care of a Patient with Myalgic Encephalomyelitis/Chronic Fatigue Syndrome (ME/CFS). *Front. Pediatr.* **2019**, *6*, 415. [CrossRef]
35. Beighton, P.; Solomon, L.; Soskolne, C.L. Articular mobility in an African population. *Ann. Rheum. Dis.* **1973**, *32*, 413–418. [CrossRef] [PubMed]
36. Bragée, B.; Michos, A.; Drum, B.; Fahlgren, M.; Szulkin, R.; Bertilson, B.C. Signs of Intracranial Hypertension, Hypermobility, and Craniocervical Obstructions in Patients with Myalgic Encephalomyelitis/Chronic Fatigue Syndrome. *Front. Neurol.* **2020**, *11*. [CrossRef] [PubMed]
37. Nacul, L.C.; Mudie, K.; Kingdon, C.C.; Clark, T.G.; Lacerda, E.M. Hand Grip Strength as a Clinical Biomarker for ME/CFS and Disease Severity. *Front. Neurol.* **2018**, *9*, 992. [CrossRef] [PubMed]
38. Hickie, I.; Davenport, T.; Vernon, S.D.; Nisenbaum, R.; Reeves, W.C.; Hadzi-Pavlovic, D.; Lloyd, A. Are chronic fatigue and chronic fatigue syndrome valid clinical entities across countries and health-care settings? *Aust. N. Z. J. Psychiatry* **2009**, *43*, 25–35. [CrossRef]
39. Boda, W.L.; Natelson, B.H.; Sisto, S.A.; Tapp, W.N. Gait abnormalities in chronic fatigue syndrome. *J. Neurol. Sci.* **1995**, *131*, 156–161. [CrossRef]
40. Twisk, F. The status of and future research into Myalgic Encephalomyelitis and Chronic Fatigue Syndrome: The need of accurate diagnosis, objective assessment, and acknowledging biological and clinical subgroups. *Front. Physiol.* **2014**, *5*, 109. [CrossRef] [PubMed]
41. Nacul, L.; De Barros, B.; Kingdon, C.C.; Cliff, J.M.; Clark, T.G.; Mudie, K.; Dockrell, H.M.; Lacerda, E.M. Evidence of Clinical Pathology Abnormalities in People with Myalgic Encephalomyelitis/Chronic Fatigue Syndrome (ME/CFS) from an Analytic Cross-Sectional Study. *Diagnostics* **2019**, *9*, 41. [CrossRef]
42. Tomas, C.; Finkelmeyer, A.; Hodgson, T.; Maclachlan, L.; Macgowan, G.A.; Blamire, A.M.; Newton, J.L. Elevated brain natriuretic peptide levels in chronic fatigue syndrome associate with cardiac dysfunction: A case control study. *Open Heart* **2017**, *4*, e000697. [CrossRef]
43. Guenther, S.; Loebel, M.; Mooslechner, A.A.; Knops, M.; Hanitsch, L.G.; Grabowski, P.; Wittke, K.; Meisel, C.; Unterwalder, N.; Volk, H.D.; et al. Frequent IgG subclass and mannose binding lectin deficiency in patients with chronic fatigue syndrome. *Hum. Immunol.* **2015**, *76*, 729–735. [CrossRef]
44. National Institute of Neurological Disorders and Stroke (NINDS). Myalgic Encephalomyelitis/Chronic Fatigue Syndrome. 2018. Available online: https://www.commondataelements.ninds.nih.gov/Myalgic%20Encephalomyelitis/Chronic%20Fatigue%20Syndrome#pane-166 (accessed on 11 April 2021).
45. Rowe, K.S. Long Term Follow up of Young People with Chronic Fatigue Syndrome Attending a Pediatric Outpatient Service. *Front. Pediatr.* **2019**, *7*, 21. [CrossRef]
46. Williams, M.V.; Cox, B.; Lafuse, W.P.; Ariza, M.E. Epstein-Barr Virus dUTPase Induces Neuroinflammatory Mediators: Implications for Myalgic Encephalomyelitis/Chronic Fatigue Syndrome. *Clin. Ther.* **2019**, *41*, 848–863. [CrossRef]
47. Shimosako, N.; Kerr, J.R. Use of single-nucleotide polymorphisms (SNPs) to distinguish gene expression subtypes of chronic fatigue syndrome/myalgic encephalomyelitis (CFS/ME). *J. Clin. Pathol.* **2014**, *67*, 1078–1083. [CrossRef] [PubMed]
48. Zhang, L.; Gough, J.; Christmas, D.; Mattey, D.L.; Richards, S.C.; Main, J.; Kerr, J.R. Microbial infections in eight genomic subtypes of chronic fatigue syndrome/myalgic encephalomyelitis. *J. Clin. Pathol.* **2010**, *63*, 156–164. [CrossRef]
49. Kerr, J.R.; Petty, R.; Burke, B.; Gough, J.; Fear, D.; Sinclair, L.I.; Mattey, D.L.; Richards, S.C.M.; Montgomery, J.; Baldwin, D.A.; et al. Gene expression subtypes in patients with chronic fatigue syndrome/myalgic encephalomyelitis. *J. Infect. Dis.* **2008**, *197*, 1171–1184. [CrossRef] [PubMed]

50. Kerr, J.R.; Burke, B.; Petty, R.; Gough, J.; Fear, D.; Mattey, D.L.; Axford, J.S.; Dalgleish, A.G.; Nutt, D.J. Seven genomic subtypes of chronic fatigue syndrome/myalgic encephalomyelitis: A detailed analysis of gene networks and clinical phenotypes. *J. Clin. Pathol.* **2008**, *61*, 730–739. [CrossRef] [PubMed]
51. Hives, L.; Bradley, A.; Richards, J.; Sutton, C.; Selfe, J.; Basu, B.; Maguire, K.; Sumner, G.; Gaber, T.; Mukherjee, A.; et al. Can physical assessment techniques aid diagnosis in people with chronic fatigue syndrome/myalgic encephalomyelitis? A diagnostic accuracy study. *BMJ Open* **2017**, *7*, e017521. [CrossRef]
52. EMERGE Australia. Pacing. Available online: https://www.emerge.org.au/Handlers/Download.ashx?IDMF=2a2287ee-b84d-428f-b72e-00da812ddd7c (accessed on 6 May 2021).
53. CureME. Samples and Data. Available online: https://cureme.lshtm.ac.uk/researchers/431-2 (accessed on 6 May 2021).
54. Lacerda, E.M.; Bowman, E.W.; Cliff, J.M.; Kingdon, C.C.; King, E.C.; Lee, J.S.; Clark, T.G.; Dockrell, H.M.; Riley, E.M.; Curran, H.; et al. The UK ME/CFS Biobank for biomedical research on Myalgic Encephalomyelitis/Chronic Fatigue Syndrome (ME/CFS) and Multiple Sclerosis. *Open J. Bioresour.* **2017**, *4*, 91. [CrossRef]
55. Hays, R.D.; Sherbourne, C.D.; Mazel, R.M. The RAND 36-Item Health Survey 1.0. *Health Econ.* **1993**, *2*, 217–227. [CrossRef]
56. Varni, J.W.; Seid, M.; Kurtin, P.S. PedsQL™ 4.0: Reliability and Validity of the Pediatric Quality of Life Inventory™ Version 4.0 Generic Core Scales in Healthy and Patient Populations. *Med. Care* **2001**, *39*, 800–812. [CrossRef]
57. Johns, M.W. A new method for measuring daytime sleepiness: The Epworth sleepiness scale. *Sleep* **1991**, *14*, 540–545. [CrossRef]
58. Northwestern University. Health Measures. 2020. Available online: https://www.healthmeasures.net/explore-measurement-systems/neuro-qol (accessed on 11 April 2021).
59. Zigmond, A.S.; Snaith, R.P. The Hospital Anxiety and Depression Scale. *Acta Psychiatr. Scand.* **1983**, *67*, 361–370. [CrossRef] [PubMed]
60. Spitzer, R.L.; Kroenke, K.; Williams, J.B.; Löwe, B. A brief measure for assessing generalized anxiety disorder: The GAD-7. *Arch. Intern. Med.* **2006**, *166*, 1092–1097. [CrossRef] [PubMed]
61. Krupp, L.B.; Larocca, N.G.; Muir-Nash, J.; Steinberg, A.D. The fatigue severity scale. Application to patients with multiple sclerosis and systemic lupus erythematosus. *Arch. Neurol.* **1989**, *46*, 1121–1123. [CrossRef]
62. Huskisson, E.C. Measurement of pain. *Lancet* **1974**, *2*, 1127–1131. [CrossRef]
63. Tseng, B.Y.; Gajewski, B.J.; Kluding, P.M. Reliability, responsiveness, and validity of the visual analog fatigue scale to measure exertion fatigue in people with chronic stroke: A preliminary study. *Stroke Res. Treat.* **2010**, 412964. [CrossRef] [PubMed]
64. Buysse, D.J.; Reynolds, C.F.; Monk, T.H.; Berman, S.R.; Kupfer, D.J. The Pittsburgh Sleep Quality Index: A new instrument for psychiatric practice and research. *Psychiatry Res.* **1989**, *28*, 193–213. [CrossRef]
65. Sletten, D.M.; Suarez, G.A.; Low, P.A.; Mandrekar, J.; Singer, W. COMPASS 31: A refined and abbreviated Composite Autonomic Symptom Score. *Mayo Clin. Proc.* **2012**, *87*, 1196–1201. [CrossRef]
66. Wolfe, F.; Clauw, D.J.; FitzCharles, M.; Goldenberger, D.; Häuser, W.; Katz, R.S.; Russell, I.J.; Mease, P.J. 2016 Revisions to the 2010/2011 Fibromyalgia Diagnostic Criteria. Abstract Number: 997. American College of Rheumatology/Association of Rheumatology Professionals Annual Meeting 2016, Washington DC, USA. Available online: https://acrabstracts.org/abstract/2016-revisions-to-the-20102011-fibromyalgia-diagnostic-criteria/ (accessed on 16 May 2021).
67. Andersson, G.; Rozental, A.; Shafran, R.; Carlbring, P. Long-term effects of internet-supported cognitive behaviour therapy. *Expert Rev. Neurother.* **2018**, *18*, 21–28. [CrossRef]
68. Geraghty, K.J.; Blease, C. Cognitive behavioural therapy in the treatment of chronic fatigue syndrome: A narrative review on efficacy and informed consent. *J. Health Psychol.* **2018**, *23*, 127–138. [CrossRef]
69. Vink, M.; Vink-Niese, A. The draft updated NICE guidance for ME/CFS highlights the unreliability of subjective outcome measures in non-blinded trials. *J. Health Psychol.* **2021**, 1359105321990810. [CrossRef]
70. Escorihuela, R.M.; Capdevila, L.; Castro, J.R.; Zaragozà, N.C.; Maurel, S.; Alegre, J.; Castro-Marrero, J. Reduced heart rate variability predicts fatigue severity in individuals with Chronic Fatigue Syndrome/Myalgic Encephalomyelitis. *J. Transl. Med.* **2020**, *18*, 4. [CrossRef] [PubMed]
71. Haß, U.; Herpich, C.; Norman, K. Anti-Inflammatory Diets and Fatigue. *Nutrients* **2019**, *11*, 2315. [CrossRef] [PubMed]
72. Jason, L.; Muldowney, K.; Torres-Harding, S. The Energy Envelope Theory and myalgic encephalomyelitis/chronic fatigue syndrome. *AAOHN J. Off. J. Am. Assoc. Occup. Health Nurses* **2008**, *56*, 189–195.

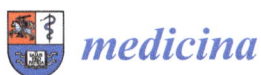

Review

Systematic Review of Mind-Body Interventions to Treat Myalgic Encephalomyelitis/Chronic Fatigue Syndrome

Samaneh Khanpour Ardestani [1], Mohammad Karkhaneh [2], Eleanor Stein [3], Salima Punja [1], Daniela R. Junqueira [1], Tatiana Kuzmyn [4], Michelle Pearson [5], Laurie Smith [6], Karin Olson [7] and Sunita Vohra [8,*]

1. Department of Pediatrics, Faculty of Medicine & Dentistry, University of Alberta, Edmonton, AB T6G 1C9, Canada; khanpour@ualberta.ca (S.K.A.); punja@ualberta.ca (S.P.); junqueir@ualberta.ca (D.R.J.)
2. Institute of Health Economics, Edmonton, AB T6X 0E1, Canada; mk4@ualberta.ca
3. Department of Psychiatry, Faculty of Medicine, University of Calgary, Calgary, AB T2T4L8, Canada; espc@eleanorsteinmd.ca
4. Patient Research Partner, Retired RN, Patient and Community Engagement Research (PaCER) Program Graduate, University of Calgary, Calgary, AB T2P 1B2, Canada; tkuzmyn@telus.net
5. Patient Research Partner, MAPC, CEO Wunjo IS, Calgary, AB T3K 4N8, Canada; michelle@wunjo-is.com
6. Patient Research Partner, Calgary, AB 95060, Canada; lauriem.smith@gmail.com
7. Faculty of Nursing, University of Alberta, Edmonton, AB T6G 1C9, Canada; karin.olson@ualberta.ca
8. Departments of Pediatrics and Psychiatry, Faculty of Medicine & Dentistry, University of Alberta, Edmonton, AB T6G 1C9, Canada
* Correspondence: svohra@ualberta.ca; Tel.: +1-780-492-6445

Abstract: *Background and Objectives*: Myalgic Encephalomyelitis/Chronic Fatigue Syndrome (ME/CFS) is a chronic condition distinguished by disabling fatigue associated with post-exertional malaise, as well as changes to sleep, autonomic functioning, and cognition. Mind-body interventions (MBIs) utilize the ongoing interaction between the mind and body to improve health and wellbeing. *Purpose*: To systematically review studies using MBIs for the treatment of ME/CFS symptoms. *Materials and Methods*: MEDLINE, EMBASE, CINAHL, PsycINFO, and Cochrane CENTRAL were searched (inception to September 2020). Interventional studies on adults diagnosed with ME/CFS, using one of the MBIs in comparison with any placebo, standard of care treatment or waitlist control, and measuring outcomes relevant to the signs and symptoms of ME/CFS and quality of life were assessed for inclusion. Characteristics and findings of the included studies were summarized using a descriptive approach. *Results*: 12 out of 382 retrieved references were included. Seven studies were randomized controlled trials (RCTs) with one including three reports (1 RCT, 2 single-arms); others were single-arm trials. Interventions included mindfulness-based stress reduction, mindfulness-based cognitive therapy, relaxation, Qigong, cognitive-behavioral stress management, acceptance and commitment therapy and isometric yoga. The outcomes measured most often were fatigue severity, anxiety/depression, and quality of life. Fatigue severity and symptoms of anxiety/depression were improved in nine and eight studies respectively, and three studies found that MBIs improved quality of life. *Conclusions*: Fatigue severity, anxiety/depression and physical and mental functioning were shown to be improved in patients receiving MBIs. However, small sample sizes, heterogeneous diagnostic criteria, and a high risk of bias may challenge this result. Further research using standardized outcomes would help advance the field.

Keywords: myalgic encephalomyelitis/chronic fatigue syndrome; mind-body interventions; systematic review; adults

Citation: Khanpour Ardestani, S.; Karkhaneh, M.; Stein, E.; Punja, S.; Junqueira, D.R.; Kuzmyn, T.; Pearson, M.; Smith, L.; Olson, K.; Vohra, S. Systematic Review of Mind-Body Interventions to Treat Myalgic Encephalomyelitis/Chronic Fatigue Syndrome. *Medicina* 2021, 57, 652. https://doi.org/10.3390/medicina57070652

Academic Editor: Derek F. H. Pheby

Received: 11 May 2021
Accepted: 17 June 2021
Published: 24 June 2021

Publisher's Note: MDPI stays neutral with regard to jurisdictional claims in published maps and institutional affiliations.

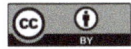

Copyright: © 2021 by the authors. Licensee MDPI, Basel, Switzerland. This article is an open access article distributed under the terms and conditions of the Creative Commons Attribution (CC BY) license (https://creativecommons.org/licenses/by/4.0/).

1. Introduction

Myalgic encephalomyelitis/chronic fatigue syndrome (ME/CFS) is a chronic condition distinguished by disabling fatigue associated with multiple symptoms including post-exertional malaise, orthostatic intolerance, pain, sleep problems, and impaired cognitive and immune functions [1]. While the true prevalence is unknown, Johnston et al., estimated the pooled prevalence of ME/CFS to be 3.28% and 0.76% according to self-reporting and clinical assessment, respectively [2]. In Canada, 1.4% of people older than 12 years old [3] suffer from ME/CFS. Patients report post-exertional malaise (69–100%), muscle pain (63–95%), impaired memory or concentration (88%), non-restorative sleep (87%), joint pain (55–85%), and sore throat (62%) [1,4]. Health-related quality of life in ME/CFS patients is consistently reported as significantly lower than otherwise healthy populations with regards to physical and mental health, self-care, and ability to perform usual activities [5,6]. Not surprisingly, ME/CFS reduces patients' abilities to carry out normal working activities leading to higher unemployment rates [7]. It is estimated that annual household and labor force productivity of ME/CFS patients are decreased by 37% and 54%, respectively, costing an approximate annual loss of $9.1 billion in the United States (US) [8]. ME/CFS patients, their families and employers endure a high financial burden estimated to be between $18 to $51 billion annually in the US [9].

Despite extensive research, the etiology and pathophysiology of ME/CFS have not yet been fully understood. Disruptions in the autonomic nervous system, hypothalamic-pituitary-adrenocortical (HPA) axis, and immune system were shown in several studies [10,11]. Metabolic and mitochondrial dysfunction and abnormal gut microbiota were also shown to be interconnected with the above dysregulation [11]. A recent systematic review of neuroimaging studies showed inconsistent but widespread abnormalities in white matter, functional connectivity, and morphological changes of the autonomic nervous system [12].

With no specific etiology, there is no gold standard method to diagnose ME/CFS to date. A recent systematic review of diagnostic methods by Haney et al., identified nine case definitions [13]. Due to the lack of a biomarker, most of the case definitions require other competing diagnoses to be ruled out [14,15]. In the literature, the term myalgic encephalomyelitis (ME) [16] was used earlier than the term chronic fatigue syndrome (CFS) [17]. The Canadian case definition published in 2003 required post-exertional malaise as an essential symptom in these patients and recommended the umbrella term ME/CFS [18], used in this systematic review.

There is no cure for ME/CFS nor any FDA or Health Canada approved medication to treat it [14,19], therefore the focus tends to be on managing and minimizing the symptoms and improving quality of life. A variety of conventional and complementary therapies have been used to mitigate the symptoms of ME/CFS. As in other chronic conditions, long-term pharmacological interventions may have significant impacts on patients and their families in terms of adverse effects and financial burden [20,21]. Non-pharmacological options are of interest to patients as they may be less expensive and have fewer associated adverse effects.

Systematic reviews have shown low strength of evidence for the effectiveness of different complementary therapies [19], cognitive-behavioral therapy (CBT), counseling and behavioral therapies [14,22], and graded exercise therapy [23] for improvement of fatigue, physical functioning, sleep, and quality of life in patients with ME/CFS.

Mind-body approaches utilize the interactions between the brain, mind, and body, and behavior to improve health and wellbeing [24]. Using these interconnections strengthens self-awareness and self-care and helps to improve mood, quality of life, and increase one's ability to cope. Examples of mind-body therapy interventions (MBIs) include progressive muscle relaxation, guided imagery, hypnosis, meditation, mindfulness, Tai chi, yoga, and biofeedback. Newer approaches are using the brain's ability to change (i.e., neuroplasticity) associated with repeated, purposeful thoughts, feelings or behaviors [25]. The science behind how mind-body therapies work is expanding. It has been shown that the brain and body communicate in multiple directions using neurotransmitters/neuropeptides, hormones, and cytokines and MBIs may be influencing physical health by affecting these interactions [24,26].

Considering the complex nature of ME/CFS and the involvement of psycho-neuroendocrine and immune systems, these patients are an ideal population for evaluating MBIs. Furthermore, by enhancing self-knowledge and patients' abilities to work through their problems and reduce stress, MBIs may improve their quality of life and wellbeing [27].

Several MBIs such as mindfulness-based stress reduction (MBSR), mindfulness-based cognitive therapy (MBCT), yoga, and Qigong have been studied in ME/CFS patients, but to our knowledge, have not yet been included in any systematic review or meta-analysis. There are some promising results to improve anxiety, fatigue, depression, quality of life, and physical functioning [28–32] in ME/CFS. In this systematic review, we evaluated the effectiveness and safety of MBIs that were studied in individuals diagnosed with ME/CFS. The results of this review will inform the design and methodology of future randomized controlled trials.

Objectives

The objectives of this study were to systematically review studies of MBIs for the treatment of ME/CFS symptoms and to report any adverse events reported for these approaches in ME/CFS patients.

2. Materials and Methods

We followed the Preferred Reporting Items for Systematic Reviews and Meta-Analysis (PRISMA) guidelines [33]. The protocol of this systematic review was registered at PROSPERO (CRD42018085981).

2.1. Population, Intervention, Control, Outcome- Study Design (PICO-S)

The population of interest was adults ($\geq$18 years old) diagnosed or symptom-matched with one of the ME/CFS case definitions (Appendix A, Table A1). Patients with any other conditions were included in this review, as long as they were diagnosed with ME/CFS. Interventions of interest included any of the MBIs listed in Table 1 and any placebo, the standard of care treatment or waiting list as a control group. To be eligible for inclusion, multiple-arm interventional studies were also required to have at least one of the control groups mentioned above.

All outcomes relevant to the signs and symptoms of ME/CFS and quality of life were considered. The outcomes included fatigue, sleep refreshment, pain, anxiety (stress, nervousness, etc.), depression (mood, hopefulness, and helplessness), quality of life, performance (physical, mental, emotional), work-related outcomes (employment, income, etc.), and physical health symptoms such as sore throat, tender lymph nodes, and muscle weakness (Table 1).

Study designs eligible for inclusion were parallel/cross-over/N-of-1 randomized controlled trials (RCTs), controlled clinical trials (CCTs), single-arm experimental (within subject control group), controlled before and after studies, or cohort studies.

2.2. Search Methods

Five electronic databases (MEDLINE, EMBASE, CINAHL, PsycINFO, and Cochrane Register of Controlled Trials (CENTRAL)) were searched from inception to September 2020. Search terms were based on those presented in Table 1; an example is found in Appendix B. No limitation was implemented in terms of publication dates. English language restriction was applied. The reference lists of included studies, and systematic reviews, were reviewed to identify additional studies.

Table 1. Criteria for selecting studies.

Population	Patients with a diagnosis of CFS, ME, and ME/CFS including: Patients who were previously treated Patients who are previously untreated Adults ($\geq$18 years)
Interventions	Mind-body interventions (alone or in combination) including: Art Therapy Autogenic training Biofeedback/neurofeedback Breathing exercise Cognitive restructuring Dynamic Neural Retraining System Emotional Freedom Techniques (EFT) Eye movement desensitization and reprocessing (EMDR) Guided imagery Hypnotherapy/self-hypnosis Meditation (mindfulness, mantra, guided, transcendental) Mindfulness-based cognitive therapy (MBCT) Mindfulness-based Stress Reduction (MBSR) Music therapy Neurolinguistic programming Prayer/spirituality Psychological flexibility Qigong Relaxation therapy (relaxation response, progressive muscle relaxation) Tai Chi Visualization Yoga
Comparators	One or more of the following control conditions including: Placebo Standard of care treatments Waitlist
Outcomes	Any single or combination of, but not limited to, the following outcomes: Fatigue (energy, motivation) Refreshing sleep Pain Anxiety (stress, nervousness, etc.,) Depression (mood, hopefulness, helplessness) Quality of life Performance (physical, mental, emotional) Work-related outcome (employment, income, etc.) Changes in physical health such as sore throat, tender lymph nodes, and muscle weakness
Study Design	Parallel/Cross-over randomized controlled trials (RCTs) Controlled clinical trials (CCTs) Controlled before and after studies Single-arm interventional studies (within subject control group) Cohort
Other	English language

2.3. Selection of Studies

Two review authors (MK, DJ) independently screened all the titles and abstracts retrieved from the search in order to identify those that may meet the inclusion criteria. They classified studies as being relevant, possibly relevant and irrelevant. Three reviewers (MK, DJ, SKA) independently assessed the full texts of all relevant and possibly relevant studies to assess inclusion. Discrepancies were resolved by referring to a senior review author (ES, SV).

2.4. Data Collection

Standardized data extraction forms were used to extract data from full-text articles. Extracted data included general characteristics of the study (first author, publication year, country, settings, design), sample size, age and sex distribution in groups, diagnosis methods, type of MBI and other relevant data including frequency and duration, control (active or passive), primary outcome, secondary outcomes, primary and secondary measurement tools, length of study, follow up period, statistically significant outcomes, and adverse events reported. Data extraction was completed by one reviewer (DJ) and independently verified by a second reviewer (SKA). Disagreements between the authors were resolved by discussion until consensus was reached; if consensus could not be reached, a senior reviewer's opinion was sought.

2.5. Data Analysis

This systematic review was conducted to determine which outcomes and outcome measures were used in the studies of MBIs for the treatment of ME/CFS patients and whether the interventions were effective. General information of the included studies along with the statistically significant and insignificant outcomes were described. We present the findings of studies using different diagnostic criteria (e.g., Oxford criteria, CDC criteria) separately. We also report whether studies assessed adverse events, their absence or presence, and frequencies. A meta-analysis was not performed due to heterogeneous interventions and outcomes used in the included studies. Cochrane risk of bias assessment tool was used by two independent review authors (SKA, SP) to assess sequence generation, allocation concealment, blinding, incomplete outcome data, selective outcome reporting, and other sources of bias [34] in RCTs. Other study designs including single-arm experimental studies were also appraised by two independent reviewers (SKA, SP) for risk of bias using Cochrane Risk of Bias Assessment Tool for Non-Randomized Studies of Intervention (ACROBAT_NRSI) which was recently renamed ROBINS-I [35]. Domains for assessing the risk of bias in these studies include bias due to confounding, selection of participants, measurement of interventions, a departure from the intended intervention, missing data, measurement of outcomes, and selection of the reported result.

2.6. Patient Involvement

Patient engagement in health research can improve the quality, relevance and impact of the research [36,37]. To recruit patient research partners in this study, a "call for patient representative" letter was developed and distributed among patients, caregivers and advocates. Three patient partners were selected based on their educational background, personal experience, and health status to participate in the study team. They did not receive any financial compensation. They participated regularly in teleconference calls and skype meetings. They also provided feedback and participated in team discussions via email. They contributed to the protocol design, development of the literature search strategy, the condition/diagnosis definitions, and outcome selection.

3. Results

Our search results yielded 382 references. After removing duplicates, 270 were screened using title and abstracts, and 47 references were considered relevant for full-text screening. Considering the a priori inclusion criteria and obtaining additional clarifying information from authors of some of the references, twelve studies (17 reports) were ultimately included [10,28–30,38–45]. The flow of studies through the screening process of the review is shown in Figure 1. The excluded studies and the reasons for exclusion are shown in Table A2.

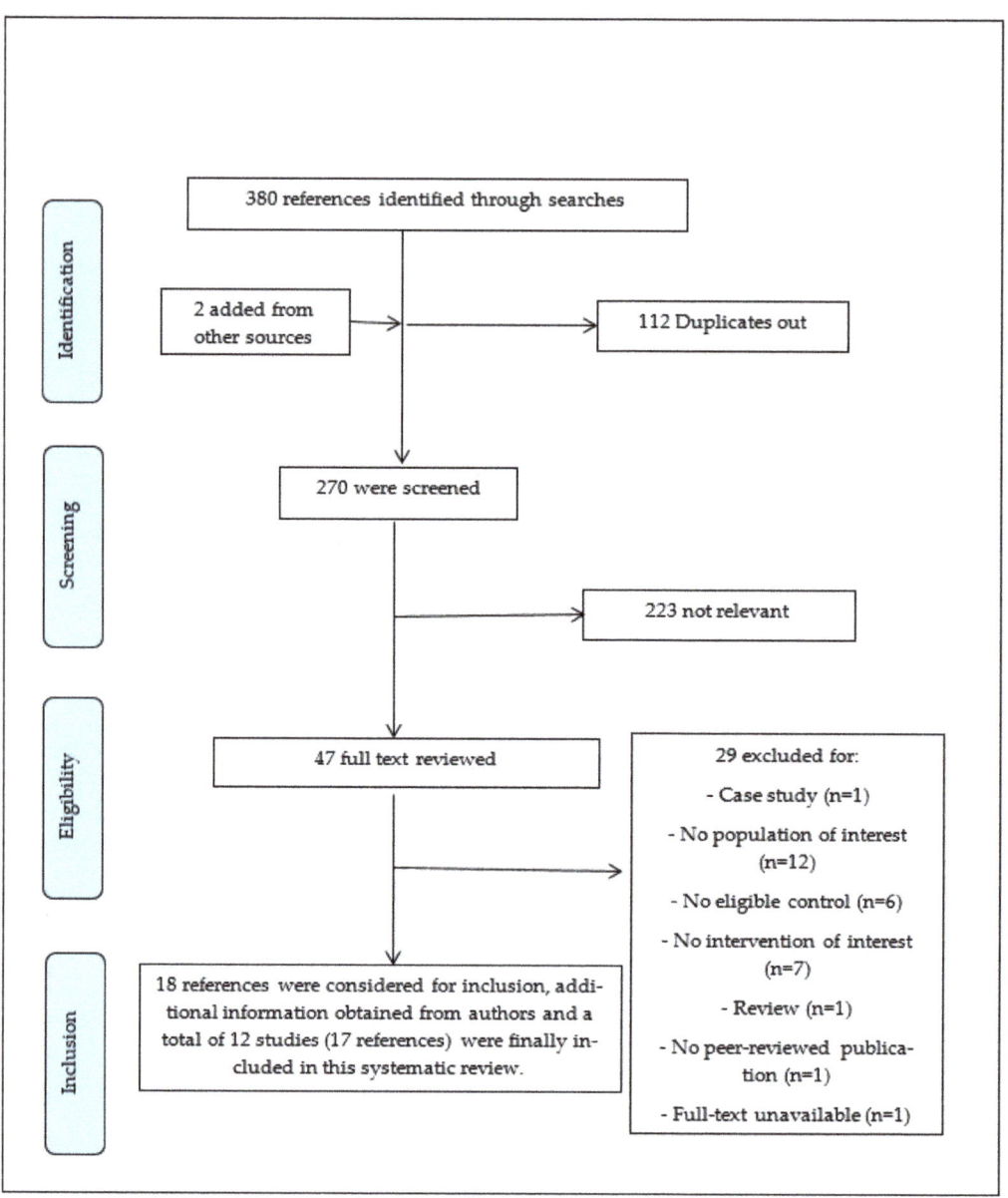

Figure 1. Adapted version of PRISMA flow diagram of study selection for the ME/CFS systematic review.

3.1. Characteristics of the Included Studies

Table 2 shows the characteristics of all the included studies.

Table 2. General characteristics of the included studies.

First Author, Year, Country	Setting	Design, Sample Size (Enrolled/Completed/Analyzed), Treatment Duration	Study Population (Diagnosis, Age, Gender)	Mind-Body Intervention, Frequency, Duration, Self-Practice	Control Group	Outcome, Measurement Tool and Validity
Surawy, Ch., 2005, UK [29]	Not reported	A series of exploratory studies: Study 1 Design: RCT, Sample size: Intervention: 9/9/9, Control: 9/8/8 Treatment duration: 8 weeks Study 2 Design: single-arm trial, Sample size: 12/9/9,Treatment duration: 8 weeks Study 3 Design: single-arm trial, Sample size: 11/9/9, Treatment duration: 8 weeks and a follow-up period of 3 months	Patients diagnosed with Oxford criteria [46] Study 1 Age range: 18–65 y/o, 56% female Study 2 Age range: 18–65 y/o, 75% female Study 3 Age range: 18–65 y/o, 64% female	MBSR/MBCT Frequency: Once a week, Duration: Not reported, Self-practice: Not reported	Study 1: Wait list Study 2: No control group Study 3: No control group	Study 1, 2, and 3 Anxiety and Depression: Hospital Anxiety and Depression Scale (HADS) [47] Fatigue Severity: Chalder's Fatigue Scale [48] Quality of Life: SF36 physical functioning [49] Study 2 and 3 Effect of fatigue on quality of life: Fatigue impact scale [50]
Thomas, M. 2006 and 2008, UK [39,51]	Outpatient clinics	Design: RCT, Sample size: Intervention (relaxation group): 14/14/14, Control: 9/9/9 Treatment duration: 10 weeks Follow-up: 6 months	Patients diagnosed with CFS by CDC diagnostic criteria for CFS [52] Age (mean ± SD): Intervention (relaxation): 45.7 ± 12.5, Control: 46.2 ± 11.04, Intervention (relaxation): 71.4% female, Control: 66.7% female	Relaxation therapy Frequency: Once a week, Duration: 1 h, Self-practice: Not reported	Standard medical care	Report 1 Illness history: Beck Depression Inventory [53] Centre for Epidemiological Studies-Depression Scale [54], Chalder Fatigue Scale [48], Cognitive Failures Questionnaire [55], Cohen–Hoberman Index of Physical Symptoms [56], Current State of Health [57], Fatigue Problem Rating Scale [58], Hospital Anxiety and Depression Scale [47], MOS SF-36 [49] Perceived Stress [56] Positive and Negative Affect [59], Profile of Fatigue Related Symptoms [60], Sleep Questionnaire [57], Symptom Check List [57] Mood testing: Alertness, hedonic tone and anxiety: measured using 18 computerized visual analogue mood scales Performance testing: Word recall, reaction time, vigilance tasks using a Viglen Dossier laptop computer connected to a simple 3-button response box [57] Report 2 Primary outcome: Functional performance: Karnofsky performance scale [61] Secondary outcome: Global measures of illness and satisfaction with treatment (including improvement and changes in fatigue and disability)

Table 2. Cont.

First Author, Year, Country	Setting	Design, Sample Size (Enrolled/Completed/Analyzed), Treatment Duration	Study Population (Diagnosis, Age, Gender)	Mind-Body Intervention, Frequency, Duration, Self-Practice	Control Group	Outcome, Measurement Tool and Validity
Bogaerts, K., 2007, Belgium [38]	University hospital clinic	Design: Single-arm trial, Sample size: 30/30/30 Treatment duration: Single time imagery trial	Patients diagnosed with CFS by CDC diagnostic criteria for CFS [52]	Relaxation imagery Frequency: once Duration: less than 5 min Self-practice: NA	No control group	Ventilatory measures: Pet CO_2 Subjective measures: Degree of fatigue, imagery vividness, concentration ability on the scripts and similarity of evoked feelings with daily life feelings: 9-point rating scale Positive and negative affectivity: Positive and Negative Affect Schedule (PANAS) [62] Hyperventilation complaints: Symptom checklist [63] Chronic fatigue acceptance: Acceptance Chronic Fatigue Test (ACFT) Tendency to worry: Penn-State Worry Questionnaire (PSWQ) [64] Valence, arousal and dominance: Self-assessment Manikin [65]
Lopez, C., 2011. USA [45]	Physician referrals, community	Design: RCT Sample size: 69/58/58 Treatment duration: 12 weeks	Patients diagnosed with CFS by CDC diagnostic criteria for CFS [52]. Age (mean ±SD): 45.9 ± 9.3 88.4% female	Cognitive-behavioral stress management Frequency: Weekly Duration: Two hours Self-practice: Workbook and relaxation tapes	Psychoeducation (half-day seminar)	Distress: Perceived Stress Scale (PSS) [66], Profile of Mood States (POMS) [67] Quality of life: Quality of Life Inventory (QOLI) [68] CFS symptoms: CDC Symptom Inventory for Chronic Fatigue Syndrome [69]
Chan, J., 2013, Hong Kong [41] (characteristics of Ho et al, 2012 [70] as the preliminary study and Li et al, 2015 [71] as the study conducted on a subset of participants suffering from bereavement are reported here as well)	Community	Design: RCT, Sample size: Ho, R., 2012 report: Intervention: 35*/27/33 Control group: 35**/25/31 Chan, J., 2013 (main report): Intervention: 77/53/72 ^ Control: 777/58/65 ^ Li, J., 2015, report: Intervention: 22/22/22 Control: 24/24/24 Treatment duration: 5 consecutive weeks training sessions + 12 weeks home-based qigong exercise (4 months in total) Li et al., however, reported their findings after three months of intervention.	Patients diagnosed with CFS by CDC diagnostic criteria for CFS [52] Age (mean ± SD), % female: Ho, R., 2012 report: Intervention: 42.1 ± 7.3, Control: 42.5 ± 5.5, Intervention: 75.8% female, Control: 83.9% female Chan, J., 2013 (main report): Intervention: 42.4 ± 6.7, Control: 42.5 ± 6.4, Intervention: 72.2% female, Control: 81.5% female Li, J., 2015, report: Patient with CFS had been bereaved within the previous 2 years. Age (median, range): Intervention: 46 (23–52), Control: 45 (32–51), Intervention: 86.4% female, Control: 87.5% female	Qigong exercise training (Wu Xing Ping Heng Gong), Frequency: twice a week, Duration: 2 h, Self-practice: 30 min, every day at home	Waitlist	Chan, J., 2013 (main report): Primary outcome: Fatigue severity: Chalder's Fatigue Scale [48,72] Secondary outcomes: Anxiety and Depression: Hospital Anxiety and Depression Scale (HADS) [47,73] Ho, R., 2012 report: In addition to fatigue severity, they measured Physical functioning and mental functioning: the Chinese version of the Medical Outcomes Study 12- Item Short-Form Health Survey [74,75] as their primary outcome and Telomerase Activity as their secondary outcome. Li, J., 2015, report: In addition to fatigue severity and anxiety and depression, they measured quality of life: Short form health survey (SF-12) [74,75] and Spiritual well-being: the "spirituality" subscale of the Body-Mind-Spirit Well-being Inventory (BMSWBE-S) [76]

Table 2. Cont.

First Author, Year, Country	Setting	Design, Sample Size (Enrolled/Completed/Analyzed), Treatment Duration	Study Population (Diagnosis, Age, Gender)	Mind-Body Intervention, Frequency, Duration, Self-Practice	Control Group	Outcome, Measurement Tool and Validity
Rimes, K., 2013, U.K. [30]	A specialist National Health Service CFS Unit	Design: RCT, Sample size: Intervention group: 19/19/19 18/16/16 Control group: 19/19/19 Treatment duration: Introductory session + 8 weeks Follow-up: at 2 months, and at 6 months for MBCT group only	Patients diagnosed with CFS by Fukuda et al. [52] criteria or Oxford criteria [46] Age (mean ± SD): Intervention: 41.4 ± 10.9, Control: 45.2 ± 9.4, Intervention:75% female, Control: 89.5% female	MBCT, Frequency: Once a week, Duration: 2.25 h, Self-practice: Home practice with the support of CDs.	Waitlist	Primary outcome: Fatigue: Chalder Fatigue Scale [48] Secondary outcomes: Impairment: The Work and Social Adjustment Scale [77] Physical Functioning: Physical Functioning (PF-10) scale) [78,79] Beliefs about Emotions: Beliefs about Emotions Scale [80] Self-Compassion: Self-Compassion Scale [81] Mindfulness: Five-Facet Mindfulness Questionnaire [82] Anxiety and Depression: Hospital Anxiety and Depression Scale (HADS) [47] All-or-Nothing Behaviour and Catastrophic Thinking about Fatigue: five-item subscale of the Cognitive and Behavior Responses to Symptoms Questionnaire (Moss-Morris and Chalder, in preparation; King's College London, UK) Acceptability and Engagement: Record of class attendance and amount of home practice undertaken
Chan, J., 2014 and 2017, Hong Kong [40,83]	Community	Design: RCT, Sample size: Report 1: Intervention: 75/57/75 Control: 75/58/75 Report 2: Intervention:46 Control: 62 Treatment duration: 9 consecutive weeks Follow-up: 3-month post-intervention.	Patients diagnosed with CFS by CDC diagnostic criteria for CFS [52] Report 1: Age (mean ± SD): Intervention: 39.1 ± 7.8, Control: 38.9 ± 8.1, Intervention: 61.3% female, Control: 82.7% female Report 2 Age (mean ± SD): 39 ± 7.9 All females	Qigong exercise: Baduanjin Qigong Frequency: 16 sessions, Duration: 1.5 h, Self-practice: 30 min, every day	Waitlist	Report 1 Primary outcomes: Sleep Quality: Pittsburgh Sleep Quality Index (PSQI) [84–86] Fatigue severity: Chalder Fatigue Scale (ChFS) [48,72] Anxiety and Depression: Hospital Anxiety and Depression Scale (HADS) [47,73] Secondary outcome: Dose-response relationship between Qigong exercise and improvements. Global Assessment, Satisfaction Report 2 Anxiety and Depression: Hospital Anxiety and Depression Scale (HADS) [47,73] Plasma Adiponectin Levels

Table 2. Cont.

First Author, Year, Country	Setting	Design, Sample Size (Enrolled/Completed/Analyzed), Treatment Duration	Study Population (Diagnosis, Age, Gender)	Mind-Body Intervention, Frequency, Duration, Self-Practice	Control Group	Outcome, Measurement Tool and Validity
Oka, T., 2014, Japan [28]	Outpatients with CFS who visited the Department of Psychosomatic Medicine of Kyushu University Hospital	Design: RCT, Sample size: Intervention: 15/15/15 Control: 15/15/15 Treatment duration: Two months	Patients diagnosed with CFS by CDC diagnostic criteria for CFS [52] Age (mean ±SD): Intervention:38.0 ±11.1, Control:39.1 ± 14.2, Intervention: 80% female, Control: 80% female	Isometric yoga Frequency: every two to three weeks, at least 4 times during the intervention period, Duration: 20 min, Self-practice: With the aid of a digital videodisk and booklet	Waitlist	Acute effects of isometric yoga on fatigue: The fatigue and vigor score of the Profile of Mood States (POMS) questionnaire [67] immediately after the final 20-min yoga session Chronic effects of isometric yoga on fatigue: Chalder's Fatigue Scale [48] Quality of Life: Medical Outcomes Study Short Form 8, standard version (SF-8) [87]
Sollie, K., 2017. Norway [43]	Community	Design: Single-arm trial Sample size: 10 Treatment duration: Eight weeks with three months follow-up	Patients diagnosed with CFS by Canada criteria [88] Age (mean ± SD):43.5 ± 9.9, 80% female	MBCT, Frequency: Weekly Duration: Two hours Self-practice: Homework with the aid of workbook and CD	No control group	Fatigue: Chalder Fatigue Scale [48] Symptom burden: Likert scale Anxiety and depression: Hospital Anxiety and Depression Scale (HADS) [47] Tendency to ruminate: Ruminative Response Scale [89] Dispositional mindfulness: Five Facet Mindfulness questionnaire [82] Quality of life: Satisfaction with Life Scale (SWLS) [90]
Oka, T., 2018 and 2019, Japan [42,91]	Outpatients with CFS who visited the Department of Psychosomatic Medicine of Kyushu University Hospital	Design: Single-arm trial Sample size: 15 Treatment duration: Eight weeks	Patients diagnosed with CFS by CDC diagnostic criteria for CFS [52], the 2011 international consensus criteria for myalgic encephalomyelitis [92] and the 2015 diagnostic criteria for systemic exertion intolerance disease [1] Age (mean ± SD): 38.0 ± 11.1 80% female	Sitting isometric yoga Frequency: Biweekly with a yoga instructor Duration: 20 min Self-practice: Daily in-home session	No control group	Report 1: Fatigue and vigor: The fatigue and vigor score of the Profile of Mood States (POMS) questionnaire [67] Autonomic nervous system (ANS) functions: Heart rate and Heart rate variability (HRV) Blood biomarkers: Serum cortisol, DHEA-S, TNF-α, IL-6, IFN-γ, PRL, total carnitine, free carnitine, and acylcarnitine, and plasma TGF-β1, BDNF, MHPG, and HVA Report 2: Fatigue severity: Chalder fatigue scale (FS) score [48] Levels of the blood biomarkers: Cortisol, DHEA-S, TNF-α, IL-6, prolactin, carnitine, TGF-β1, BDNF, MHPG, HVA, and α-MSH The autonomic nervous functions: Heart rate (HR) and HR variability Alexithymia: The 20-item Toronto Alexithymia Scale (TAS-20) [93] Anxiety and depression: Japanese version of the Hospital Anxiety and Depression Scale (HADS) [47]

Table 2. Cont.

First Author, Year, Country	Setting	Design, Sample Size (Enrolled/Completed/Analyzed), Treatment Duration	Study Population (Diagnosis, Age, Gender)	Mind-Body Intervention, Frequency, Duration, Self-Practice	Control Group	Outcome, Measurement Tool and Validity
Jonsjo, M., 2019, Sweden [44]	Tertiary specialist clinic	Design: Single-arm trial Sample size: 40/32/32 Treatment duration: 13 sessions with three- and six-month follow-up	Patients diagnosed with CFS according to CDC [52] and 2003 Canadian criteria for ME/CFS [88] Age (mean ± SD): 49.02 ± 10.78 76.7% female	Acceptance and commitment therapy Frequency: Weekly to biweekly depending on illness severity (13 sessions) Duration: 45 min Self-practice: Home assignments	No control group	Primary outcomes: Disability: The pain disability index [94] Psychological inflexibility: The Psychological Inflexibility in Fatigue Scale (PIFS) [95] Secondary outcomes: ME/CFS symptoms and severity: 5-point scale Fatigue: The Multidimensional Fatigue Inventory (MFI-20) [96] Anxiety and depression: The Hospital Anxiety and Depression Scale (HADS) [47] Dimensions of mental and physical health: SF-36 Health Survey [79] Health-related quality of life: EQ-5D-3L [97]
Takakura, S., 2019, Japan [10]	Outpatients with CFS who visited the Department of Psychosomatic Medicine of Kyushu University Hospital	Design: Single-arm trial Sample size: 9 Treatment duration: Three months	Patients diagnosed with CFS according to the 1994 Fukuda case definition of CFS [52], the 2011 International Consensus Criteria for ME [92], and the 2015 diagnostic criteria for systemic exertion intolerance disease [1] Age (mean ± SD): 37.2 ± 9.9 All female	Recumbent isometric yoga Frequency: Every two to four weeks Duration: 20–30 min depending on patient's preference Self-practice: In-home daily sessions	No control group	Fatigue: Japanese version of 11 item Chalder Fatigue Scale [98,99] Human microRNA

* 2 dropped out before the intervention ** 4 dropped out before the intervention ^ 5 dropped out before the intervention ^^ 12 dropped out before the intervention.

3.2. Design

Six studies were prospective RCTs with at least one eligible control group [28,30,39–41,45]. One manuscript presented a brief report of three studies in which one was a prospective RCT and the other two were single-arm experimental studies [29]. Five additional publications were also single-arm experimental studies [10,38,42–44].

3.3. Population

Participants were all adults diagnosed with ME/CFS (n = 564 total; sample size range n = 9–150). Six studies used the Center for Disease Control and Prevention (CDC) criteria for the diagnosis of their patients [28,39–41,45,51]. One study used the 2003 Canadian criteria [43]. One study used Oxford criteria [29], one study used both CDC and Oxford criteria [30] and three studies used a combination of CDC criteria with 2003 or 2005 versions of Canadian criteria and 2011 international consensus criteria [10,42,44].

The healthcare settings included outpatient settings [28,39], community [40,41,43,45], a university hospital clinic [38], department of psychosomatic medicine [10,42] and a specialist ME/CFS unit [30,44]. One study did not report the setting from which their patients were recruited [29].

Three studies were conducted in the United Kingdom [29,30,39], three in Japan [10,28,42], two were conducted in Hong Kong, China [40,41], and one each in Belgium [38], Norway, Sweden, and USA [43–45].

3.4. Intervention

A variety of different interventions were implemented in the included studies comprising mindfulness-based stress reduction/mindfulness-based cognitive therapy (MBSR/MBCT) [29], MBCT [30,43], relaxation therapy [39], relaxation imagery [38], Qigong exercise training [41], Baduanjin Qigong [40], and isometric yoga [28], seated isometric yoga [42], recumbent isometric yoga [10], acceptance and commitment therapy [44] and cognitive-behavioral stress management [45]. Treatment duration ranged between 5–12 weeks.

3.5. Comparison

Participants assigned to the control group were either placed on the waiting list [28–30,40,41] or received standard medical care [39]. They were advised to keep their usual lifestyle activities including seeking general medical care but not to participate in any activities similar to the intervention of interest.

3.6. Outcomes

Many different outcomes and outcome measures were reported in the included studies. Four studies clearly stated their primary and secondary outcomes/objectives [30,39–41]. Fatigue severity was measured by seven studies using Chalder fatigue scale [10,28–30,40,41,43]. One study (published as two reports), listed Chalder fatigue scale in one of the reports as the administered questionnaire [51]. In the other report, however, they measured fatigue using patient-rated Likert-type scales [39]. Other studies used either profile of mood state (POMS) [42,45] or multidimensional fatigue inventory (MFI-20) [44].

Eight studies measured anxiety and depression using the Hospital Anxiety and Depression Scale (HADS) [29,30,40,41,43,44,51,91]. Six studies measured quality of life or physical and/or mental functioning using different quality of life outcome measures [28–30,41,45,51]. Seven studies measured objective outcomes including ventilatory parameters [38], performance testing by computer programs [51], telomerase activity [70], autonomic nervous system functions, blood biomarkers [42,91], adiponectin levels [83], and microRNA changes [10]. Table 2 describes the details of these outcome measures and the other outcomes measured in the included studies.

3.7. Effects of Interventions

Due to heterogeneous interventions and outcome measures used in the included studies, a meta-analysis was not performed. The statistically significant outcomes reported by these studies are presented in Tables 3 and 4. Tables A3 and A4 show the statistically insignificant outcomes.

Table 3. Significant outcomes in the included studies using CDC, Canadian and international consensus criteria for diagnosing CFS.

Intervention Type	First Author, Year		Outcome (Assessed by)	Comparison Groups	Comparison Time Point	p-Value
Relaxation-based	Thomas, M., 2006 and 2008 [39,51]	Report 1 (2006)	Alertness (as part of a subjective mood scale)	Relaxation group (pre-post)	Post follow-up (6 months)	<0.027
			Anxiety (as part of a subjective mood scale)	Relaxation group (pre-post)	Post follow-up (6 months)	<0.002
			Current state of health (self-reporting scale)	Relaxation group (pre-post)	Post-treatment (10 weeks)	Reported significant (value not reported)
			Performance score-10% improvement (Karnofsky scale)	Relaxation group (pre-post)	Post-treatment (10 weeks)	Reported significant (value not reported)
			Global measures of health: overall condition (Likert-type scale)	Relaxation group (pre-post)	Post-treatment (10 weeks)	Reported significant (value not reported)
		Report 2 (2008)	Global measures of health: Fatigue levels (Likert-type scale)	Relaxation group (pre-post)	Post-treatment (10 weeks)	Reported significant (value not reported)
			Global measures of health: Fatigue levels (Likert-type scale)	Relaxation group (pre-post)	Post follow-up (6 months)	Reported significant (value not reported)
			Global measures of health: reduction in disability (Likert-type scale)	Relaxation group (pre-post)	Post-treatment (10 weeks)	Reported significant (value not reported)
			Global measures of health: reduction in disability (Likert-type scale)	Relaxation group (pre-post)	Post follow-up (6 months)	Reported significant (value not reported)
	Bogaerts K., 2007 [38]		$PetCO_2$	Relaxation imagery (pre-post)	Post intervention	<0.01
Cognitive-based	Lopez C., 2011 [45] (Cognitive restructuring)		Distress (Perceived stress scale)	CBSM compared to control	Time X group **	0.03
			Total mood disturbance (Profile of Mood States (POMS))	CBSM compared to control	Time X group **	0.05
			Quality of life (QOLI Category)	CBSM compared to control	Time X group **	0.002
			Quality of life (QOLI Raw score)	CBSM compared to control	Time X group **	0.05
			Quality of life (QOLI Total score)	CBSM compared to control	Time X group **	0.05
			CFS symptoms (Total CDC symptom severity)	CBSM compared to control	Time X group **	0.04

Table 3. *Cont.*

Intervention Type	First Author, Year	Outcome (Assessed by)	Comparison Groups	Comparison Time Point	p-Value
	Sollie K., 2017 [43] (Mindfulness-based cognitive therapy)	Fatigue (Chalder Fatigue Scale)	MBCT (pre-post)	Post intervention (8 weeks)	p value not reported, medium effect size was reported (d = 0.56)
		Anxiety (HADS)	MBCT (pre-post)	Post intervention (8 weeks)	p value not reported, medium to large effect size was reported (d = 0.68)
		Anxiety (HADS)	MBCT (pre-post)	Post follow-up (3 months)	p value not reported, medium effect size was reported (d = 0.48)
		Dispositional mindfulness (Five Facet Mindfulness questionnaire)	MBCT (pre-post)	Post follow-up (3 months)	p value not reported, large effect size was reported (d = 0.77)
		Disability (Pain disability index)	ACT (pre-post)	Post intervention (after 13 sessions)	0.000
		Psychological flexibility (Psychological inflexibility fatigue scale)	ACT (pre-post)	Post intervention (after 13 sessions)	0.000
		CFS symptoms	ACT (pre-post)	Post intervention (after 13 sessions)	0.017
		Anxiety (HADS)	ACT (pre-post)	Post intervention (after 13 sessions)	0.001
	Jonsjo, M., 2019 [44] (Psychological flexibility)	General fatigue (MFI-20)	ACT (pre-post)	Post intervention (after 13 sessions)	0.024
		General fatigue (MFI-20)	ACT (pre-post)	Post intervention to post follow-up (3 months)	0.049
		Physical fatigue (MFI-20)	ACT (pre-post)	Post intervention (after 13 sessions)	0.046
		Mental fatigue (MFI-20)	ACT (pre-post)	Post intervention (after 13 sessions)	0.004
		Reduced activity (MFI-20)	ACT (pre-post)	Post intervention (after 13 sessions)	0.041
		Reduced motivation (MFI-20)	ACT (pre-post)	Post intervention (after 13 sessions)	0.043

Table 3. Cont.

Intervention Type	First Author, Year	Outcome (Assessed by)	Comparison Groups	Comparison Time Point	p-Value
Movement-based	Chan J., 2013 [41]	SF-36 physical	ACT (pre-post)	Post intervention (after 13 sessions)	0.009
	Ho, R., 2012 (Preliminary report)	Quality of life: Mental functioning score (MOS SF-12)	Qigong (pre-post)	Post-training (5 weeks)	<0.01
		Quality of life: Mental functioning score (MOS SF-12)	Qigong (pre-post)	Post intervention (4 months)	<0.01
		Quality of life: Mental functioning score (MOS SF-12)	Qigong compared to control	Time X group **	0.001
		Telomerase activity * (Telomerase PCR ELISA)	Qigong (pre-post)	Post intervention (4 months)	<0.05
		Telomerase activity * (Telomerase PCR ELISA)	Qigong compared to control	Time X group **	0.029
	Chan J., 2013 (main report)	Total fatigue score (ChFS)	Qigong (pre-post)	Post intervention (4 months)	<0.001
		Total fatigue score (ChFS)	Qigong compared to control	Time X group **	0.000
		Physical fatigue score (ChFS)	Qigong (pre-post)	Post intervention (4 months)	<0.001
		Physical fatigue score (ChFS)	Qigong compared to control	Time X group **	0.000
		Mental fatigue score (ChFS)	Qigong (pre-post)	Post intervention (4 months)	<0.001
		Mental fatigue score (ChFS)	Qigong compared to control	Time X group **	0.050
		Anxiety score (HADS)	Qigong (pre-post)	Post intervention (4 months)	<0.001
		Depression score (HADS)	Qigong (pre-post)	Post intervention (4 months)	<0.001
		Depression score (HADS)	Qigong compared to control	Time X group **	0.002
	Li J., 2015 (Subset study report)	Spirituality (the spirituality subscale of BMSWBI-S)	Qigong compared to control	Post intervention (3 months)	0.013
		Quality of life: mental component summary (MOS SF-12)	Qigong compared to control	Post intervention (3 months)	0.002
		Quality of life: mental component summary (MOS-SF 12)	Qigong compared to control	Post intervention (change score from baseline to 3 months)	0.002

Table 3. Cont.

Intervention Type	First Author, Year	Outcome (Assessed by)	Comparison Groups	Comparison Time Point	p-Value
	Chan, J. 2014 [40] and Chan, J. 2017 [83] Report 1 (2014)	Sleep quality: total score (PSQI)	Baduanjin Qigong compared to waitlist	Post intervention (change score from baseline to 9 weeks)	<0.05
		Subjective sleep quality (PSQI)	Baduanjin Qigong compared to waitlist	Post intervention (change score from baseline to 9 weeks)	<0.01
		Subjective sleep quality (PSQI)	Baduanjin Qigong compared to waitlist	Post follow-up (change score from baseline to 3 months)	<0.01
		Subjective sleep quality (PSQI)	Baduanjin Qigong compared to wait list	Time X group **	0.002
		Sleep latency (PSQI)	Baduanjin Qigong compared to waitlist	Post intervention (change score from baseline to 9 weeks)	<0.05
		Sleep latency (PSQI)	Baduanjin Qigong compared to waitlist	Time X group **	0.044
		Sleep duration (PSQI)	Baduanjin Qigong compared to waitlist	Post intervention (change score from baseline to 9 weeks)	<0.05
		Total fatigue score (ChFS)	Baduanjin Qigong compared to waitlist	Post intervention (change score from baseline to 9 weeks)	<0.001
		Total fatigue score (ChFS)	Baduanjin Qigong compared to waitlist	Post follow-up (change score from baseline to 3 months)	<0.001
		Total fatigue score (ChFS)	Baduanjin Qigong compared to waitlist	Time X group **	<0.001
		Physical fatigue score (ChFS)	Baduanjin Qigong compared to waitlist	Post intervention (change score from baseline to 9 weeks)	<0.001
		Physical fatigue score (ChFS)	Baduanjin Qigong compared to waitlist	Post follow-up (change score from baseline to 3 months)	<0.001

Table 3. Cont.

Intervention Type	First Author, Year	Outcome (Assessed by)	Comparison Groups	Comparison Time Point	p-Value
		Physical fatigue score (ChFS)	Baduanjin Qigong compared to waitlist	Time X group **	<0.001
		Mental fatigue score (ChFS)	Baduanjin Qigong compared to waitlist	Post intervention (change score from baseline to 9 weeks)	<0.001
		Mental fatigue score (ChFS)	Baduanjin Qigong compared to waitlist	Post follow-up (change score from baseline to 3 months)	<0.01
		Mental fatigue score (ChFS)	Baduanjin Qigong compared to waitlist	Time X group **	<0.001
		Anxiety (HADS)	Baduanjin Qigong compared to waitlist	Post intervention (change score from baseline to 9 weeks)	<0.01
		Anxiety (HADS)	Baduanjin Qigong compared to waitlist	Post follow-up (change score from baseline to 3 months)	<0.05
		Anxiety (HADS)	Baduanjin Qigong compared to waitlist	Time X group **	0.016
		Depression (HADS)	Baduanjin Qigong compared to waitlist	Post intervention (change score from baseline to 9 weeks)	<0.001
		Depression (HADS)	Baduanjin Qigong compared to waitlist	Time X group **	<0.001
	Report 2 (2017)	Increase in adiponectin levels	Baduanjin Qigong compared to waitlist	Post intervention (change score from baseline to 9 weeks)	<0.05
		Depression (HADS)	Baduanjin Qigong compared to waitlist	Post intervention (change score from baseline to 9 weeks)	<0.001
		Anxiety (HADS)	Baduanjin Qigong compared to waitlist	Post intervention (9 weeks)	<0.05

Table 3. Cont.

Intervention Type	First Author, Year	Outcome (Assessed by)	Comparison Groups	Comparison Time Point	p-Value
	Oka T, 2014 [28]	Fatigue score - acute effect (POMS)	Isometric yoga (pre-post)	Before to after the final 20-min session	<0.001
		Vigor score - acute effect (POMS)	Isometric yoga (pre-post)	Before to after the final 20-min session	<0.01
		Physical fatigue score (ChFS)	Isometric yoga (pre-post)	Post intervention (2 months)	0.004
		Physical fatigue score (ChFS)	Isometric yoga compared to control	Time X group **	0.009
		Mental fatigue score (ChFS)	Isometric yoga (pre-post)	Post intervention (2 months)	0.004
		Mental fatigue score (ChFS)	Isometric yoga compared to control	Time X group **	0.007
		Total fatigue score (ChFS)	Isometric yoga (pre-post)	Post intervention (2 months)	0.002
		Total fatigue score (ChFS)	Isometric yoga compared to control	Time X group **	0.003
		Quality of life: bodily pain (SF-8)	Isometric yoga (pre-post)	Post intervention (2 months)	0.0001
		Quality of life: general health perception (SF-8)	Isometric yoga (pre-post)	Post intervention (2 months)	0.0021
		Quality of life: Physical component summary (SF-8)	Isometric yoga (pre-post)	Post intervention (2 months)	0.024
	Oka, T., 2018 and Oka, T., 2019 [42,91] Report 1 (2018)	Fatigue (POMS)	Acute effects of sitting isometric yoga (pre-post)	Before to after the final 20-min session	0.001
		Vigor (POMS)	Acute effects of sitting isometric yoga (pre-post)	Before to after the final 20-min session	0.002
		Decreased heart rate	Acute effects of sitting isometric yoga (pre-post)	Before to after the final 20-min session	0.047
		Increased high-frequency power of HR variability	Acute effects of sitting isometric yoga (pre-post)	Before to after the final 20-min session	0.028
		Increased serum levels of DHEA-S	Acute effects of sitting isometric yoga (pre-post)	Before to after the final 20-min session	0.012

Table 3. *Cont.*

Intervention Type	First Author, Year	Outcome (Assessed by)	Comparison Groups	Comparison Time Point	p-Value
		Decreased levels of cortisol	Acute effects of sitting isometric yoga (pre-post)	Before to after the final 20-min session	0.016
		Decreased level of TNF-α	Acute effects of sitting isometric yoga (pre-post)	Before to after the final 20-min session	0.035
	Report 2 (2019)	Fatigue (POMS)	Longitudinal effects of sitting isometric yoga (pre-post)	Post intervention (2 months)	0.002
		Depression (HADS)	Longitudinal effects of sitting isometric yoga (pre-post)	Post intervention (2 months)	0.02
	Takakura, S., 2019 [10]	Fatigue (11 score Chalder's fatigue scale)	Recumbent isometric yoga (pre-post)	Post intervention (3 months)	<0.0001
		Changes in miRNA expression	Recumbent isometric yoga (pre-post)	Post intervention (3 months)	<0.05 (Four miRNAs significantly upregulated and 42 were significantly downregulated)

BMSWBI-S: Body-Mind-Spirit Well-being Inventory, ChFS: Chalder's Fatigue Scale, HADS: Hospital Anxiety and Depression Scale, MOS SF-12: Medical Outcomes Study 12- Item Short-Form Health Survey, POMS: Profile of Mood States, PSQI: Pittsburgh Sleep Quality Index, SF-8: Medical Outcomes Study Short Form 8, QOLI: Quality of life inventory, MFI-20: Multidimensional fatigue inventory-20, ACT: Acceptance and commitment therapy, MBCT: Mindfulness-based cognitive therapy, CBSM: Cognitive-based stress management. * measure of stress-related damage at a cellular level. ** to test the interaction effect of time and group.

Table 4. Significant outcomes in the included studies using Oxford criteria for diagnosing CFS.

Intervention Type	First Author, Year	Study	Outcome (Assessed by)	Comparison Groups	Comparison Time Point	p-Value
Mindfulness and cognitive-based	Surawy, Ch., 2005 [29]	Study 1 (RCT)	Anxiety (HADS)	MBSR/MBCT compared to controls	Post treatment (8 weeks)	0.010
		Study 2 (single-arm experimental study)	Anxiety (HADS)	MBCT/MBSR (pre-post)	Post treatment (8 weeks)	0.000
			Fatigue impact: total score (FIS)	MBCT/MBSR (pre-post)	Post treatment (8 weeks)	0.010
			Anxiety (HADS)	MBCT/MBSR (pre-post)	Post treatment (8 weeks)	0.010
			Anxiety (HADS)	MBCT/MBSR (pre-post)	Post follow-up (3 months)	0.010
			Depression (HADS)	MBCT/MBSR (pre-post)	Post-treatment (8 weeks)	0.010
			Depression (HADS)	MBCT/MBSR (pre-post)	Post follow-up (3 months)	0.050
		Study 3 (single-arm experimental study)	Fatigue score (ChFS)	MBCT/MBSR (pre-post)	Post treatment (8 weeks)	0.010
			Fatigue score (ChFS)	MBCT/MBSR (pre-post)	Post follow-up (3 months)	0.000
			Quality of life: physical functioning (SF-36)	MBCT/MBSR (pre-post)	Post treatment (8 weeks)	0.010
			Quality of life: physical functioning (SF-36)	MBCT/MBSR (pre-post)	Post follow-up (3 months)	0.000
			Fatigue impact: total score (FIS)	MBCT/MBSR (pre-post)	Post treatment (8 weeks)	0.020
			Fatigue impact: total score (FIS)	MBCT/MBSR (pre-post)	Post follow-up (3 months)	0.050
	Rimes, K., 2013 [30]		Fatigue (ChFS)	MBCT compared to waitlist	Post treatment (8 weeks)	0.014
			Fatigue (ChFS)	MBCT compared to waitlist	Post follow-up (2 months)	0.033
			Fatigue (ChFS)	MBCT (pre-post)	Post follow-up (6 months)	0.010
			Impairment (The work and social adjustment scale)	MBCT compared to wait list	Post-treatment (8 weeks)	0.04
			Impairment (The work and social adjustment scale)	MBCT compared to waitlist	Post follow-up (2 months)	0.054
			Impairment (The work and social adjustment scale)	MBCT (pre-post)	Post follow-up (6 months)	0.004
			Impairment (The work and social adjustment scale)	MBCT (pre-post)	Between 2- and 6-month follow-up	0.004
			Beliefs about Emotions (Self-reporting scale)	MBCT compared to waitlist	Post treatment (8 weeks)	0.01
			Beliefs about Emotions (Self-reporting scale)	MBCT compared to waitlist	Post follow-up (2 months)	0.012
			Beliefs about Emotions (Self-reporting scale)	MBCT (pre-post)	Post follow-up (6 months)	0.004
			Self-Compassion (Self-reporting scale)	MBCT compared to waitlist	Post treatment (8 weeks)	0.007
			Self-Compassion (Self-reporting scale)	MBCT compared to waitlist	Post follow-up (2 months)	0.006

Table 4. *Cont.*

Intervention Type	First Author, Year	Outcome (Assessed by)	Comparison Groups	Comparison Time Point	p-Value
		Self-Compassion (Self-reporting scale)	MBCT (pre-post)	Post follow-up (6 months)	0.003
		Mindfulness (5 facet mindfulness questionnaire)	MBCT compared to waitlist	Post follow-up (2 months)	0.035
		Mindfulness (5 facet mindfulness questionnaire)	MBCT (pre-post)	Post follow-up (6 months)	0.006
		Mindfulness (5 facet mindfulness questionnaire)	MBCT (pre-post)	Between 2- and 6-month follow-up	0.017
		Catastrophizing (Self-reporting scale)	MBCT compared to waitlist	Post treatment (8 weeks)	0.004
		Catastrophizing (Self-reporting scale)	MBCT (pre-post)	Post follow-up (6 months)	0.012
		All-or-nothing behavior (Self-reporting scale)	MBCT compared to waitlist	Post treatment (8 weeks)	0.005
		All-or-nothing behavior (Self-reporting scale)	MBCT (pre-post)	Post follow-up (6 months)	0.017
		Depression (HADS)	MBCT compared to waitlist	Post-treatment (8 weeks)	0.038

ChFS: Chalder's Fatigue Scale, HADS: Hospital Anxiety and Depression Scale, MBSR: Mindfulness-based stress reduction, MBCT: Mindfulness-based cognitive therapy, SF-36: 36- Item Short-Form Health Survey.

In comparison to the control group, both mental and physical fatigue scores improved significantly in four included studies using MBCT [30], isometric yoga [28], Qigong exercise [41] and Baduanjin Qigong [40]. Two studies showed within-group fatigue improvement in participants receiving an 8-week mindfulness therapy [29] and in participants receiving a 10-week relaxation program [39] (Tables 3 and 4)

Anxiety and depression were improved in participants receiving Baduanjin Qigong compared to the controls after 16 sessions (9 weeks) of therapy [40]. Depression was improved in participants after 4 months of Qigong exercise [41] and 8 weeks of MBCT [30] compared to the control groups. Surawy et al. [29] also showed improvement of anxiety after 8 weeks of MBSR/MBCT intervention compared to the control group.

In comparison to the control group, quality of life improved in participants receiving Qigong exercise [41,70,71] and cognitive-behavioral stress management [45].

Tables 3 and 4 show the details of all the significant outcomes of the included studies according to the diagnosis of ME/CFS (Oxford or CDC criteria).

3.8. Adverse Events

Seven studies assessed adverse events: Four did not identify any adverse events [30,39,41,43]; and three studies recorded adverse events such as deterioration of their symptoms, muscle ache, palpitation, dizziness, knee pain, backache, fatigue, and nervousness [28,40,44]. Five studies did not report if they assessed adverse events [10,29,38,42,45]

3.9. Risk of Bias in the Included Studies

All the included RCT studies were assessed at a high risk of bias in relation to the lack of blinding of participants and personnel. We were not able to assess the risk of bias in many areas as most of the studies were poorly reported (Figure 2). The risk of bias assessment for the single-arm experimental studies using the ROBINS-I assessment tool is shown in Table A5.

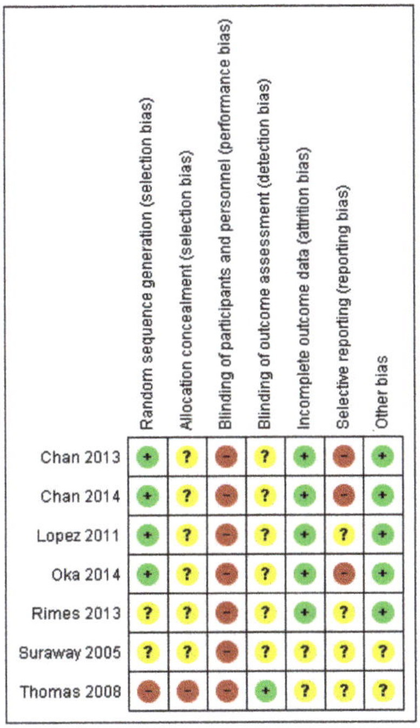

Figure 2. Risk of bias summary: review authors' judgments about each risk of bias item for each included study.

4. Discussion

This is the first systematic review of studies using MBIs in patients with ME/CFS. The MBIs used in these studies were mindfulness-based stress reduction and mindfulness-based cognitive therapy, relaxation, Qigong, and yoga.

The etiology and pathogenesis of ME/CFS are still unknown [1]. Researchers have shown changes in some biological markers [100–103]. Other studies highlight changes in the hypothalamic-pituitary-adrenal (HPA) axis in these patients [104].

It was also suggested that ME/CFS may be a neurophysiological disorder in the brain caused by repeated incidental or unnecessary stimuli in the limbic system, which is known as the threat response/protection center. These stimuli can be emotional, psychological, chemical, and/or physiological and they can keep the threat response center on a continuous high alert [105]. Connections between the amygdala and sympathetic, hypothalamic and other limbic brain systems can initiate a series of stimulations and uncontrolled reactions throughout the whole body, which could be considered as the root cause of CFS symptoms [105].

With increasing knowledge based on neuroplasticity and the impact of limbic function on somatic symptoms, the potential mechanisms of MBIs might be explained. There is growing interest in using MBIs and many programs are being offered directly to the public to assist with mental and physical health. One of these programs developed specifically for ME/CFS (25) has shown modest success in functional ability in a clinical audit. Because patients are accessing MBI programs, there is an urgent need for evidence as to whether these programs are having an impact on the core symptoms of ME/CFS or mainly address the secondary dissatisfaction that comes with having a chronic, poorly understood disease for which there is no cure. In this review, the MBIs used in the included studies were quite heterogenous. Two studies used relaxation techniques, five studies used movement-based therapies including different forms of yoga and Qigong and the remaining ones used various forms of mindfulness and cognitive-based approaches. Table A6 describes these interventions briefly.

In this systematic review, we found the most commonly measured outcomes were fatigue severity, anxiety and depression, and quality of life or its components (e.g., physical and mental functioning). When compared to the control group, fatigue severity, mental functioning and anxiety/depression mostly improved in patients receiving MBIs. However, poor reporting, small sample sizes, different diagnostic criteria, and a high risk of bias may challenge this result. It is also worth noting that these symptoms are not specific and can be found not only in some individuals with ME/CFS but also in individuals with many other physical and mental health conditions.

According to the 2015 Institute of Medicine report [1], impaired function, post-exertional malaise and unrefreshing sleep are the core symptoms in ME/CFS patients. None of our included studies, however, measured post-exertional malaise. One study measured sleep using a self-reporting scale which improved after 9 weeks of Qigong exercise [40]. Physical or mental functioning and functional performance were mostly measured using self-report scales and only one study measured performance using objective measures [51].

In contrast, anxiety and depression and some cognitive constructs were commonly measured in the included studies. While these symptoms are important, they are secondary and not the key features of ME/CFS. Reporting secondary outcomes while omitting measurement of the core symptoms of a disease may lead to inaccurate conclusions about treatment effectiveness.

Previous studies have used a variety of definitions for the diagnosis of ME/CFS. Lack of consensus and competing definitions act as a barrier for research in this field. Most of the studies in this systematic review used the 1994 CDC criteria for the diagnosis of ME/CFS and two studies used Oxford criteria.

The Oxford criteria were developed at a consensus meeting [46]. They do not require the presence of any symptom other than disabling fatigue. The presence of other symptoms such as immune, autonomic and mood symptoms differentiate ME/CFS from other common medical and psychiatric conditions including major depression. It has long been suspected that the Oxford criteria may therefore fail to exclude individuals with other fatiguing conditions [14,19].

To address this concern, the Agency for Healthy Research and Quality (AHRQ) in the United States conducted a sensitivity analysis in which the outcomes of treatment studies using the Oxford criteria were compared with studies using other criteria (mostly the 1994 CDC Criteria) [14]. They found that whereas most studies using the Oxford criteria showed some benefits for CBT, studies using the CDC criteria were mixed with no overall benefit. With regards to graded exercise therapy, exclusion of the trials using the Oxford case definition left insufficient evidence about the effectiveness of graded exercise therapy on any outcome. Studies of other therapies were not affected as primary studies had small sample sizes and a high risk of bias. These findings confirm that the choice of inclusion criteria impacts study outcomes. The AHRQ concluded that future research should retire the use of the Oxford case definition. The National Institutes of Health held a consensus workshop to guide the future of ME/CFS research [19]. For similar reasons as the AHRQ, they also recommended that the Oxford Criteria should be retired.

The 1994 CDC criteria also have significant drawbacks. They require four out of eight criteria but none are mandatory. This means two subjects identified with these criteria may have no symptoms in common with each other—one might have four and the other, another four. Moreover, minor symptoms may overlap with the symptoms of psychiatric disorders including major depression [14].

The Institute of Medicine [1] has proposed diagnostic criteria which are very similar to the Canadian Consensus Criteria [88]. They require patients to have moderate, substantial or severe disabling fatigue, post-exertional malaise and unrefreshing sleep for at least half of the time and one of the cognitive impairments or orthostatic intolerance symptoms. Conclusions about the effectiveness of interventions will be possible once studies use the same diagnostic criteria and measure core outcomes using standardized measures.

4.1. Strengths and Limitations

Assessment of a broad range of mind-body approaches and outcomes in a systematic fashion was one of the main strengths of this systematic review. Engaging patients in the process of designing the review protocol and in reviewing the findings increase the applicability and relevance of the findings of this study.

As we found a diverse range of interventions and outcomes across the included studies; we were not able to perform a meta-analysis. We also may have missed some relevant information by including only studies published in the English language.

4.2. Research Implications

1. As recommended by the Institute of Medicine report, using objective measures is a priority in studies of ME/CFS. There are several symptoms such as post-exertional malaise, cognitive dysfunction, orthostatic intolerance, and changes including impaired immune function and abnormal brain functions that could be measured objectively.
2. Future RCTs will benefit from larger sample sizes. Investigators must use an appropriate randomization method and ensure outcome assessors are blinded to the group identity of the participants. They should measure and report the outcomes specified in their protocol in order to avoid selective reporting.

5. Conclusions

In this systematic review, we described the current literature on MBIs for the treatment of ME/CFS. Future clinical trials will benefit from the findings of this study in terms of what outcomes and outcome measures are mostly used in previous studies. We showed that the included studies did not report measuring post-exertional malaise as a core outcome of ME/CFS. On the other hand, fatigue severity, anxiety/depression and mental functioning were shown to be improved in the patients receiving MBIs. However, poor reporting, small sample sizes, different diagnostic criteria, and a high risk of bias may challenge this result. We highlight the need for further research to use objective and standardized outcomes and outcome measures for making definitive conclusions.

Author Contributions: Conceptualization, S.V., E.S., and K.O; methodology, S.K.A., M.K., E.S., S.P., D.R.J., T.K., M.P., L.S., K.O. and S.V.; validation, S.K.A., M.K., E.S., D.R.J., S.P. and S.V.; formal analysis, S.K.A.; investigation, S.K.A., M.K., D.R.J. and E.S.; resources, S.V.; data curation, S.K.A.; writing—original draft preparation, S.K.A., M.K. and E.S.; writing—review and editing, S.P., E.S. and S.V.; visualization, S.K.A.; supervision, S.V.; project administration, S.P.; funding acquisition, S.V. All authors have read and agreed to the published version of the manuscript.

Funding: This research was funded by the University of Calgary.

Acknowledgments: The authors thank Susanne King-Jones for her help in the search strategy and contributions to the project.

Conflicts of Interest: The authors declare no conflict of interest. The funders had no role in the design of the study; in the collection, analyses, or interpretation of data; in the writing of the manuscript, or in the decision to publish the results.

Appendix A

Table A1. Case definitions for the diagnosis of ME/CFS over time.

Advisor Group, Year	Identifier	Case Definition and Required Symptom(s)
For Adults		
Holmes et al., 1988 (CDC) [17]	CFS	Major criteria New onset of persistent or relapsing, debilitating fatigue or easy fatigability in a person who has no previous history of similar symptoms, that does not resolve with bedrest, and that is severe enough to reduce or impair average daily activity below 50% of the patient's premorbid activity level for a period of at least 6 months Minor criteria Mild fever Sore throat Painful lymph node in the anterior or posterior cervical or axillary distribution Unexplained generalized muscle weakness Muscle discomfort or myalgia Prolonged generalized fatigue ($\geq$24 h) after normal level of exercise Migratory arthralgia without joint swelling or redness Neurological complains one or more of: photophobia, transient visual scotomata, forgetfulness, excessive irritability, confusion, difficulty thinking, inability to concentrate, depression Sleep disturbances
Sharp et al., 1991 (Oxford) [46]	CFS	Fatigue as the principal symptom A definite onset that is not lifelong The fatigue is severe, disabling, and affects physical and mental functioning The fatigue should have been present for a minimum of 6 months during which it was present for more than 50% of the time Other symptoms may be present, particularly myalgia, mood and sleep disturbance.
Fukuda et al., 1994, (CDC) [52]	CFS	Clinically evaluated, "unexplained", persistent or relapsing fatigue for $\geq$6 months. Not the result of ongoing exertion Not substantially alleviated by rest Resulting in a substantial reduction in previous activity level. Four or more of the following concurrently present for $\geq$ 6 months: impaired memory or concentration sore throat tender cervical or axillary lymph nodes muscle pain multi-joint pain new headaches unrefreshing sleep post-exertion malaise

Table A1. Cont.

Advisor Group, Year	Identifier	Case Definition and Required Symptom(s)
London criteria-V2, (Dowsett et al., 1994) [106]		These three criteria must all be present for a diagnosis of M.E./PVFS Exercise-induced fatigue precipitated by trivially small exertion -physical or mental -relative to the patient's previous exercise tolerance Impairment of short-term memory and loss of powers of concentration, usually coupled with other neurological and psychological disturbances such as emotional lability, nominal dysphasia, disturbed sleep patterns, disequilibrium or tinnitus Fluctuation of symptoms, usually precipitated by either physical or mental exercise
Canadian Consensus Criteria, (Carruthers et al., 2003) [88]	ME/PVFS	For a diagnosis of CFS/ME, a patient must meet the following criteria 1–6 and adhere to item 7: Fatigue Post-exertional malaise and/or fatigue Sleep dysfunction Pain Two or more of the following neurological/cognitive manifestations: Confusion Impairment of concentration and short-term memory consolidation Disorientation difficulty with information processing categorizing and word retrieval perceptual and sensory disturbances One or more symptoms from two of the following categories: Autonomic manifestation (e.g., orthostatic intolerance, postural orthostatic tachycardia syndrome, ...) Neuroendocrine manifestation (e.g., loss of thermostatic stability, sweating episode, ...) Immune manifestation (e.g., tender lymph nodes, recurrent sore throat, ...) Illness lasting ≥6 months
Revised Canadian Consensus Criteria, (Jason et al., 2010) [107]	ME/CFS	Definition of Research CFS/ME criteria: Over the past 6 months, persistent or recurring chronic fatigue that is not lifelong and results in substantial reductions in previous levels of occupational, educational, social and personal activities Post-exertional malaise and/or fatigue Unrefreshing sleep or disturbance of sleep quantity or rhythm disturbance Pain (or discomfort) that is often widespread and migratory in nature. At least one symptom from any of the following: Myofascial and/or joint pain (e.g., deep pain, abdomen/stomach pain, or achy and sore muscles. Pain, stiffness, or tenderness may occur in any joint but must be present in more than one joint and lacking edema or other signs of inflammation) Abdominal and/or head pain (e.g., stomach pain or chest pain). Headaches often described as localized behind the eyes or in the back of the head (includes headaches localized elsewhere, including migraines; headaches would need to be more frequent than they were before, which would indicate a new pattern of a new type as compared to headaches previously experienced (i.e., location of pain has changed, nature of pain has changed), or different in severity type as compared to headaches previously experienced by the patient) Two or more of the following neurological/cognitive manifestations: Impaired memory (self-reported or observable disturbance in the ability to recall information or events on a short-term basis) Difficulty focusing vision and attention (disturbed concentration may impair the ability to remain on task, to screen out extraneous/excessive stimuli) Loss of depth perception Difficulty finding the right word Frequently forget what wanted to say Absent-mindedness Slowness of thought Difficulty recalling information Need to focus on one thing at a time Trouble expressing thought Difficulty comprehending information Frequently lose train of thought Sensitivity to bright lights or noise Muscle weakness/muscle twitches At least one symptoms from two of the following categories: Autonomic manifestation: Neurally mediated hypotension, postural orthostatic tachycardia, delayed postural hypotension, palpitations with or without cardiac arrhythmias, dizziness or fainting, feeling unsteady on the feet–disturbed balance, shortness of breath, nausea, bladder dysfunction, or irritable bowel syndrome Neuroendocrine manifestation: Recurrent feelings of feverishness and cold extremities, subnormal body temperature and marked diurnal fluctuations, sweating episodes, intolerance of extremes of heat and cold, marked weight change-loss of appetite or abnormal appetite Immune manifestation: Recurrent flu-like symptoms, non-exudative sore or scratchy throat, repeated fevers and sweats, lymph nodes tender to palpitation–generally minimal swelling observed, new sensitivities to food, odors, or chemicals

Table A1. Cont.

Advisor Group, Year	Identifier	Case Definition and Required Symptom(s)

International Consensus Criteria, (Carruthers et al., 2011) [90]	ME	Myalgic encephalomyelitis is an acquired neurological disease with complex global dysfunctions. Pathological dysregulation of the nervous, immune and endocrine systems, with impaired cellular energy metabolism and ion transport, are prominent features. Although signs and symptoms are dynamically interactive and causally connected, the criteria are grouped by regions of pathophysiology to provide general focus. A patient will meet the following criteria
		A. Post-exertional neuro-immune exhaustion (PENEpen'-e): Compulsory
		This cardinal feature is a pathological inability to produce sufficient energy on demand with prominent symptoms primarily in the neuro-immune regions. Characteristics are as follows:
		1. Marked, rapid physical and/or cognitive fatigability in response to exertion, which may be minimal such as activities of daily living or simple mental tasks, can be debilitating and cause a relapse
		2. Post-exertional symptom exacerbation: e.g., acute flu-like symptoms, pain and worsening of other symptoms.
		3. Post-exertional exhaustion may occur immediately after activity or be delayed by hours or days.
		4. Recovery period is prolonged, usually taking 24-h or longer. A relapse can last days, weeks or longer.
		5. Low threshold of physical and mental fatigability (lack of stamina) results in a substantial reduction in pre-illness activity level.
		B. Neurological impairments: At least one symptom from three of the following four symptom categories
		1. Neuro-cognitive impairments
		  a. Difficulty processing information: slowed thought, impaired concentration, e.g., confusion, disorientation, cognitive overload, difficulty with making decisions, slowed speech, acquired or exertional dyslexia
		  b. Short-term memory loss: e.g., difficulty remembering what one wanted to say, what one was saying, retrieving words, recalling information, poor working memory
		2. Pain
		  a. Headaches: e.g., chronic, generalized headaches often involve aching of the eyes, behind the eyes or back of the head that may be associated with cervical muscle tension; migraine; tension headaches
		  b. Significant pain can be experienced in muscles, muscle-tendon junctions, joints, abdomen or chest. It is non-inflammatory in nature and often migrates, e.g., generalized hyperalgesia, widespread pain (may meet fibromyalgia criteria), myofascial or radiating pain
		3. Sleep disturbance
		  a. Disturbed sleep patterns: e.g., insomnia, prolonged sleep including naps, sleeping most of the day and being awake most of the night, frequent awakenings, awaking much earlier than before illness onset, vivid dreams/nightmares
		  b. Unrefreshed sleep: e.g., awaken feeling exhausted regardless of the duration of sleep, day-time sleepiness
		4. Neuro-sensory, perceptual and motor disturbances
		  a. Neurosensory and perceptual: e.g., inability to focus vision, sensitivity to light, noise, vibration, odor, taste and touch; impaired depth perception
		  b. Motor: e.g., muscle weakness, twitching, poor coordination, feeling unsteady on feet, ataxia
		  c. Immune, gastro-intestinal and genitourinary Impairments: At least one symptom from three of the following five symptom categories
		    1. Flu-like symptoms may be recurrent or chronic and typically activate or worsen with exertion. e.g., sore throat, sinusitis, cervical and/or axillary lymph nodes may enlarge or be tender on palpitation
		    2. Susceptibility to viral infections with prolonged recovery periods
		    3. Gastro-intestinal tract: e.g., nausea, abdominal pain, bloating, irritable bowel syndrome
		    4. Genitourinary: e.g., urinary urgency or frequency, nocturia
		    5. Sensitivities to food, medications, odors or chemicals
		  d. Energy production/transportation impairments: At least one symptom
		    1. Cardiovascular: e.g., inability to tolerate an upright position—orthostatic intolerance, neurally mediated hypotension, postural orthostatic tachycardia syndrome, palpitations with or without cardiac arrhythmias, light-headedness/dizziness
		    2. Respiratory: e.g., air hunger, labored breathing, fatigue of chest wall muscles
		    3. Loss of thermostatic stability: e.g., subnormal body temperature, marked diurnal fluctuations; sweating episodes, recurrent feelings of feverishness with or without low-grade fever, cold extremities
		    4. Intolerance of extremes of temperature

Table A2. Excluded studies.

Primary Author, Publication Year	Reason for Exclusion
Aaron L. 2003	Review study
Arroll M. 2012	Not intervention of interest
Arroll MA. 2014	Not eligible control group
Benor D. 2017	Not population of interest
Bentler S. 2005	Not population of interest
Craske N. 2009	Not population of interest
Crawley E. 2017	Not population of interest
Deale A. 1997	Not intervention of interest
Deale A. 2001	Not eligible control group
Densham S. 2016	Not population of interest
Fjorback LO. 2012	Not population of interest
Fjorback LO. 2013	Not population of interest
Fjorback LO. 2013	Not population of interest
Guthlin C. 2012	Not intervention of interest
Hlavaty LE. 2011	Not intervention of interest
Hall DL. 2017	Not eligible control group
Jacobson HB. 2017	Not population of interest
James, L. 1996	Case study
Jason L. 2007	Not intervention of interest
Kos D. 2015	Not eligible control group
Lee J. 2015	Not population of interest
Nijs J. 2008	Not intervention of interest
Oka T. 2017	Not eligible control group
Pauzano-Slamm N. 2005	Not peer-reviewed publication
Ryan M. 2004	Not population of interest
Sampalli T. 2009	Not population of interest
Stevens MW. 1999	Full-text not available
Toussaint L. 2012	Not population of interest
Walach H. 2008	Not intervention of interest
Windthorst P. 2017	Not eligible control group

Table A3. Statistically insignificant outcomes in the included studies using CDC, Canadian and international consensus criteria for diagnosing CFS.

Intervention Type	First Author, Year		Outcome (Assessed by)	Comparison Groups	Comparison Time Point	p-Value
Relaxation-based	Thomas, M., 2006 and 2008 [39,51]	Report 1 (2006)	Anxiety (as part of a self-report subjective mood scale)	Relaxation group (pre-post)	Post treatment (10 weeks)	Non-significant
			Performance (word recall, reaction time and vigilance tasks)	Relaxation group (pre-post)	Post follow-up (6 months)	Non-significant
		Report 2 (2008)	Performance score–10% improvement or 80% attainment (Karnofsky scale)	Relaxation group compared to MCT and control groups	Post treatment (10 weeks)	Non-significant
Cognitive-based	Lopez C., 2011 [45] (Cognitive restructuring)		Fatigue (Profile of Mood States (POMS)	CBSM compared to control	Time X group **	0.06
	Sollie K., 2017 [43] (Mindfulness-based cognitive therapy)		Fatigue (Chalder Fatigue Scale)	MBCT (pre-post)	Post follow-up (3 months)	p value not reported, small effect size was reported (d = 0.26)
			Depression (HADS)	MBCT (pre-post)	Post intervention (8 weeks)	p value not reported, small effect size was reported (d = 0.32)
			Depression (HADS)	MBCT (pre-post)	Post follow-up (3 months)	p value not reported, small effect size was reported (d = 0.33)
			Dispositional mindfulness (Five Facet Mindfulness questionnaire)	MBCT (pre-post)	Post intervention (8 weeks)	p value not reported, small effect size was reported (d = 0.11)
			Rumination (Ruminative Response Scale)	MBCT (pre-post)	Post intervention (8 weeks)	p value not reported, small effect size was reported (d = 0.26)
			Rumination (Ruminative Response Scale)	MBCT (pre-post)	Post follow-up (3 months)	p value not reported, small effect size was reported (d = 0.32)
			CFS symptom burden	MBCT (pre-post)	Post intervention (8 weeks)	p value not reported, small effect size was reported (d = 0.07)
			CFS symptom burden	MBCT (pre-post)	Post follow-up (3 months)	p value not reported, small effect size was reported (d = 0.04)

Table A3. *Cont.*

Intervention Type	First Author, Year	Outcome (Assessed by)	Comparison Groups	Comparison Time Point	*p*-Value
		Satisfaction with life (Satisfaction With Life Scale)	MBCT (pre-post)	Post intervention (8 weeks)	*p* value not reported, small effect size was reported (d = −0.09)
		Satisfaction with life (Satisfaction With Life Scale)	MBCT (pre-post)	Post follow-up (3 months)	*p* value not reported, small effect size was reported (d = 0.09)
		Disability (Pain disability index)	ACT (pre-post)	Post intervention to post follow-up (3 months)	0.608
		Psychological flexibility (Psychological inflexibility fatigue scale)	ACT (pre-post)	Post intervention to post follow-up (3 months)	0.775
		CFS symptoms	ACT (pre-post)	Post intervention to post follow-up (3 months)	0.652
		Anxiety (HADS)	ACT (pre-post)	Post intervention to post follow-up (3 months)	0.922
		Depression (HADS)	ACT (pre-post)	Post intervention (after 13 sessions)	0.574
	Jonsjo, M., 2019 [44] (Psychological flexibility)	Depression (HADS)	ACT (pre-post)	Post intervention to post follow-up (3 months)	0.066
		Physical fatigue (MFI-20)	ACT (pre-post)	Post intervention to post follow-up (3 months)	0.352
		Mental fatigue (MFI-20)	ACT (pre-post)	Post intervention to post follow-up (3 months)	0.943
		Reduced activity (MFI-20)	ACT (pre-post)	Post intervention to post follow-up (3 months)	0.449
		Reduced motivation (MFI-20)	ACT (pre-post)	Post intervention to post follow-up (3 months)	0.918
		SF-36 physical	ACT (pre-post)	Post intervention to post follow-up (3 months)	0.325
		SF-36 mental	ACT (pre-post)	Post intervention (after 13 sessions)	0.520

Table A3. Cont.

Intervention Type	First Author, Year	Outcome (Assessed by)	Comparison Groups	Comparison Time Point	p-Value
Movement-based	Chan J., 2013 [41]	SF-36 mental	ACT (pre-post)	Post intervention to post follow-up (3 months)	0.301
		EQ. 5D-Index	ACT (pre-post)	Post intervention (after 13 sessions)	0.065
		EQ. 5D-Index	ACT (pre-post)	Post intervention to post follow-up (3 months)	0.524
		Quality of life: physical functioning score (MOS SF-12)	Qigong (pre-post)	Post training (5 weeks)	Non-significant
		Quality of life: physical functioning score (MOS SF-12)	Qigong (pre-post)	Post intervention (4 months)	Non-significant
		Quality of life: physical functioning score (MOS SF-12)	Qigong compared to control	Time X group **	0.484
	Ho, R., 2012 (Preliminary report)	Quality of life: physical functioning score (MOS SF-12)	Control (pre-post)	Post training (5 weeks)	Non-significant
		Quality of life: physical functioning score (MOS SF-12)	Control (pre-post)	Post intervention (4 months)	Non-significant
		Quality of life: mental functioning score (MOS SF-12)	Control (pre-post)	Post training (5 weeks)	Non-significant
		Quality of life: mental functioning score (MOS SF-12)	Control (pre-post)	Post intervention (4 months)	Non-significant
		Telomerase activity* (Telomerase PCR ELISA)	Control (pre-post)	Post intervention (4 months)	Non-significant
	Chan J., 2013 (main report)	Anxiety score (HADS)	Qigong (pre-post)	Time X group **	0.584
		Depression score (HADS)	Control (pre-post)	Post-intervention (4 months)	0.365
	Li J., 2015 (Subset study report)	Quality of life: physical component summary (MOS SF-12)	Qigong compared to control	Post intervention (change score from baseline to 3 months)	0.451

Table A3. Cont.

Intervention Type	First Author, Year	Outcome (Assessed by)	Comparison Groups	Comparison Time Point	p-Value
	Chan, J. 2014 [40] and Chan, J. 2017 [83]	Sleep quality: total score (PSQI)	Baduanjin Qigong compared to waitlist	Time X group **	0.064
	Report 1 (2014)	Sleep duration (PSQI)	Baduanjin Qigong compared to waitlist	Time X group **	0.151
		Sleep efficacy (PSQI)	Baduanjin Qigong compared to wait list	Time X group **	0.522
		Sleep disturbance (PSQI)	Baduanjin Qigong compared to waitlist	Time X group **	0.062
		Use of sleep medication (PSQI)	Baduanjin Qigong compared to waitlist	Time X group **	0.803
		Daytime dysfunction (PSQI)	Baduanjin Qigong compared to waitlist	Time X group **	0.253
	Report 2 (2017)	Adiponectin levels	Baduanjin Qigong compared to waitlist	Post intervention (change score from baseline to 3-month)	Non-significant
		Depression (HADS)	Baduanjin Qigong compared to waitlist	Post intervention (change score from baseline to 3-month)	Non-significant
		Anxiety (HADS)	Baduanjin Qigong compared to waitlist	Post intervention (change score from baseline to 9 weeks)	Non-significant
		Anxiety (HADS)	Baduanjin Qigong compared to waitlist	Post intervention (change score from baseline to 3-month)	Non-significant

Table A3. Cont.

Intervention Type	First Author, Year	Outcome (Assessed by)	Comparison Groups	Comparison Time Point	p-Value
	Oka T, 2014 [28]	Quality of life: vitality (SF-8)	Isometric yoga (pre-post)	Post intervention (2 months)	Non-significant
		Quality of life: role emotional (SF-8)	Isometric yoga (pre-post)	Post intervention (2 months)	Non-significant
		Quality of life: mental health (SF-8)	Isometric yoga (pre-post)	Post intervention (2 months)	Non-significant
		Quality of life: physical functioning (SF-8)	Isometric yoga (pre-post)	Post intervention (2 months)	Non-significant
		Quality of life: mental component summary (SF-8)	Isometric yoga (pre-post)	Post intervention (2 months)	Non-significant
		Quality of life: role physical (SF-8)	Isometric yoga (pre-post)	Post intervention (2 months)	Non-significant
		Quality of life: social functioning (SF-8)	Isometric yoga (pre-post)	Post intervention (2 months)	Non-significant
	Oka, T., 2018 and Oka, T., 2019 [42,91] Report 1 (2018)	Autonomic function indices (low-frequency power of HR variability, CVR-R: Coefficient of variation of R-R intervals)	Acute effects of sitting isometric yoga (pre-post)	Before to after the final 20-min session	Non-significant
		Serum biomarkers (IL-6, prolactin, Free carnitine, total carnitine, acylcarnitine)	Acute effects of sitting isometric yoga (pre-post)	Before to after the final 20-min session	Non-significant
		Plasma biomarkers (Transforming growth factor-beta1; Brain-derived Neurotrophic factor, Homovanillic acid, 3-methoxy-4-hydroxyphenylglycol)	Acute effects of sitting isometric yoga (pre-post)	Before to after the final 20-min session	Non-significant

Table A3. Cont.

Intervention Type	First Author, Year	Outcome (Assessed by)	Comparison Groups	Comparison Time Point	p-Value
	Report 2 (2019)	Autonomic function tests, serum, and blood biomarkers	Longitudinal effects of sitting isometric yoga (pre-post)	Post intervention (2 months)	Non-significant
		Anxiety (HADS)	Seated isometric yoga compared to controls	Time X group **	0.786
		Depression (HADS)	Seated isometric yoga compared to controls	Time X group **	0.008
		Alexithymia (TAS-20)	Seated isometric yoga compared to controls	Time X group **	0.950

BMSWBI-S: Body-Mind-Spirit Well-being Inventory, ChFS: Chalder's Fatigue Scale, HADS: Hospital Anxiety and Depression Scale, MCT: Multi-convergent therapy, MOS SF-12: Medical Outcomes Study 12- Item Short-Form Health Survey, POMS: Profile of Mood States, PSQI: Pittsburgh Sleep Quality Index, SF-8: Medical Outcomes Study Short Form 8, QOLI: Quality of life inventory, MFI-20: Multidimensional fatigue inventory-20, ACT: Acceptance and commitment therapy, MBCT: Mindfulness-based cognitive therapy, CBSM: Cognitive-based stress management, TAS: 20-item Toronto alexithymia scale. ** to test the interaction effect of time and group.

Table A4. Statistically insignificant outcomes in the included studies using Oxford criteria for diagnosing CFS.

Intervention Type	First Author, Year		Outcome (Assessed by)	Comparison Groups	Comparison Time Point	p-Value
Mindfulness and cognitive-based	Surawy, Ch., 2005 [29]	Study 1 (RCT)	Depression (HADS)	MBSR/MBCT compared to controls	Post treatment (8 weeks)	0.28
			Fatigue score (ChFS)	MBSR/MBCT compared to controls	Post treatment (8 weeks)	0.08
		Study 2 (single-arm experimental study)	Depression (HADS)	MBCT/MBSR (pre-post)	Post treatment (8 weeks)	0.16
			Fatigue score (ChFS)	MBCT/MBSR (pre-post)	Post treatment (8 weeks)	0.06
			Quality of life: physical functioning (SF-36)	MBCT/MBSR (pre-post)	Post treatment (8 weeks)	0.69

Table A4. Cont.

Intervention Type	First Author, Year	Outcome (Assessed by)	Comparison Groups	Comparison Time Point	p-Value
	Rimes, K., 2013 [30]	Mindfulness (5 facet mindfulness questionnaire)	MBCT compared to waitlist	Post treatment (8 weeks)	0.067
		Catastrophizing (Self-reporting scale)	MBCT compared to waitlist	Post follow-up (2 months)	0.152
		All-or-nothing behavior (Self-reporting scale)	MBCT compared to waitlist	Post follow-up (2 months)	0.089
		Depression (HADS)	MBCT compared to waitlist	Post follow-up (2 months)	0.153
		Anxiety (HADS)	MBCT compared to waitlist	Post treatment (8 weeks)	0.173
		Anxiety (HADS)	MBCT compared to waitlist	Post follow-up (2 months)	0.296
		Quality of life: physical functioning (SF-36)	MBCT compared to waitlist	Post treatment (8 weeks)	0.124
		Quality of life: physical functioning (SF-36)	MBCT compared to waitlist	Post follow-up (2 months)	0.345
		Impairment (The work and social adjustment scale)	MBCT compared to waitlist	Post follow-up (2 months)	0.054
		Fatigue (ChFS)	MBCT (pre-post)	Between 2- and 6-month follow-up	0.089
		Depression (HADS)	MBCT (pre-post)	Between 2- and 6-month follow-up	0.069
		Catastrophizing (Self-reporting scale)	MBCT (pre-post)	Between 2- and 6-month follow-up	0.063
		All-or-nothing behavior (Self-reporting scale)	MBCT (pre-post)	Between 2- and 6-month follow-up	0.082
		Self-Compassion (Self-reporting scale)	MBCT (pre-post)	Between 2- and 6-month follow-up	0.110
		Anxiety (HADS)	MBCT (pre-post)	Between 2- and 6-month follow-up	0.211
		Quality of life: physical functioning (SF-36)	MBCT (pre-post)	Between 2- and 6-month follow-up	0.164
		Beliefs about Emotions (Self-reporting scale)	MBCT (pre-post)	Between 2- and 6-month follow-up	0.84
		Quality of life: physical functioning (SF-36)	MBCT (pre-post)	Post follow-up (6 months)	0.051
		Depression (HADS)	MBCT (pre-post)	Post follow-up (6 months)	0.051
		Anxiety (HADS)	MBCT (pre-post)	Post follow-up (6 months)	0.206

ChFS: Chalder's Fatigue Scale, HADS: Hospital Anxiety and Depression Scale, MBSR: Mindfulness-based stress reduction, MBCT: Mindfulness-based cognitive therapy, SF-36: 36- Item Short-Form Health Survey.

Table A5. Risk of Bias (ROBINS-I).

Domains	Bogaerts 2007	Surawy 2005 Study 2	Surawy 2005 Study 3	Sollie 2017	Oka 2018 and 2019	Jonsjo 2019	Takakura 2019
Confounding	No information	No information	No information	Low	Low	Low	Low
Selection bias	Low	Serious	Serious	Low	Moderate	Low	Low
Measurement of intervention	Low	Low	Low	Low	Low	Low	Low
Deviation from the intended intervention	Low	Low	Low	Low	Low	Low	Low
Missing data	Low	Low	Low	Low	Low	Low	Low
Measurement of outcomes	Moderate	Serious	Serious	Moderate	Moderate	Moderate	Moderate
Reported results	No information	No information	No information	Low	Low	Low	Low
Overall	Moderate	Serious	Serious	Moderate	Moderate	Moderate	Moderate

Low risk of bias (the study is comparable to a well-performed randomized trial with regard to this domain), Moderate risk of bias (the study is sound for a nonrandomized study with regard to this domain but cannot be considered comparable to a well-performed randomized trial), Serious risk of bias (the study has some important problems).

Table A6. Brief descriptions of mind-body interventions used in the included studies.

MBIs	Definition
Relaxation therapies	https://www.nccih.nih.gov/health/relaxation-techniques-for-health (accessed on 13 June 2021). "Relaxation techniques include a number of practices such as progressive relaxation, guided imagery, biofeedback, self-hypnosis, and deep breathing exercises. The goal is similar in all: to produce the body's natural relaxation response, characterized by slower breathing, lower blood pressure, and a feeling of increased well-being".
Movement-based interventions	https://www.nccih.nih.gov/health/yoga-what-you-need-to-know (accessed on 13 June 2021). "Although classical yoga also includes other elements, yoga as practiced in the United States typically emphasizes physical postures (asanas), breathing techniques (pranayama), and meditation (dyana). There are many different yoga styles, ranging from gentle practices to physically demanding ones. Differences in the types of yoga used in research studies may affect study results. This makes it challenging to evaluate research on the health effects of yoga. Yoga and two practices of Chinese origin—tai chi and qi gong—are sometimes called "meditative movement" practices. All three practices include both meditative elements and physical ones".
	https://www.nccih.nih.gov/health/tai-chi-and-qi-gong-in-depth (accessed on 13 June 2021). "Tai chi and qi gong are centuries-old practices that involve certain postures and gentle movements with mental focus, breathing, and relaxation. The movements can be adapted or practiced while walking, standing, or sitting. In contrast to qi gong, tai chi movements, if practiced quickly, can be a form of combat or self-defense".

Table A6. *Cont.*

MBIs	Definition
Mindfulness and cognitive-based	Mindfulness-based stress reduction (MBSR): "The program is conducted as an 8- to 10-week course for groups of up to 30 participants who meet weekly for 2—2.5 hr for instruction and practice in mindfulness meditation skills, together with a discussion of stress, coping, and homework assignments". [1]
	Mindfulness-based cognitive therapy (MBCT): "MBCT incorporates elements of cognitive therapy that facilitate a detached or de-centered view of one's thoughts, including statements such as "thoughts are not facts" and "I am not my thoughts." This decentered approach also is applied to emotions and bodily sensations". [1]
	Cognitive-behavioral stress management (CBSM) is based on cognitive restructuring: "CBSM interventions reduce distress by teaching relaxation techniques; modifying patients' outlook, cognitive appraisals, and coping strategies; and when performed in a group format may also improve their perceptions of social support". [2]
	Acceptance commitment therapy (ACT) is based on psychological flexibility. "This is defined as the ability to act in line with important long-term goals or values in life, even in the presence of negative experiences (e.g., non-acute somatic symptoms or psychological distress). Psychological flexibility is a complex overarching behavioral construct that includes several behavioral processes such as acceptance/non-acceptance and cognitive fusion/diffusion". [3]

[1] Baer RA. Mindfulness training as a clinical intervention: A conceptual and empirical review. Clinical psychology: Science and practice. June 2003, 10,125–143. [2] Lopez C, Antoni M, Penedo F, Weiss D, Cruess S, Segotas M-C, et al. A pilot study of cognitive-behavioral stress management effects on stress, quality of life, and symptoms in persons with chronic fatigue syndrome. Journal of psychosomatic research. 2011, 70, 328–334. [3] Jonsjö MA, Wicksell RK, Holmström L, Andreasson A, Olsson GL. Acceptance and commitment therapy for ME/CFS (Chronic Fatigue Syndrome)–a feasibility study. Journal of Contextual Behavioral Science. 2019, 12, 89–97.

Appendix B

Medline Search Strategy

1. Fatigue Syndrome, Chronic/
2. Myalgic Encephalomyelitis.mp.
3. exp Encephalomyelitis/
4. Fatigue/
5. 3 and 4
6. 1 or 2 or 5
7. (chronic$ adj3 fatig$ adj3 syndrom$).mp.
8. (myalg$ adj3 encephal$).mp.
9. 6 or 7 or 8
10. exp Mind-Body Therapies/
11. exp Biofeedback, Psychology/
12. exp Neurofeedback/
13. exp "Imagery (Psychotherapy)"/
14. exp Hypnosis/
15. exp Relaxation Therapy/
16. exp Mindfulness/
17. exp Meditation/
18. exp Yoga/
19. exp Tai Ji/
20. (Mindfulness-based adj2 cognitive adj2 therapy).mp.
21. self-hypnosis.mp.
22. Guided imagery.mp.
23. exp Art Therapy/
24. mindfulness-based stress reduction.mp.

25. guided meditation.mp.
26. exp Autogenic Training/
27. (progressive adj2 muscle adj2 relaxation).mp.
28. exp Breathing Exercises/
29. Chi Gong.mp.
30. exp Qigong/
31. Psychological flexibility.mp.
32. Relaxation Response.mp.
33. exp Spirituality/
34. Mindful meditation.mp.
35. Mantra.mp.
36. Transcendental Meditation.ti,ab.
37. Mindfulness-based cognitive therapy.ti,ab.
38. Prayer.ti,ab.
39. Visualization.ti,ab.
40. Neurolinguistic programming.ti,ab.
41. Cognitive restructuring.ti,ab.
42. exp Music Therapy/
43. (Eye movement desensitization and reprocessing).ti,ab.
44. Emotional Freedom Techniques.ti,ab.
45. Dynamic Neural Retraining System.ti,ab.
46. or/10–45
47. 9 and 46
48. limit 47 to English language

References

1. Institute of Medicine. *Beyond Myalgic Encephalomyelitis/Chronic Fatigue Syndrome: Redefining an Illness, Committe on the Diagnosis for ME/CFS.*; The National Academies Pres: Washington, DC, USA, 2015.
2. Johnston, S.; Brenu, E.W.; Staines, D.; Marshall-Gradisnik, S. The prevalence of chronic fatigue syndrome/myalgic encephalomyelitis: A meta-analysis. *Clin. Epidemiol.* **2013**, *5*, 105–110. [CrossRef] [PubMed]
3. Rusu, C.; Gee, M.E.; Lagacé, C.; Parlor, M. Chronic fatigue syndrome and fibromyalgia in Canada: Prevalence and associations with six health status indicators. *Chronic Dis. Inj. Can.* **2015**, *35*, 1678508400. [CrossRef]
4. Jason, L.A.; Richman, J.A.; Rademaker, A.W.; Jordan, K.M.; Plioplys, A.V.; Taylor, R.R.; McCready, W.; Huang, C.F.; Plioplys, S. A community-based study of chronic fatigue syndrome. *Arch. Intern. Med.* **1999**, *159*, 2129–2137. [CrossRef] [PubMed]
5. Hvidberg, M.F.; Brinth, L.S.; Olesen, A.V.; Petersen, K.D.; Ehlers, L. The Health-Related Quality of Life for Patients with Myalgic Encephalomyelitis/Chronic Fatigue Syndrome (ME/CFS). *PLoS ONE* **2015**, *10*, e0132421. [CrossRef]
6. Nacul, L.C.; Lacerda, E.M.; Campion, P.; Pheby, D.; Drachler, M.d.L.; Leite, J.C.; Poland, F.; Howe, A.; Fayyaz, S.; Molokhia, M. The functional status and well being of people with myalgic encephalomyelitis/chronic fatigue syndrome and their carers. *BMC Public Health* **2011**, *11*, 402. [CrossRef] [PubMed]
7. Bombardier, C.H.; Buchwald, D. Chronic fatigue, chronic fatigue syndrome, and fibromyalgia. Disability and health-care use. *Med. Care* **1996**, *34*, 924–930. [CrossRef] [PubMed]
8. Reynolds, K.J.; Vernon, S.D.; Bouchery, E.; Reeves, W.C. The economic impact of chronic fatigue syndrome. *Cost Eff. Resour. Alloc.* **2004**, *2*, 1–4. [CrossRef]
9. Centers for Diseases Control and Prevention. Chronic Fatigue Syndrome Awareness Day: CDC. 2018. Available online: http://www.cdc.gov/Features/cfsawarenessday/ (accessed on 21 August 2018).
10. Takakura, S.; Oka, T.; Sudo, N. Changes in circulating microRNA after recumbent isometric yoga practice by patients with myalgic encephalomyelitis/chronic fatigue syndrome: An explorative pilot study. *Bio. Psycho. Soc. Med.* **2019**, *13*, 1–10. [CrossRef] [PubMed]
11. Missailidis, D.; Annesley, S.J.; Fisher, P.R. Pathological mechanisms underlying myalgic encephalomyelitis/chronic fatigue syndrome. *Diagnostics* **2019**, *9*, 80. [CrossRef] [PubMed]
12. Maksoud, R.; du Preez, S.; Eaton-Fitch, N.; Thapaliya, K.; Barnden, L.; Cabanas, H.; Staines, D.; Marshall-Gradisnik, S. A systematic review of neurological impairments in myalgic encephalomyelitis/chronic fatigue syndrome using neuroimaging techniques. *PLoS ONE* **2020**, *15*, e0232475. [CrossRef]

13. Haney, E.; Smith, M.E.B.; McDonagh, M.; Pappas, M.; Daeges, M.; Wasson, N.; Nelson, H.D. Diagnostic Methods for Myalgic Encephalomyelitis/Chronic Fatigue Syndrome: A Systematic Review for a National Institutes of Health Pathways to Prevention WorkshopDiagnostic Methods for Myalgic Encephalomyelitis/Chronic Fatigue Syndrome. *Ann. Intern. Med.* **2015**, *162*, 834–840. [CrossRef]
14. Smith, M.; Nelson, H.D.; Haney, E.; Pappas, M.; Daeges, M.; Wasson, N.; McDonagh, M. Diagnosis and Treatment of Myalgic Encephalomyelitis/Chronic Fatigue Syndrome. Agency for Healthcare Research and Quality Evidence Report/Technology Assessment No 219 (Prepared by the Pacific Northwest Evidence-based Practice Center under Contract No 290-2012-00014-I) Rockville, MD: AHRQ Publication No. 15-E001-EF. Available online: www.effectivehealthcare.ahrq.gov/reports/final.cfm (accessed on 20 June 2021).
15. Holgate, S.T.; Komaroff, A.L.; Mangan, D.; Wessely, S. Chronic fatigue syndrome: Understanding a complex illness. *Nat. Rev. Neurosci.* **2011**, *12*, 539–544. [CrossRef] [PubMed]
16. Acheson, E.D. The clinical syndrome variously called benign myalgic encephalomyelitis, Iceland disease and epidemic neuromyasthenia. *Am. J. Med.* **1959**, *26*, 569–595. [CrossRef]
17. Holmes, G.P.; Kaplan, J.E.; Gantz, N.M.; Komaroff, A.L.; Schonberger, L.B.; Straus, S.E.; Jones, J.F.; Dubois, R.E.; Cunningham-Rundles, C.; Pahwa, S.; et al. Chronic Fatigue Syndrome: A Working Case Definition. *Ann. Intern. Med.* **1988**, *108*, 387–389. [CrossRef] [PubMed]
18. Jason, L.A.; Brown, A.; Evans, M.; Sunnquist, M.; Newton, J.L. Contrasting Chronic Fatigue Syndrome versus Myalgic Encephalomyelitis/Chronic Fatigue Syndrome. *Fatigue: Biomedicine, health & behavior. Ann. Intern. Med.* **2013**, *1*, 168–183. [CrossRef]
19. Smith, M.E.B.; Haney, E.; McDonagh, M.; Pappas, M.; Daeges, M.; Wasson, N.; Fu, R.; Nelson, H.D. Treatment of Myalgic Encephalomyelitis/Chronic Fatigue Syndrome: A Systematic Review for a National Institutes of Health Pathways to Prevention WorkshopTreatment of Myalgic Encephalomyelitis/Chronic Fatigue Syndrome. *Ann. Intern. Med.* **2015**, *162*, 841–850. [CrossRef]
20. Toward Optimal Practice. *Identification and Symptom Management of ME/CFS.*; Clinical Practice Guideline: Calgary, AB, Canada, 2016.
21. McCrone, P.; Darbishire, L.; Ridsdale, L.; Seed, P. The economic cost of chronic fatigue and chronic fatigue syndrome in UK primary care. *Psychol. Med.* **2003**, *33*, 253–261. [CrossRef] [PubMed]
22. Price, J.R.; Mitchell, E.; Tidy, E.; Hunot, V. Cognitive behaviour therapy for chronic fatigue syndrome in adults. *Cochrane Database Syst. Rev.* **2008**. [CrossRef]
23. Larun, L.; Brurberg, K.G.; Odgaard-Jensen, J.; Price, J.R. Exercise therapy for chronic fatigue syndrome. *Cochrane Database Syst. Rev.* **2015**. [CrossRef]
24. Wahbeh, H.; Elsas, S.-M.; Oken, B.S. Mind–body interventions: Applications in neurology. *Neurology* **2008**, *70*, 2321–2328. [CrossRef] [PubMed]
25. Gupta, A. Can amygdala retraining techniques improve the wellbeing of patients with chronic fatigue syndrome. *J. Holist. Healthc.* **2010**, *7*, 12–15.
26. Vitetta, L.; Anton, B.; Cortizo, F.; Sali, A. Mind-body medicine: Stress and its impact on overall health and longevity. *Ann. N. Y. Acad. Sci.* **2005**, *1057*, 492–505. [CrossRef]
27. Theadom, A.; Cropley, M.; Smith, H.E.; Feigin, V.L.; McPherson, K. Mind and body therapy for fibromyalgia. *Cochrane Database Syst. Rev.* **2015**, *1057*, 492–505. [CrossRef] [PubMed]
28. Oka, T.; Tanahashi, T.; Chijiwa, T.; Lkhagvasuren, B.; Sudo, N.; Oka, K. Isometric yoga improves the fatigue and pain of patients with chronic fatigue syndrome who are resistant to conventional therapy: A randomized, controlled trial. *BioPsychoSocial Med.* **2014**, *8*, 1–9. [CrossRef]
29. Surawy, C.; Roberts, J.; Silver, A. The Effect of Mindfulness Training on Mood and Measures of Fatigue, Activity, and Quality of Life in Patients with Chronic Fatigue Syndrome on a Hospital Waiting List: A Series of Exploratory Studies. *Behav. Cogn. Psychother.* **2005**, *33*, 103–109. [CrossRef]
30. Rimes, K.A.; Wingrove, J. Mindfulness-Based Cognitive Therapy for People with Chronic Fatigue Syndrome Still Experiencing Excessive Fatigue after Cognitive Behaviour Therapy: A Pilot Randomized Study. *Clin. Psychol. Psychother.* **2013**, *20*, 107–117. [CrossRef] [PubMed]
31. Collinge, W.; Yarnold, P.R.; Raskin, E. Use of mind/body selfhealing practice predicts positive health transition in chronic fatigue syndrome: A controlled study. *Subtle Energ. Energy Med. J. Arch.* **1998**, *9*, 107–117.
32. Dybwad, M.; Frøslie, K.; Stanghelle, J. *Work Capacity, Fatigue and Health Related Quality of Life in Patients with Myalgic Encephalopathy or Chronic Fatigue Syndrome, before and after Qigong Therapy, a Randomized Controlled Study*; Sunnaas Rehabilitation Hospital: Nesoddtangen, Norway, 2007.
33. Moher, D.; Hopewell, S.; Schulz, K.F.; Montori, V.; Gotzsche, P.C.; Devereaux, P.J.; Elbourne, D.; Egger, M.; Altman, D.G.; Consolidated Standards of Reporting Trials Group. CONSORT 2010 Explanation and Elaboration: Updated guidelines for reporting parallel group randomised trials. *J. Clin. Epidemiol.* **2010**, *63*, e1-37. [CrossRef] [PubMed]
34. Higgins, J.P.T.; Altman, D.G.; Gøtzsche, P.C.; Júni, P.; Moher, D.; Oxman, A.D.; Savović, J.; Schulz, K.F.; Weeks, L.; Sterne, J.A. The Cochrane Collaboration's tool for assessing risk of bias in randomised trials. *BMJ* **2011**, *343*, d5928. [CrossRef]

35. Sterne, J.A.; Hernán, M.A.; Reeves, B.C.; Savović, J.; Berkman, N.D.; Viswanathan, M.; Henry, D.; Altman, D.G.; Ansari, M.T.; Boutron, I.; et al. ROBINS-I: A tool for assessing risk of bias in non-randomised studies of interventions. *BMJ* **2016**, *355*, i4919. [CrossRef]
36. Domecq, J.P.; Prutsky, G.; Elraiyah, T.; Wang, Z.; Nabhan, M.; Shippee, N.; Brito, J.P.; Boehmer, K.; Hasan, R.; Firwana, B.; et al. Patient engagement in research: A systematic review. *BMC Health Serv. Res.* **2014**, *14*, 89. [CrossRef]
37. Pollock, A.; Campbell, P.; Struthers, C.; Synnot, A.; Nunn, J.; Hill, S.; Goodare, H.; Morris, J.; Watts, C.; Morley, R. Stakeholder involvement in systematic reviews: A scoping review. *Syst. Rev.* **2018**, *7*, 208. [CrossRef] [PubMed]
38. Bogaerts, K.; Hubin, M.; Van Diest, I.; De Peuter, S.; Van Houdenhove, B.; Van Wambeke, P.; Crombez, G.; Van den Bergh, O. Hyperventilation in patients with chronic fatigue syndrome: The role of coping strategies. *Behav. Res. Ther.* **2007**, *45*, 2679–2690. [CrossRef] [PubMed]
39. Thomas, M.A.; Sadlier, M.J.; Smith, A.P. A multiconvergent approach to the rehabilitation of patients with chronic fatigue syndrome: A comparative study. *Physiotherap* **2008**, *94*, 35–42. [CrossRef]
40. Chan, J.S.; Ho, R.T.; Chung, K.-F.; Wang, C.-W.; Yao, T.-J.; Ng, S.-M.; Chan, C.L. Qigong exercise alleviates fatigue, anxiety, and depressive symptoms, improves sleep quality, and shortens sleep latency in persons with chronic fatigue syndrome-like illness. *Evid. Based Complementary Altern. Med.* **2014**, *2014*, 106048. [CrossRef]
41. Chan, J.S.; Ho, R.T.; Wang, C.-W.; Yuen, L.P.; Sham, J.S.; Chan, C.L. Effects of qigong exercise on fatigue, anxiety, and depressive symptoms of patients with chronic fatigue syndrome-like illness: A randomized controlled trial. *Evid. Based Complementary Altern. Med.* **2013**, *2013*, 1–8. [CrossRef]
42. Oka, T.; Tanahashi, T.; Sudo, N.; Lkhagvasuren, B.; Yamada, Y. Changes in fatigue, autonomic functions, and blood biomarkers due to sitting isometric yoga in patients with chronic fatigue syndrome. *BioPsychoSocial Med.* **2018**, *12*, 3. [CrossRef] [PubMed]
43. Sollie, K.; Næss, E.T.; Solhaug, I.; Thimm, J. Mindfulness training for chronic fatigue syndrome: A pilot study. *Health Psychol. Rep.* **2017**, *3*, 240–250. [CrossRef]
44. Jonsjö, M.A.; Wicksell, R.K.; Holmström, L.; Andreasson, A.; Olsson, G.L. Acceptance & commitment therapy for ME/CFS (Chronic Fatigue Syndrome)–a feasibility study. *J. Contextual Behav. Sci.* **2019**, *12*, 89–97.
45. Lopez, C.; Antoni, M.; Penedo, F.; Weiss, D.; Cruess, S.; Segotas, M.-C.; Helder, L.; Siegel, S.; Klimas, N.; Fletcher, M.A. A pilot study of cognitive behavioral stress management effects on stress, quality of life, and symptoms in persons with chronic fatigue syndrome. *J. Psychosom. Res.* **2011**, *70*, 328–334. [CrossRef] [PubMed]
46. Sharpe, M.C.; Archard, L.C.; Banatvala, J.E.; Borysiewicz, L.K.; Clare, A.W.; David, A.; Edwards, R.H.; Hawton, K.E.; Lambert, H.P.; Lane, R.J. A report—Chronic fatigue syndrome: Guidelines for research. *J. R. Soc. Med.* **1991**, *84*, 118–121. [CrossRef]
47. Zigmond, A.S.; Snaith, R.P. The hospital anxiety and depression scale. *Acta Psychiatr. Scand.* **1983**, *67*, 361–370. [CrossRef] [PubMed]
48. Chalder, T.; Berelowitz, G.; Pawlikowska, T.; Watts, L.; Wessely, S.; Wright, D.; Wallace, E.P. Development of a fatigue scale. *J. Psychosom. Res.* **1993**, *37*. [CrossRef]
49. Ware, J.E., Jr.; Sherbourne, C.D. The MOS 36-item short-form health survey (SF-36): I. Conceptual framework and item selection. *Med. Care* **1992**, *30*, 473–483. [CrossRef] [PubMed]
50. Fisk, J.D.; Ritvo, P.G.; Ross, L.; Haase, D.A.; Marrie, T.J.; Schlech, W.F. Measuring the functional impact of fatigue: Initial validation of the fatigue impact scale. *Clin. Infect. Dis.* **1994**, *18* (Suppl. 1), S79–S83. [CrossRef]
51. Thomas, M.; Sadlier, M.; Smith, A. The effect of Multi Convergent Therapy on the psychopathology, mood and performance of Chronic Fatigue Syndrome patients: A preliminary study. *Couns. Psychother. Res.* **2006**, *6*, 91–99. [CrossRef]
52. Fukuda, K.; Straus, S.E.; Hickie, I.; Sharpe, M.C.; Dobbins, J.G.; Komaroff, A. The Chronic Fatigue Syndrome: A Comprehensive Approach to Its Definition and Study. *Ann. Intern. Med.* **1994**, *121*, 953–959. [CrossRef] [PubMed]
53. Beck, A.T.; Ward, C.H.; Mendelson, M.; Mock, J.; Erbaugh, J. An inventory for measuring depression. *Arch. Gen. Psychiatry* **1961**, *4*, 561–571. [CrossRef]
54. Radloff, L. The center for epidemiologic studies depression index. *Appl. Psychol. Meas.* **1977**, *1*, 385–401. [CrossRef]
55. Broadbent, D.E.; Cooper, P.F.; FitzGerald, P.; Parkes, K.R. The cognitive failures questionnaire (CFQ) and its correlates. *Br. J. Clin. Psychol.* **1982**, *21*, 1–16. [CrossRef] [PubMed]
56. Cohen, S.; Hoberman, H.M. Positive events and social supports as buffers of life change stress1. *J. Appl. Soc. Psychol.* **1983**, *13*, 99–125. [CrossRef]
57. Smith, A.; Pollock, J.; Thomas, M.; Llewelyn, M.; Borysiewicz, L. The relationship between subjective ratings of sleep and mental functioning in healthy subjects and patients with chronic fatigue syndrome. *Hum. Psychopharmacol. Clin. Exp.* **1996**, *11*, 161–167. [CrossRef]
58. Marks, I.M. *Behavioural Psychotherapy: Maudsley Pocket Book of Clinical Management*; Wright/IOP Publishing: Bristol, UK, 1986.
59. Zevon, M.A.; Tellegen, A. The structure of mood change: An idiographic/nomothetic analysis. *J. Personal. Soc. Psychol.* **1982**, *43*, 111. [CrossRef]
60. Ray, C.; Weir, W.; Stewart, D.; Miller, P.; Hyde, G. Ways of coping with chronic fatigue syndrome: Development of an illness management questionnaire. *Soc. Sci. Med.* **1993**, *37*, 385–391. [CrossRef]
61. Karnofsky, D.; Abelmann, W.; Craver, L. The use of the nitrogen mustards in the palliative treatment of carcinoma. With particular reference to bronchogenic carcinoma. *Cancer* **1948**, *1*, 634–656. [CrossRef]

62. Watson, D.; Clark, L.A.; Tellegen, A. Development and validation of brief measures of positive and negative affect: The PANAS scales. *J. Personal. Soc. Psychol.* **1988**, *54*, 1063. [CrossRef]
63. Wientjes, C.J.; Grossman, P. Overreactivity of the psyche or the soma? Interindividual associations between psychosomatic symptoms, anxiety, heart rate, and end-tidal partial carbon dioxide pressure. *Psychosom. Med.* **1994**, *56*, 533–540. [CrossRef]
64. Meyer, T.J.; Miller, M.L.; Metzger, R.L.; Borkovec, T.D. Development and validation of the Penn State Worry Questionnaire. *Behav. Res. Ther.* **1990**, *28*, 487–495. [CrossRef]
65. Bradley, M.M.; Lang, P.J. Measuring emotion: The self-assessment manikin and the semantic differential. *J. Behav. Ther. Exp. Psychiatry* **1994**, *25*, 49–59. [CrossRef]
66. Cohen, S.; Kamarck, T.; Mermelstein, R. A global measure of perceived stress. *J. Health Soc. Behav.* **1983**, *24*, 385–396. [CrossRef]
67. McNair, D.; Lorr, M.; DroppLemn, L. *Manual for the Profile of Mood States (POMS)*; Educational and Industrial Testing Service: San Diego, CA, USA, 1971.
68. Frisch, M.B. *Quality of Life Inventory (QOLI)*; National Computer Systems: Minneapolis, MN, USA, 1994.
69. Wagner, D.; Nisenbaum, R.; Heim, C.; Jones, J.F.; Unger, E.R.; Reeves, W.C. Psychometric properties of the CDC symptom inventory for assessment of Chronic Fatigue Syndrome. *Popul. Health Metr.* **2005**, *3*. [CrossRef] [PubMed]
70. Ho, R.T.; Chan, J.S.; Wang, C.-W.; Lau, B.W.; So, K.F.; Yuen, L.P.; Sham, J.S.; Chan, C.L. A randomized controlled trial of qigong exercise on fatigue symptoms, functioning, and telomerase activity in persons with chronic fatigue or chronic fatigue syndrome. *Ann. Behav. Med.* **2012**, *44*, 160–170. [CrossRef]
71. Li, J.; Chan, J.S.; Chow, A.Y.; Yuen, L.P.; Chan, C.L. From body to mind and spirit: Qigong exercise for bereaved persons with chronic fatigue syndrome-like illness. *Evid. Based Complementary Altern. Med.* **2015**, *2015*, 1–7. [CrossRef]
72. Wong, W.S.; Fielding, R. Construct validity of the Chinese version of the Chalder Fatigue Scale in a Chinese community sample. *J. Psychosom. Res.* **2010**, *68*, 89–93. [CrossRef] [PubMed]
73. Leung, C.; Wing, Y.; Kwong, P.; Shum, A.L.K. Validation of the Chinese-Cantonese version of the Hospital Anxiety and Depression Scale and comparison with the Hamilton Rating Scale of Depression. *Acta Psychiatr. Scand.* **1999**, *100*, 456–461. [CrossRef]
74. Ware, J.E., Jr.; Kosinski, M.; Keller, S.D. A 12-Item Short-Form Health Survey: Construction of scales and preliminary tests of reliability and validity. *Med. Care* **1996**, *34*, 220–233. [CrossRef]
75. Lam, C.L.; Eileen, Y.; Gandek, B. Is the standard SF-12 health survey valid and equivalent for a Chinese population? *Qual. Life Res.* **2005**, *14*, 539–547. [CrossRef] [PubMed]
76. Ng, S.; Yau, J.K.; Chan, C.L.; Chan, C.H.; Ho, D.Y. The measurement of body-mind-spirit well-being: Toward multidimensionality and transcultural applicability. *Soc. Work Health Care* **2005**, *41*, 33–52. [CrossRef]
77. Mundt, J.C.; Marks, I.M.; Shear, M.K.; Greist, J.M. The Work and Social Adjustment Scale: A simple measure of impairment in functioning. *Br. J. Psychiatry* **2002**, *180*, 461–464. [CrossRef]
78. Stewart, A.L.; Hays, R.D.; Ware, J.E. The MOS short-form general health survey: Reliability and validity in a patient population. *Med. Care* **1988**, *26*, 724–735. [CrossRef]
79. McHorney, C.A.; Ware, J.E., Jr.; Lu, J.R.; Sherbourne, C.D. The MOS 36-item Short-Form Health Survey (SF-36): III. Tests of data quality, scaling assumptions, and reliability across diverse patient groups. *Med. Care* **1994**, *32*, 40–66. [CrossRef]
80. Rimes, K.A.; Chalder, T. The Beliefs about Emotions Scale: Validity, reliability and sensitivity to change. *J. Psychosom. Res.* **2010**, *68*, 285–292. [CrossRef]
81. Neff, K.D. The development and validation of a scale to measure self-compassion. *Self Identity* **2003**, *2*, 223–250. [CrossRef]
82. Baer, R.A.; Smith, G.T.; Hopkins, J.; Krietemeyer, J.; Toney, L. Using self-report assessment methods to explore facets of mindfulness. *Assessment* **2006**, *13*, 27–45. [CrossRef]
83. Chan, J.S.; Li, A.; Ng, S.-M.; Ho, R.T.; Xu, A.; Yao, T.-J.; Wang, X.M.; So, K.F.; Chan, C.L. Adiponectin potentially contributes to the antidepressive effects of Baduanjin Qigong exercise in women with chronic fatigue syndrome-like illness. *Cell Transpl.* **2017**, *26*, 493–501. [CrossRef]
84. Buysse, D.J.; Reynolds, C.F., III; Monk, T.H.; Berman, S.R.; Kupfer, D.J. The Pittsburgh Sleep Quality Index: A new instrument for psychiatric practice and research. *Psychiatry Res.* **1989**, *28*, 193–213. [CrossRef]
85. Chong, A.M.; Cheung, C.-K. Factor structure of a Cantonese-version Pittsburgh Sleep Quality Index. *Sleep Biol. Rhythms.* **2012**, *10*, 118–125. [CrossRef]
86. Ho, R.T.; Fong, T.C. Factor structure of the Chinese version of the Pittsburgh Sleep Quality Index in breast cancer patients. *Sleep Med.* **2014**, *15*, 565–569. [CrossRef]
87. Fukuhara, S.; Suzukamo, Y. Manual of the SF-8 Japanese version. Kyoto: Institute for Health Outcomes & Process Evaluation Research. *Environ. Health Prev. Med.* **2011**, *16*, 97–105.
88. Carruthers, B.M.; Jain, A.K.; De Meirleir, K.L.; Peterson, D.L.; Klimas, N.G.; Lerner, A.M.; Bested, A.C.; Flor-Henry, P.; Joshi, P.; Powles, A.P.; et al. Myalgic Encephalomyelitis/Chronic Fatigue Syndrome. *J. Chronic Fatigue Syndr.* **2003**, *11*, 7–115. [CrossRef]
89. Nolen-Hoeksema, S.; Morrow, J. A prospective study of depression and posttraumatic stress symptoms after a natural disaster: The 1989 Loma Prieta Earthquake. *J. Personal. Soc. Psychol.* **1991**, *61*, 115. [CrossRef]
90. Diener, E.; Emmons, R.A.; Larsen, R.J.; Griffin, S. The life satisfaction scale. *J. Personal. Assess.* **1985**, *49*, 71–75. [CrossRef] [PubMed]

91. Oka, T.; Tanahashi, T.; Lkhagvasuren, B.; Yamada, Y. The longitudinal effects of seated isometric yoga on blood biomarkers, autonomic functions, and psychological parameters of patients with chronic fatigue syndrome: A pilot study. *BioPsychoSocial Med.* **2019**, *13*, 1–13. [CrossRef] [PubMed]
92. Carruthers, B.M.; van de Sande, M.I.; De Meirleir, K.L.; Klimas, N.G.; Broderick, G.; Mitchell, T.; Staines, D.; Powles, A.P.; Speight, N.; Vallings, R.; et al. Myalgic encephalomyelitis: International Consensus Criteria. *J. Intern. Med.* **2011**, *270*, 327–338. [CrossRef] [PubMed]
93. Komaki, G. The reliability and factorial validity of the Japanese version of the 20-item Toronto Alexithymia Scale. *J. Psychosom. Res.* **2003**, *55*, 143. [CrossRef]
94. Tait, R.C.; Pollard, C.A.; Margolis, R.B.; Duckro, P.N.; Krause, S.J. The Pain Disability Index: Psychometric and validity data. *Arch. Phys. Med. Rehabil.* **1987**, *68*, 438–441.
95. Wicksell, R.K.; Renöfält, J.; Olsson, G.L.; Bond, F.W.; Melin, L. Avoidance and cognitive fusion–central components in pain related disability? Development and preliminary validation of the Psychological Inflexibility in Pain Scale (PIPS). *Eur. J. Pain* **2008**, *12*, 491–500. [CrossRef] [PubMed]
96. Smets, E.; Garssen, B.; Bonke, B.; De Haes, J. The Multidimensional Fatigue Inventory (MFI) psychometric qualities of an instrument to assess fatigue. *J. Psychosom. Res.* **1995**, *39*, 315–325. [CrossRef]
97. Rabin, R.; Charro, F.D. EQ-SD: A measure of health status from the EuroQol Group. *Ann. Med.* **2001**, *33*, 337–343. [CrossRef]
98. Tanaka, M.; Fukuda, S.; Mizuno, K.; Imai-Matsumura, K.; Jodoi, T.; Kawatani, J.; Takano, M.; Miike, T.; Tomoda, A.; Watanabe, Y. Reliability and validity of the Japanese version of the Chalder Fatigue Scale among youth in Japan. *Psychol. Rep.* **2008**, *103*, 682–690. [CrossRef]
99. Jackson, C. The Chalder fatigue scale (CFQ 11). *Occup. Med.* **2015**, *65*, 86. [CrossRef] [PubMed]
100. Hornig, M.; Montoya, J.G.; Klimas, N.G.; Levine, S.; Felsenstein, D.; Bateman, L.; Peterson, D.L.; Gottschalk, C.G.; Schultz, A.F.; Che, X.; et al. Distinct plasma immune signatures in ME/CFS are present early in the course of illness. *Sci. Adv.* **2015**, *1*. [CrossRef] [PubMed]
101. Landi, A.; Broadhurst, D.; Vernon, S.D.; Tyrrell, D.L.J.; Houghton, M. Reductions in circulating levels of IL-16, IL-7 and VEGF-A in myalgic encephalomyelitis/chronic fatigue syndrome. *Cytokine* **2016**, *78*, 27–36. [CrossRef]
102. Maes, M.; Mihaylova, I.; Kubera, M.; Leunis, J.C.; Twisk, F.N.M.; Geffard, M. IgM-mediated autoimmune responses directed against anchorage epitopes are greater in Myalgic Encephalomyelitis/Chronic Fatigue Syndrome (ME/CFS) than in major depression. *Metab. Brain Dis.* **2012**, *27*, 415–423. [CrossRef]
103. Strayer, D.R.; Victoria, S.; William, C. Low NK Cell Activity in Chronic Fatigue Syndrome (CFS) and Relationship to Symptom Severity. *J. Clin. Cell. Immunol.* **2015**, *1*. [CrossRef]
104. Papadopoulos, A.S.; Cleare, A.J. Hypothalamic–pituitary–adrenal axis dysfunction in chronic fatigue syndrome. *Nat. Rev. Endocrinol.* **2011**, *8*. [CrossRef] [PubMed]
105. Gupta, A. Unconscious amygdalar fear conditioning in a subset of chronic fatigue syndrome patients. *Med. Hypotheses* **2002**, *59*, 727–735. [CrossRef]
106. Dowsett, E.; Goudsmit, E.; Macintyre, A.; Shepherd, C. London criteria for ME. In *Report from the National Task Force on Chronic Fatigue Syndrome (CFS), Post Viral Fatigue Syndrome (PVFS), Myalgic Encephalo-myelitis (ME); An Initiative of the Registered Charity Westcare*; Department of Health and with Financial Assistance from the Wellcome Trust: Westcare, UK, 1994; pp. 96–98.
107. Jason, L.; Evans, M.; Porter, N.; Brown, M.; Brown, A.; Hunnell, J.; Biotechnol, A.J. The development of a revised Canadian myalgic encephalomyelitis chronic fatigue syndrome case definition. *Am. J. Biochem. Biotechnol.* **2010**, *6*, 120–135. [CrossRef]

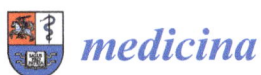

Opinion

The Role of Prevention in Reducing the Economic Impact of ME/CFS in Europe: A Report from the Socioeconomics Working Group of the European Network on ME/CFS (EUROMENE)

Derek F. H. Pheby [1,*], Diana Araja [2], Uldis Berkis [3], Elenka Brenna [4], John Cullinan [5], Jean-Dominique de Korwin [6,7], Lara Gitto [8], Dyfrig A. Hughes [9], Rachael M. Hunter [10], Dominic Trepel [11] and Xia Wang-Steverding [12]

1. Society and Health, Buckinghamshire New University, High Wycombe HP11 2JZ, UK
2. Department of Dosage Form Technology, Faculty of Pharmacy, Riga Stradins University, Dzirciema Street 16, LV-1007 Riga, Latvia; Diana.Araja@rsu.lv
3. Institute of Microbiology and Virology, Riga Stradins University, Dzirciema Street 16, LV-1007 Riga, Latvia; Uldis.Berkis@rsu.lv
4. Department of Economics and Finance, Università Cattolica del Sacro Cuore, Largo Agostino Gemelli 1, 20123 Milan, Italy; elenka.brenna@unicatt.it
5. School of Business & Economics, National University of Ireland Galway, University Road, H91 TK33 Galway, Ireland; john.cullinan@nuigalway.ie
6. Internal Medicine Department, University of Lorraine, 34, Cours Léopold CS 25233, F-54052 Nancy, France; jean-dominique.dekorwin@univ-lorraine.fr
7. University Hospital of Nancy, Rue du Morvan, 54511 Vandoeuvre-Les-Nancy, France
8. Department of Economics, University of Messina, Piazza Pugliatti 1, 98122 Messina, Italy; lara.gitto@unime.it
9. Centre for Health Economics & Medicines Evaluation, Bangor University, Bangor LL57 2PZ, UK; d.a.hughes@bangor.ac.uk
10. Department of Primary Care and Population Health, Royal Free Medical School, University College London, London NW3 2PF, UK; r.hunter@ucl.ac.uk
11. Global Brain Health Institute, School of Medicine, Trinity College Dublin, College Green, D02 PN40 Dublin, Ireland; trepeld@tcd.ie
12. Warwick Medical School, University of Warwick, Coventry CV4 7AL, UK; xiasteverding@gmail.com
* Correspondence: derekpheby@btinternet.com

Abstract: This report addresses the extent to which there may be scope for preventive programmes for Myalgic Encephalomyelitis/Chronic Fatigue Syndrome (ME/CFS), and, if so, what economic benefits may accrue from the implementation of such programmes. We consider the economic case for prevention programmes, whether there is scope for preventive programmes for ME/CFS, and what are the health and economic benefits to be derived from the implementation of such programmes. We conclude that there is little scope for primary prevention programmes, given that ME/CFS is attributable to a combination of host and environmental risk factors, with host factors appearing to be most prominent, and that there are few identified modifiable risk factors that could be the focus of such programmes. The exception is in the use of agricultural chemicals, particularly organophosphates, where there is scope for intervention, and where Europe-wide programmes of health education to encourage safe use would be beneficial. There is a need for more research on risk factors for ME/CFS to establish a basis for the development of primary prevention programmes, particularly in respect of occupational risk factors. Secondary prevention offers the greatest scope for intervention, to minimise diagnostic delays associated with prolonged illness, increased severity, and increased costs.

Keywords: prevention; economic impact; chronic fatigue syndrome; myalgic encephalomyelitis; ME/CFS

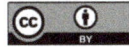

1. Introduction

Myalgic Encephalomyelitis/Chronic Fatigue Syndrome (ME/CFS) is a complex, serious, multi-system disorder, which is very disabling, with marked diminutions in function in quality of life. Its symptoms include severe fatigue, which is disabling and not improved by rest, and in particular, post-exertional malaise. Other symptoms include sleep disturbance, muscle pain, and cognitive dysfunction [1–4]. Symptoms, many of which are autonomic in nature, persist for at least six months. There is marked variation in the severity, symptoms, and clinical course of the disease. About three quarters of all patients are female. It occurs in all age groups, but most frequently arises in the 20 to 50 age group [5–7]. There may be around two million people with ME/CFS throughout Europe.

The European Network on ME/CFS (EUROMENE) was created to facilitate collaborative research, through working groups on epidemiology, biomarkers, and diagnostic criteria, clinical research, and socioeconomics, Europe-wide, to meet substantial gaps in scientific knowledge. Researchers from twenty-two countries now participate in the network. Working Group 3 (socioeconomics) focuses on the economic and social aspects of ME/CFS, with the objective of estimating the societal burden of ME/CFS.

UK experience suggests that the total cost of ME/CFS in Europe, including direct and indirect healthcare and other costs and productivity losses, may be in the region of €40 billion per annum [8], so even a 1% reduction achieved through programmes of prevention would be a substantial sum, though would need to be compared to the costs of such programmes. This report addresses the extent to which there may be scope for preventive programmes for ME/CFS, and what economic benefits may accrue therefrom.

2. The Economic Case for Prevention

There is evidence showing that many preventive programmes represent value for money [9] and that, therefore, there is a strong economic case for implementing them. Such programmes include, for example, targeted supervised tooth brushing and smoking cessation services [10]. Investments in prevention can produce value in terms of reduced healthcare spending, increased productivity, and improved quality of life, particularly when directed at chronic diseases that are major drivers of healthcare costs [11,12]. There are also benefits, in terms of both health and economic consequences of illness, from programmes that are effective, either in preventing illness or in treating it at an early stage, and there is empirical evidence to support this for certain conditions, such as colorectal cancer [13].

Thus, in many cases, there are numerous good reasons to invest in a well-defined package of preventive services that are recognised as effective in preventing disease and offer good economic value. The economic case can be demonstrated by cost-effectiveness or cost-utility analyses and/or the calculation of social return on investment (a quasi-cost-benefit analysis), or, where applicable, by cost-minimisation for two or more equivalent services. A review of economic evaluations of public health (PH) interventions assessed by the National Institute for Health and Care Excellence (NICE) found that three-quarters of preventative interventions were cost-effective at a threshold of £20,000 per quality-adjusted life year (QALY) [9].

There is evidence indicating that health promotion and primary prevention programmes are cost-effective [14,15], especially when the role of the recipients is passive, as in immunisation programmes, or when the programme is designed to deliver a public good to a whole community, such as fluoridation [16]. In the context of heart disease, as one example, and based on 19 economic evaluations informed by 15 randomised controlled trials, exercise therapy is cost-effective in patients with coronary heart disease, chronic heart failure, intermittent claudication, or with a body mass index (BMI) ≥ 25 kg/m^2 [17]. Treatments for heart disease are less cost-effective, with the majority of interventions (pharmacological and non-pharmacological) for heart failure associated with incremental cost-effectiveness ratios exceeding USD30,000 per QALY gained [18]. Preventive care, particularly for chronic diseases, can help patients and reduce costs and impacts on economic activity [19]. A study of the impact on healthcare utilisation and expenditure trends of a programme of prevention through behaviour modification found that a primary care model based on the doctor–patient relationship can have a positive impact in improving health, reducing the prevalence of chronic disease and disability, and reducing expenditure [20]. This is confirmed by a Report of the Surgeon General, which concluded that a water fluoridation programme, coupled with other dental initiatives, would improve dental health and cut costs [21]. Another review concluded that there was indeed potential for preventive services to delay or avoid distressing medical conditions that are expensive to treat [22]. Preventive care, particularly for chronic diseases, can help patients and reduce costs and impacts on economic activity [23].

3. Impediments to Prevention

A major challenge to successful implementation of programmes of prevention and demonstration of its economic value lies in the innate conservatism of people, and their unwillingness to change behaviour, as well as reticence when it comes to paying for such programmes [24], particularly as they require both a long-term view and intersectoral cooperation, and it can take many years for benefits of prevention to emerge [25]. For example, there is a significant gap in the availability of full economic evaluation studies focused on primary prevention of mental health problems among the elderly, and some patients do not appreciate the benefits of preventive programmes [14]. The evidence base regarding prevention programmes is very limited. In addition, the empirical evidence on individual prevention activities is rarely precise or definitive and there is a lack of high-quality studies. The economic benefits diffuse and appear abstract, and it is not always clear which individuals benefit [22]. In some cases, prevention (e.g., fitness, organic food, and clothing) can cause a prohibitive burden to individual and family budgets.

4. The Content of Prevention

Prevention may be primary, secondary, or tertiary. Primary prevention is designed to stop the onset of disease, often through behaviour modification, while secondary prevention consists of early detection when the disease is asymptomatic, in order to 'nip it in the bud'. Tertiary prevention is designed to mitigate the consequences of disease through disability limitation and rehabilitation. All three have the potential to reduce the costs of disease [11,24]. Prevention should address the causes of illness, be they social, economic, or environmental, including housing, education, and employment [25]. A focus on health behaviour and environmental and occupational risks is directed towards the main causes of preventable ill health, and important factors to consider in developing prevention programmes include lifestyle, social and community influences, living and working conditions, as well as socioeconomic, cultural, and environmental circumstances [26].

5. Evaluation of Prevention

Economic efficiency does not imply that cost should be minimised, or benefit maximised, but rather that cost be compared with benefit, and that net health benefits (the incremental cost divided by the opportunity cost threshold) be maximised [24]. The focus of investigation should be to determine whether the benefits accruing for the minority who benefit from a preventive intervention offset the costs (that is, the health benefits foregone) to the population as a whole.

The studies required to support evidence-based decisions on funding preventive programmes include effectiveness studies, simulation modelling, and economic evaluations [11]. In evaluating prevention programmes, aspects to consider include long-term impacts, non-health and non-monetary impacts, differential impacts across groups, and time preference [27]. Methodologically robust economic evaluations are needed to support decision-making in the allocation of healthcare resources, but especially in the context of prevention, where there are significant uncertainties in determining effectiveness, challenges in the measurement and valuation of outcomes, and often a lack of consideration of inter-sectoral costs, consequences, and equity implications [14,25].

There is a variety of possible approaches to evaluating the health and economic impacts of preventive programmes. Some are of more use to decision makers than others, particularly where they cover a long time-span [21]. Interventions for the prevention of chronic non-communicable diseases (NCDs) and certain types of injuries mainly address programmes designed to modify health-related behaviours and their interaction with environmental influences [28]. Research conducted in the UK since the 1970s stressed the relationship between socioeconomic position and health [26]. The World Health Organization (WHO) Commission on the Social Determinants of Health worked on the basis of a conceptual framework in which two main groups of determinants were identified, structural (e.g., socioeconomic and political contexts, social structures, and socioeconomic position) and intermediary factors (e.g., biological, behavioural, health system and psychosocial factors, living and working conditions) [29].

There is a need to elucidate the nature and extent of the evidence that demonstrates cost-effectiveness of disease and injury prevention programmes and clinical prevention services [11]. Estimating the cost-effectiveness of prevention, generally, is problematic, because such an evaluation may combine interventions of proven effectiveness with others—the effectiveness of which is less certain [23]. Recent reviews of economic evaluations of prevention programmes highlight the methodological limitations and challenges [9,25]. The choice of discount rate, as one example, to account for time preference, can impact significantly on the cost-effectiveness of prevention programmes, as even large future health benefits may result in low net present value.

In considering approaches to evaluation, it is necessary to consider the extent to which modelling methods could be used to project the clinical and spending impact of prevention programmes and whether wider impacts on employment should be taken into account. There is also a need to determine appropriate time horizons for evaluations, to consider how health benefits, including health-related quality of life, should be measured, and the extent to which it is possible to evaluate prevention programmes using traditional economic models [21,29].

Methods for quantifying the (social) return on investment of a proposed prevention programme are gaining popularity. These are consistent, in the UK, with the National Institute for Health and Care Excellence public health guidance, which comments on the appropriateness of cost-benefit analysis for public health programmes. Social return on investment analyses incorporate considerations of effectiveness and its time period, as well as of cost and perspective (i.e., which costs and benefits are included in the analysis) [30,31]. As public health has impacts extending beyond health alone, a broader perspective is often warranted. The pertinent question for prevention is whether it offers good value, in terms of return on investment, bearing in mind that addressing a single risk factor can impact on a broad range of conditions, and that the long-time horizon creates an opportunity for the compounding of health benefits [23].

Taking into account the above considerations, two main questions should be addressed: first, as to whether there is scope for preventive programmes for ME/CFS, and secondly, if so, whether there are health and economic benefits to be derived from the implementation of such programmes [32]. The answer to the first question depends on whether there are risk factors for ME/CFS which are capable of modification by means of such programmes, and this is considered next.

6. Risk Factors for ME/CFS

Although the exact pathogenesis of ME/CFS is still unknown, the most plausible hypothesis is that it is a complex multifactorial syndrome in which immunological and environmental factors play a crucial role [33,34].

7. Infections

Viral infections are involved in the aetiology of most cases of ME/CFS [35,36]. Various viral illnesses have been implicated, including for example the Epstein–Barr virus [37–40], and various sites of infection, including gastrointestinal infections [41]. Whether or not a viral infection creates a risk of ME/CFS depends on a number of parameters, including virus burden, strain, patterns of replication, and life cycle [42]. Cases may be epidemic or sporadic, with epidemic cases appearing to have a better prognosis [43].

Other infections which have been implicated as causes of ME/CFS include the Ross River virus and Coxiella burnetti [36]. Infections studied which have not been shown to cause ME/CFS include human herpesvirus 6, enterovirus, rubella, Candida albicans, bornaviruses, mycoplasma, and human immunodeficiency virus (HIV). An increase in the titre of anti-HHV-6 IgG and IgM antibodies in the sera of CFS patients has been demonstrated in comparison with a control population, but this was unspecific, with increases also in antibodies to other viruses, so this may simply reflect underlying immune dysfunction [44].

8. Immunological Factors

In addition, ME/CFS has some features in common with autoimmune illnesses and several studies have identified immunologic biomarkers [33]. Thus, both are more common in women and demonstrate increased inflammation. Other ways in which the immune system might contribute to ME/CFS include production of cytokines affecting the body's ability to respond to stress, low-functioning natural killer (NK) cells, and differences in markers of T-cell activation. Physical or emotional stress causing derangement of the hypothalamic-pituitary-adrenal axis (HPA axis), leading to low levels of cortisol, may thus lead to an increase in inflammation and chronic activation of the immune system. Finally, possible causative factors include immune suppression, increased intestinal permeability, impaired mitochondrial performance, changes in energy production, and a possible genetic link [34,40].

9. Occupational Exposures

Most of the concern about chemical exposures as a possible cause of ME/CFS centres on the agricultural use of organophosphates (OPs) and, to a lesser extent, of organochlorines. Fatigue syndromes may be secondary to occupational exposures to organochlorine or organophosphate compounds [45]. Fernández-Solà et al. [46] described a series of twenty-six patients, nine of whom were exposed to organophosphates alone, who developed chronic fatigue following insecticide exposure. Thamaz et al. [47] observed a dose–response relationship between chronic fatigue scores and levels of exposure to organophosphate pesticides.

The EU's Scientific Steering Committee reviewed the role of organophosphates as agricultural insecticides, used to control arthropod pests, including parasites, such as grub, horn fly, and other cattle exoparasites. It did not consider, however, the possible role of organophosphate exposure as a risk factor for ME/CFS, as their concern was the cause of bovine spongiform encephalopathy (BSE), in respect of which they concluded that there was no evidence to support the hypothesis that organophosphate exposure might be involved [48].

UK press reports assert involvement of organophosphates in the development of ME/CFS, and the risk to highly exposed agricultural workers cannot be disregarded [49]. A study of reports to the UK Veterinary Medicines Directorate of ill health attributed to pesticide exposure among agricultural workers found that ME/CFS-like symptoms were frequently mentioned, and questionnaire responses indicated an association with organophosphate exposure [47]. It appears that the major hazards of pesticide use are poisonings associated with exposure of operators as a result of misuse. This is supported by a study supported by the UK Health and Safety Executive, in which a comparison of 146 sheep dippers exposed to OPs and 143 non-exposed controls (quarry workers) found significant differences between the groups in various neuropsychological tests, such as simple reaction time, symbol-digit substitution, and syntactic reasoning, and also on neurological examination and the General Health Questionnaire. There were no observable differences on tests of memory or psychomotor function. There was evidence of sensory neuropathy of hands and feet among the sheep dippers. The authors concluded that "although the effects identified are not severe, the results of the investigation suggest that further efforts should be made to reduce exposure to organophosphates in terms of identifying the most appropriate protective clothing and dipping equipment and encouraging its use" [50].

Another study found that patients with a fatigue syndrome following organophosphate exposure manifested some differences in symptoms compared with sporadic cases of ME/CFS [51], but both groups conformed to the CDC-94 (Fukuda) case definition [52]. This is confirmed by a study comparing patients with Gulf War syndrome (GWS), ME/CFS, and the fatigue syndrome associated with organophosphate exposure, which found many similarities between the three conditions, but only patients with ME/CFS manifested peripheral cholinergic abnormalities in vascular endothelium, perhaps indicating a different aetiology [52]. Similarly, a study comparing agricultural workers who had been exposed to organophosphates with ME/CFS patients found that the two groups were identical in terms of mode of onset of illness, symptoms, and the results of neuroendocrine studies [53]. Kennedy et al. [51] described patients meeting the diagnostic criteria for CFS/ME following exposure to OPs. Another study compared forearm skin blood flow responses to iontophoresis of acetylcholine that were measured using laser Doppler imaging in patients with ME/CFS, GWS, illness following organophosphate exposure, and matched healthy controls. The acetylcholine response was higher in patients with CFS than in controls, but normal in GWS patients and those exposed to organophosphates, which may suggest aetiological differences [42]. Since ME/CFS is a syndrome, defined by its clinical features rather than underlying pathology [52], it is reasonable to regard the illness which may be a long-term outcome of OP exposure as ME/CFS, since the two conditions have many clinical features in common [53]. This is underlined by another study, which found that similar reproducible abnormalities of gene expression were found in ME/CFS patients and in patients following OP exposure [54].

Various studies have identified a range of long-term neurological abnormalities following OP exposure. These include significantly impaired performance in neuro-behavioural tests and peripheral neuropathy, with impaired memory and concentration, depressed mood [55], delayed neuropathy characterised by weakness or paralysis, and paraesthesia of the extremities, an intermediate syndrome muscular weakness, predominantly involving muscles of the face, neck, and limbs, with cranial nerve palsies and depressed reflexes. These may be related to neuromuscular transmission dysfunction [56], prolonged cognitive processing of visual stimuli [57], and neurocognitive, fibromyalgic, and chronic fatigue manifestations [45]. Acute OP poisoning due to acetylcholinesterase inhibition can lead to permanent disability or delayed peripheral neuropathy. Long-term low-dose effects are not necessarily due to acetylcholinesterase inhibition, however, but may indicate targeting of brain proteins [58]. The long-term consequences of OP exposure observed in humans are also apparent in animal experiments. Thus, repeated exposures of rats to two OPs (chlorpyrifos and diisopropylfluorophosphate) in low doses may lead to chronic deficits in spatial learning and memory [59].

Organochlorines have also been implicated in the development of fatigue syndromes. One study found that patients with unexplained, persistent fatigue had higher levels of DDE (1,1-dichloro-2,2-bis (p-chlorophenyl) ethane—an organochlorine) compared with controls [60]. A study of chlorinated hydrocarbon levels in patients with chronic fatigue syndrome concluded that organochlorines may indeed be involved in the aetiology of ME/CFS [61], and it could be that this involvement of such environmental chemicals is in combination with genetic factors [62]. There have been reports of an outbreak of ME/CFS in Nevada at the same time as an increased incidence of non-Hodgkin's lymphoma [63,64].

A causal relationship has been suggested [65], but both conditions may be attributable to exposure to agrichemicals, particularly organochlorines [66].

In conclusion, most of the studies considered were not population-based, had small sample sizes, or achieved very small response rates, and variations in diagnostic criteria make it difficult to draw general conclusions. A review of the research literature on the role of chemical exposures in the aetiology of ME/CFS concluded that the evidence of possible associations was inconclusive, so more research is needed [67]. However, there are sufficient pointers to conclude that, in respect of OPs, there is sufficient reason to at least adopt a precautionary principle and minimise exposure as far as possible.

10. Psychological Factors

Much of the research on risk factors has focused on psychology. Psychological risk factors reported include perfectionism, self-sacrificial tendencies, unhelpful beliefs about emotions, and perceived stress [68], personality disorders, and childhood traumatic experiences [69]. Other psychosocial risk factors proposed include functional somatic syndromes [70], cultural factors [71], other conditions labelled as somatisation disorders such as irritable bowel syndrome [72], socioeconomic deprivation [73], maladaptive personality and personality disorders [74], premorbid stress [75], premorbid distress and depression [76], maternal overprotection [77], and childhood trauma [78,79]. Membership of minority ethnic groups has been identified as another possible risk factor for ME/CFS. However, this may be associated with higher levels of anxiety, depression, physical inactivity, social strain, and lack of social support, rather than being part of an ethnic minority per se [80]. Psychiatric disorders, or shared risk factors for psychiatric disorders, it is asserted may have an aetiological role in some cases of CFS/ME [81], but the evidence for this and the other psychological factors reported here, is equivocal, to say the least.

11. Children and Adolescents

In children and adolescents, identified risk factors include family adversity [82], maternal anxiety, or depression [83]. It is more common in those who are socially deprived [84], and also among adolescents who experience anxiety and decreased physical activity [85]. However, other authors have found no relationship between childhood trauma and ME/CFS [86], and much of the evidence for psychosocial risk factors for ME/CFS is conjectural and unconfirmed. A systematic scoping review failed to reveal definitive evidence of risk factors for ME/CFS [87]. Another study failed to find any association between maternal or child psychological distress, academic ability, parental illness, atopy, or birth order and lifetime risk of CFS/ME, which was increased by sedentary behaviour [88]. Another study found physical factors such as disability and fatigue to be more prominent as risk factors for ME/CFS than psychosocial factors such as stress and coping [89]. The studies listed above for the most part identified associations rather than causal relationships, and Hickie et al. concluded that psychological disturbance was likely to be a consequence of ME/CFS, rather than a risk factor for it [90].

12. Other Possible Risk Factors

Other possible risk factors have also been suggested but remain unconfirmed. Thus, the risk of ME/CFS is increased if a close family member also has the illness, suggesting a role for genetic factors [91,92]. A questionnaire-based study found that the prevalence of CFS was higher in genetically unrelated household contacts and in non-resident genetic relatives than in the community, indicating that both household contact and genetic relationship are risk factors for CFS [93]. Other proposed factors include female gender, age, previous exposure to stress or toxins, occupational exposures, and infectious diseases, poorer health status [94], gynaecological conditions and surgery [95], ethnic minority status [96], and premorbid persistent unexplained severe fatigue [97,98]. The mechanism through which such risk factors take effect could be oxidative stress [99], while the increased risk of ME/CFS due to profound inactivity, deconditioning, or sleep abnormalities may be mediated via neuroendocrine dysregulation [100].

Two reports from the UK ME/CFS Biobank confirmed that little was known about risk factors for ME/CFS. A cross-sectional study of participants assessed the prevalence of cognitive and sleep symptoms in ME/CFS patients, in comparison with MS patients also participating in the Biobank. Cognitive symptoms included problems with short-term memory, attention, and executive function. Sleep symptoms included unrefreshing sleep and poor quality or inadequate duration of sleep. Such problems were more prevalent in the ME/CFS group than among the MS patients. Older ME/CFS patients (i.e., over 50) were much more likely to experience severe symptoms than younger ones (less than 30) (Odds ratio (OR) 3.23, p = 0.031). Severe symptoms were much more common among smokers and those with household incomes below £15,000 per year [101].

A further report found that a previous history of frequent infections, including colds and influenza, were the factors most strongly associated with a higher risk of ME/CFS compared to healthy controls. Other factors were being single, having lower income, and a family history of anxiety. Lower age at onset was associated with more severe disease, as also was a family history of neurological illness, which suggests that genetic and environmental factors may be involved. However, the authors concluded that there was little consistency in published reports [102].

This conclusion was borne out by a recent systematic scoping review of causal factors for CFS/ME. This examined 1161 studies published between 1979 and June 2019. Most were case-control studies, with under 100 participants. Potential factors studied were many and varied and ranged from environmental through to genetic factors. The categories of potential factors most frequently studied were immunological, psychological/psychosocial, socioeconomic, infections, and neuroendocrinal/hormonal/metabolic, with the greatest variety of possible risk factors being examined in the infections category. Studies of viruses predominated, particularly the Epstein–Barr virus, human herpes virus, and xenotropic murine leukaemia-related virus. No one possible causal factor was dominant, indicating much uncertainty in the field. The authors concluded that the quality of the evidence was too low to draw conclusions about causal factors, especially as there was a preponderance of weak study designs, with small numbers of participants and insufficient power to detect small effect sizes [94].

13. Perpetuating Factors

As regards perpetuating factors for ME/CFS and outcomes, a systematic review asserted that factors associated with worse prognosis included old age, chronic illness, comorbid psychiatric disorders, and, controversially, belief in a physical cause for the illness [103]. Severity of fatigue and psychiatric morbidity at baseline were associated with persistence twelve months later [104]. Among adolescents, risk factors for prolonged illness include older age at the outset, pain, and poor mental health and self-esteem [105]. Cardiovascular morbidity and mortality are increased in ME/CFS. Oxidative damage to DNA is found both in severe depression and ME/CFS [106], and is also a risk factor for atherosclerosis, hence the increased cardiovascular morbidity in ME/CFS [107]. In addition, reduced coenzyme Q10 may be the cause of chronic heart failure and increased cardiovascular mortality in ME/CFS [108]. In conclusion, it is likely that ME/CFS is attributable to a combination of host and environmental risk factors [109]. In most cases, a number of factors may be involved, of which host factors appear to be most prominent [110].

UK study of risk factors for severe ME/CFS (i.e., being housebound or bedbound) found that early management of the illness appeared to be an important determinant of prolonged, severe disease. This observational, questionnaire-based study was designed to identify risk factors for severe (i.e., housebound or bedbound) disease. Exposure to potential risk factors, including familial risks, personality, and early management of the illness, was compared in 124 people with severe disease and 619 mildly ill controls. Severity was determined by self-report and the Barthel (activities of daily living) Index. Premorbid personality was assessed using the Neuroticism and Conscientiousness domains of the International Personality Item Pool (IPIP) scale. Analysis was performed by tests of association and logistic regression. Early management of the illness appeared the most important determinant of severity. Having a mother with ME/CFS was also important. Smoking and personality were not risk factors, neurotic traits being more frequent among the less severely ill. Conscientiousness overall was not related to severity [111]. This confirmed the findings of an earlier population-based study, which showed that shorter illness duration was a significant predictor of sustained remission, and thus early detection of CFS is of utmost importance [112], as well as removal of barriers to healthcare utilisation, which is a serious problem [113].

14. Scope for Prevention in ME/CFS

This review has demonstrated that there is little consensus about the nature and impact of risk factors for ME/CFS and, as regards those risk factors about which there is general agreement, few are modifiable. Therefore, there is little scope for programmes of primary prevention, with the exception of organophosphate exposure.

Secondly prevention is a different matter, however. As detailed above, there are modifiable risk factors for severe and prolonged disease, in particular in mismanagement of the early stages of the illness, including diagnostic delays [111,112] and barriers to healthcare utilisation [113]. Previous work undertaken by the Working Group has considered the reasons for delay in diagnosis, which is a major barrier to healthcare utilisation. We reviewed the literature on knowledge and understanding of ME/CFS among GPs and concluded that between a third and a half of all GPs either disbelieved in the existence of ME/CFS as a genuine clinical entity or had little understanding of it, while a similar proportion of ME/CFS patients expressed dissatisfaction with the primary care that had received, and that these proportions occurred across a wide geographical area and had changed little over many years [114]. We also conducted a survey of how GP knowledge and understanding of ME/CFS was perceived among EUROMENE participants and found that similar misgivings were encountered across Europe [115]. Overall, it appears that, in Europe, a high proportion of GPs, upwards of 50%, do not recognise ME/CFS as a genuine clinical entity and therefore never diagnose it. Among those GPs who do recognise its existence, there is a marked lack of confidence in making the diagnosis and managing the condition. Therefore, estimates of the public health burden of the illness and of its economic impact are likely to be substantial underestimates [7].

Vink and Vink-Niese have demonstrated further scope for secondary prevention within the occupational setting. They demonstrated that patients required to rest at the outset of their illness have the best prognosis and that, on return to work, not pressurising such patients to over-perform could minimise relapses, long-term sick leave, and retirement on medical grounds [116]. Others have pointed out that many ME/CFS patients, particularly the most ill, are neglected by the healthcare system, often due to impediments to diagnosis and associated stigma, and argue for a holistic model of care leading to more supportive interactions between patients and practitioners [117,118].

In children, the experience of an Italian treatment and support initiative in education underlines the importance of early intervention in achieving successful outcomes in ME/CFS [119].

15. Associated Features

There may be scope to minimise some of the clinical features of ME/CFS, such as associated orthostatic intolerance, and hence thereby to reduce its economic impact. Thus, cardiovascular symptoms are common in ME/CFS patients. Cardiac dysfunction with low cardiac output due to small left ventricle may contribute to the development of chronic fatigue as a constitutional factor in a considerable number of ME/CFS patients [120], is most marked in patients with orthostatic intolerance [121], and it may be the consequence of a co-morbid hypovolaemic condition [122]. Many ME/CFS patients have a small heart, and this may predispose them to fatigue [123], and to the development of ME/CFS in a well-defined subgroup of ME/CFS patients [124]. A cross-sectional survey found that treatment of orthostatic symptoms in ME/CFS could improve functional capacity and quality of life [125]. Approaches to minimising the impact of orthostatic intolerance include the avoidance of factors that make symptoms worse, including hot surroundings and standing for prolonged periods. Insufficient salt and fluid intake may be a contributory factor to orthostatic intolerance in ME/CFS patients, so should be increased in the absence of contraindications including hypertension, congestive cardiac failure, and renal failure. Support stockings may also help [126]. Pharmacological treatment may help in patients who fail to respond to such conservative measures, including, for example, midodrine, and the mineralocorticoid fludrocortisone [127].

16. Conclusions and Recommendations

There is little scope for primary prevention programmes for ME/CFS, because there is little knowledge of, or consensus about, the modifiable risk factors that could be addressed by such a programme. The exception to this is in the use of agrichemicals, particularly organophosphates, where a precautionary principle suggests that Europe-wide programmes of health education to encourage safe use could be beneficial. There is a need for more research on such risk factors for ME/CFS, in order to establish a basis for the development of primary prevention programmes, and there are increasing opportunities for such research to be undertaken. For example, the European Human Biomonitoring programme creates a window opportunity to develop consistent mapping of the distribution of agricultural risk factors, which in turn could enable ecological studies of the distribution of ME/CFS in rural areas [128].

However, by contrast, there is considerable scope for secondary prevention, as improving the management of ME/CFS in the early stages of illness could have an impact in reducing the incidence and prevalence of severe prolonged disease, and thereby also its economic impact. Far too frequently, the primary care management of the illness is characterised by disbelief, lack of knowledge, and misunderstanding. Major benefits could be achieved by improving knowledge and understanding of ME/CFS in general practice, in order to minimise the diagnostic delays that are associated with prolonged illness and increased severity, and hence with increased costs. In addition, further benefits may be achievable through amelioration of associated features such as orthostatic intolerance.

Author Contributions: Conceptualisation—D.F.H.P., D.A., U.B., E.B., J.C., J.-D.d.K., L.G., D.A.H., R.M.H., D.T. and X.W.-S.; methodology—D.F.H.P., D.A., U.B., E.B., J.C., J.-D.d.K., L.G., D.A.H., R.M.H., D.T. and X.W.-S.; validation—D.F.H.P., D.A., U.B., E.B., J.C., J.-D.d.K., L.G., D.A.H., R.M.H., D.T. and X.W.-S.; investigation—D.F.H.P., D.A., U.B., E.B., J.C., J.-D.d.K., L.G., D.A.H., R.M.H., D.T. and X.W.-S.; writing—original draft preparation—D.F.H.P.; writing—review and editing—D.F.H.P., D.A.H., J.-D.d.K., D.A., J.C., L.G. and X.W.-S.; project administration—D.F.H.P. All authors have read and agreed to the published version of the manuscript.

Funding: This research received no external funding. EUROMENE receives funding for networking activities from the COST programme (COST Action 15111), via the COST Association.

Institutional Review Board Statement: Not applicable.

Informed Consent Statement: Not applicable.

Data Availability Statement: No new data were created or analysed in this study. Data sharing is not applicable to this article.

Conflicts of Interest: The authors declare no conflict of interest.

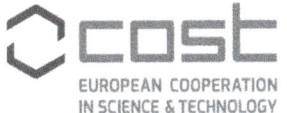
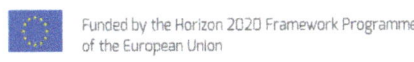

This article/publication is based upon work from the COST Action "European network on Myalgic Encephalomyelitis/Chronic Fatigue Syndrome", EUROMENE, supported by COST (European Cooperation in Science and Technology). COST is a funding agency for research and innovation networks. Its Actions help connect research initiatives across Europe and enable scientists to grow their ideas by sharing them with their peers. This boosts their research, careers and innovation. www.cost.eu (accessed on 15 April 2021).

References

1. Lindan, R. Benign Myalgic Encephalomyelitis. *Can. Med. Assoc. J.* **1956**, *75*, 596–597.
2. Acheson, E.D. The clinical syndrome variously called myalgic encephalomyelitis, Iceland disease and epidemic neurom-yasthenis. *Am. Med.* **1959**, *26*, 589–595. [CrossRef]
3. Carruthers, B.M.; Jain, A.K.; De Meirleir, K.L.; Peterson, D.L.; Klimas, N.G.; Lerner, A.M.; Bested, A.C.; Flor-Henry, P.; Joshi, P.; Powles, A.C.P.; et al. Myalgic encephalomyelitis/chronic fatigue syndrome: Clinical working case definition, diagnostic and treatment protocols. *J. Chronic Fatigue Syndr.* **2003**, *11*, 7–116. [CrossRef]
4. Institute of Medicine (IOM). *Beyond Myalgic Encephalomyelitis/Chronic Fatigue Syndrome: Redefining an Illness*; The National Academies Press: Washington, DC, USA, 2015.
5. Johnstone, S.C.; Staines, D.R.; Marshall-Gradisnik, S.M. Epidemiological characteristics of chronic fatigue syndrome/myalgic encephalomyelitis in Australian patients. *Clin. Epidemiol.* **2016**, *8*, 97–107. [CrossRef] [PubMed]
6. Pheby, D.; Lacerda, E.; Nacul, L.; Drachler, M.D.L.; Campion, P.; Howe, A.; Poland, F.; Curran, M.; Featherstone, V.; Fayyaz, S.; et al. A Disease Register for ME/CFS: Report of a Pilot Study. *BMC Res. Notes* **2011**, *4*, 139. [CrossRef]
7. Lloyd, A.R.; Hickie, I.; Boughton, C.R. Prevalence of chronic fatigue syndrome in an Australian population. *Med. J. Aust.* **1990**, *153*, 522–528. [CrossRef] [PubMed]
8. Pheby, D.F.; Araja, D.; Berkis, U.; Brenna, E.; Cullinan, J.; De Korwin, J.-D.; Gitto, L.A.; Hughes, D.; Hunter, R.M.; Trepel, D.; et al. The Development of a Consistent Europe-Wide Approach to Investigating the Economic Impact of Myalgic Encephalomyelitis (ME/CFS): A Report from the European Network on ME/CFS (EUROMENE). *Healthcare* **2020**, *8*, 88. [CrossRef]
9. Owen, L.; Fischer, A. The cost-effectiveness of public health interventions examined by the National Institute for Health and Care Excellence from 2005 to 2018. *Public Health* **2019**, *169*, 151–162. [CrossRef]
10. Newton, J.; Ferguson, B. 6 September 2017-Health Economics. Available online: www.gov.uk (accessed on 18 March 2020).
11. Benson, B.L.; Storey, E.; Huntington, C.G.; Eberle, M.U.; Ferris, A.M. The Economic Impact of Prevention: A report prepared by The Center for Public Health and Health Policy at The University of Connecticut Health Center and The University of Connecticut, Storrs, Niger. *J. Clin. Pract.* **2008**, *19*, 161.
12. Edwards, R.T.; McIntosh, E. *Handbooks in Health Economic Evaluation*; Oxford University Press: Oxford, UK, 2019.
13. Goede, S.L.; Kuntz, K.M.; van Ballegooijen, M.; Knudsen, A.B.; Lansdorp-Vogelaar, I.; Tangka, F.K.; Howard, D.H.; Chin, J.; Zauber, A.G.; Seeff, L.C. Cost-Savings to Medicare From Pre-Medicare Colorectal Cancer Screening. *Med. Care* **2015**, *53*, 630–638. [CrossRef]
14. Dubas-Jakóbczyk, K.; Kocot, E.; Kissimova-Skarbek, K.; Huter, K.; Rothgang, H. Economic evaluation of health promotion and primary prevention actions for older people—A systematic review. *Eur. J. Public Health* **2017**, *27*, 670–679. [CrossRef]
15. Masters, R.; Anwar, E.; Collins, B.; Cookson, R.; Capewell, S. Return on investment of public health interventions: A systematic review. *J. Epidemiol. Community Health* **2017**, *71*, 827–834. [CrossRef]
16. Warner, K.E. The economic implications of preventive health care. *Soc. Sci. Med. Part. C Med. Econ.* **1979**, *13*, 227–237. [CrossRef]
17. Oldridge, N.; Taylor, R.S. Cost-effectiveness of exercise therapy in patients with coronary heart disease, chronic heart failure and associated risk factors: A systematic review of economic evaluations of randomized clinical trials. *Eur. J. Prev. Cardiol.* **2020**, *27*, 1045–1055. [CrossRef] [PubMed]
18. Rohde, L.E.; Bertoldi, E.G.; Goldraich, L.; Polanczyk, C.A. Cost-effectiveness of heart failure therapies. *Nat. Rev. Cardiol.* **2013**, *10*, 338–354. [CrossRef] [PubMed]
19. Beaton, T. How Preventive Healthcare Services Reduce Spending for Payers. In *Value-Based Care News*; Health Payer Intelligence: Danvers, MA, USA, 2017.
20. Musich, S.; Wang, I.S.; Hawkins, J.K.; Klemes, A. The Impact of Personalized Preventive Care on Health Care Quality, Utilization, and Expenditures. *Popul. Health Manag.* **2016**, *19*, 389–397. [CrossRef]
21. Sharon, S.C.; Connolly, I.M.; Murphree, K.R. A review of the literature: The economic impact of preventive dental hygiene services. *J. Dent. Hyg. JDH* **2005**, *79*, 11.

22. Miller, W.; Rein, D.; O'Grady, M.; Yeung, J.-E.; Eichner, J.; McMahon, M. A review and analysis of economic models of prevention benefits. In *April 2013 U.S. Department of Health & Human Services. ASPE: Office of the Assistant Secretary for Planning and Evaluation*. Available online: https://aspe.hhs.gov/basic-report/review-and-analysis-economic-models-prevention-benefits (accessed on 15 April 2021).
23. Woolf, S.H.; Husten, C.G.; Lewin, L.S.; Marks, J.S.; Fielding, J.E.; Sanchez, E.J. The Economic Argument for Disease Prevention: Distinguishing Between Value and Savings. A Prevention Policy Paper Commissioned by Partnership for Prevention (on behalf of the National Commission on Prevention Priorities (NCPP)). 2009. Available online: https://www.coursehero.com/file/66910396/EconomicValue-Preventionpdf/ (accessed on 8 March 2021).
24. Pauly, M.V.; Sloan, F.A.; Sullivan, S.D. An Economic Framework for Preventive Care Advice. *Health Aff.* **2014**, *33*, 2034–2040. [CrossRef]
25. Weatherly, H.; Drummond, M.; Claxton, K.; Cookson, R.; Ferguson, B.; Godfrey, C.; Rice, N.; Sculpher, M.; Sowden, A. Methods for assessing the cost-effectiveness of public health interventions: Key challenges and recommendations. *Health Policy* **2009**, *93*, 85–92. [CrossRef]
26. Marmot, M. *The Status Syndrome*; Henry Holt: New York, NY, USA, 2004.
27. Marshall, L. The Economic Case for Preventing Ill Health. The Health Foundation. 2016. Available online: https://www.health.org.uk/blogs/the-economic-case-for-preventing-ill-health (accessed on 15 April 2001).
28. McDaid, D.; Sassi, F.; Merkur, S. *Promoting Health, Preventing Disease: The Economic Case*; Open University Press: Maidenhead, UK, 2015; pp. 3–18.
29. World Health Organization (WHO). *Preventing Chronic Diseases: A Vital Investment*; World Health Organization: Geneva, Switzerland, 2005.
30. Drummond, M.; Sculpher, M.; Claxton, K.; Stoddart, G.L.; Torrance, G. *Methods for the Economic Evaluation of Health Care Programmes*; Oxford University Press: Oxford, UK, 2015.
31. Jones, C.; Hartfiel, N.; Brocklehurst, P.; Lynch, M.; Edwards, R.T. Social Return on Investment Analysis of the Health Precinct Community Hub for Chronic Conditions. *Int. J. Environ. Res. Public Health* **2020**, *17*, 5249. [CrossRef] [PubMed]
32. National Institute for Health and Care Excellence. *Methods for the Development of NICE Public Health Guidance*, 3rd ed.; National Institute for Health and Care Excellence: London, UK, 2012.
33. Scheibenbogen, C.; Freitag, H.; Blanco, J.; Capelli, E.; Lacerda, E.; Authier, J.; Meeus, M.; Marrero, J.C.; Nora-Krukle, Z.; Oltra, E.; et al. The European ME/CFS Biomarker Landscape project: An initiative of the European network EUROMENE. *J. Transl. Med.* **2017**, *15*, 162. [CrossRef] [PubMed]
34. Morris, G.; Maes, M.; Berk, M.; Puri, B.K. Myalgic encephalomyelitis or chronic fatigue syndrome: How could the illness develop? *Metab. Brain Dis.* **2019**, *34*, 385–415. [CrossRef] [PubMed]
35. Miller, G. Molecular approaches to epidemiologic evaluation of viruses as risk factors for patients who have chronic fatigue syndrome. *Rev. Infect. Dis.* **1991**, *13*, 22–119. [CrossRef]
36. Rasa, S.; Nora-Krukle, Z.; Henning, N.; Eliassen, E.; Shikova, E.; Harrer, T.; Scheibenbogen, C.; Murovska, M.; Prusty, B.K. Chronic viral infections in myalgic encephalomyelitis/chronic fatigue syndrome (ME/CFS). *J. Transl. Med.* **2018**, *16*, 1–25. [CrossRef] [PubMed]
37. Katz, B.Z.; Shiraishi, Y.; Mears, C.J.; Binns, H.J.; Taylor, R. Chronic fatigue syndrome after infectious mononucleosis in adolescents. *Pediatrics* **2009**, *124*, 189–193. [CrossRef]
38. Candy, B.; Chalder, T.; Cleare, A.J.; Wessely, S.; White, P.D.; Hotopf, M. Recovery from infectious mononucleosis: A case for more than symptomatic therapy? A systematic review. *Br. J. Gen. Pract.* **2002**, *52*, 844–851.
39. White, P.D.; Thomas, J.M.; Amess, J.; Crawford, D.H.; Grover, S.A.; Kangro, H.O.; Clare, A.W. Incidence, risk and prognosis of acute and chronic fatigue syndromes and psychiatric disorders after glandular fever. *Br. J. Psychiatry* **1998**, *173*, 475–481. [CrossRef]
40. Possible Causes | Myalgic Encephalomyelitis/Chronic Fatigue Syndrome (ME/CFS) | CDC. Available online: https://www.cdc.gov/me-cfs/about/possible-causes.html#:~{}:text=People%20with%20ME%2FCFS%20often%20have%20their%20illness%20begin,of%20symptoms%20that%20meet%20the%20criteria%20for%20ME%2FCFS. (accessed on 8 January 2021).
41. Donnachie, E.; Schneider, A.; Mehring, M.; Enck, P. Incidence of irritable bowel syndrome and chronic fatigue following GI infection: A population-level study using routinely collected claims data. *Gut* **2017**, *67*, 1078–1086. [CrossRef]
42. Khan, F.; Kennedy, G.; Spence, V.A.; Newton, D.J.; Belch, J.J.F. Peripheral cholinergic function in humans with chronic fatigue syndrome, Gulf War syndrome and with illness following organophosphate exposure. *Clin. Sci.* **2004**, *106*, 183–189. [CrossRef]
43. Levine, P.H.; Snow, P.G.; Ranum, A.B.; Paul, C.; Holmes, M.J. Epidemic neuromyasthenia and chronic fatigue syndrome in west Otago, New Zealand. A 10-year follow-up. *Arch. Intern. Med.* **1997**, *157*, 750–754. [CrossRef]
44. Manian, F.A. Simultaneous measurement of antibodies to Epstein–Barr virus, human herpesvirus 6, herpes simplex virus types 1 and 2, and 14 enteroviruses in chronic fatigue syndrome: Is there evidence of activation of a nonspecific polyclonal immune response? *Clin. Infect. Dis.* **1994**, *19*, 448–453. [CrossRef] [PubMed]
45. Corrigan, F.; Macdonald, S.; Brown, A.; Armstrong, K.; Armstrong, E. Neurasthenic fatigue, chemical sensitivity and GABAa receptor toxins. *Med. Hypotheses* **1994**, *43*, 195–200. [CrossRef]

46. Fernandez-Sola, J.; Lluis Padierna, M.; Nogue Xarau, S.; Munne Mas, P. Chronic fatigue syndrome and multiple chemical hypersensitivity after insecticide exposure. *Med. Clin.* **2005**, *124*, 451–453.
47. Tahmaz, N.; Soutar, A.; Cherrie, J. Chronic fatigue and organophosphate pesticides in sheep farming: A retrospective study amongst people reporting to a UK pharmacovigilance scheme. *Ann. Occup. Hyg.* **2003**, *47*, 261–267. [CrossRef] [PubMed]
48. Opinion on Possible Links between BSE and Organophosphates Used as Pesticides against Ecto- and Endoparasites in Cattle Report and Opinion Adopted at the Scientific Steering Committee Meeting of 25–26 June 1998. Available online: https://ec.europa.eu/food/sites/food/files/safety/docs/sci-com_ssc_out18_en.pdf. (accessed on 6 January 2021).
49. Ray, E.D. Pesticide neurotoxicity in Europe: Real risks and perceived risks. *NeuroToxicology* **2000**, *21*, 219–221. [PubMed]
50. Jackson, C.A.; Spurgeon, A. Symptom-Reporting Following Occupational Exposure to Organophosphate Pesticides in Sheep Dip (Institute of Occupational Health University of Birmingham). Available online: https://www.hse.gov.uk/research?crr_pdf/1995/crr95074.pdf (accessed on 6 January 2021).
51. Kennedy, G.; Abbot, N.C.; Spence, V.; Underwood, C.; Belch, J.J. The specificity of the CDC-1994 criteria for chronic fatigue syndrome: Comparison of health status in three groups of patients who fulfill the criteria. *Ann. Epidemiol.* **2004**, *14*, 95–100. [CrossRef] [PubMed]
52. Fukuda, K.; Straus, S.E.; Hickie, I.; Sharpe, M.C.; Dobbins, J.G.; Komaroff, A. The chronic fatigue syndrome: A comprehensive approach to its definition and study. International Chronic Fatigue Syndrome Study Group. *Ann. Intern Med.* **1994**, *15*, 953–959. [CrossRef] [PubMed]
53. Behan, P.O. Chronic Fatigue Syndrome as a Delayed Reaction to Chronic Low-dose Organophosphate Exposure. *J. Nutr. Environ. Med.* **1996**, *6*, 341–350. [CrossRef]
54. Kaushik, N.; Fear, D.; Richards, S.C.M.; McDermott, C.R.; Nuwaysir, E.F.; Kellam, P.; Harrison, T.J.; Wilkinson, R.J.; Tyrrell, D.A.J.; Holgate, S.T.; et al. Gene expression in peripheral blood mononuclear cells from patients with chronic fatigue syndrome. *J. Clin. Pathol.* **2005**, *58*, 826–832. [CrossRef] [PubMed]
55. Recognition and Management of Pesticide Poisonings: Sixth Edition: 2013: Chapter 5 Organophosphates (epa.gov). Available online: https://www.epa.gov/sites/production/files/documents/rmpp_6thed_ch5_organophosphates.pdf (accessed on 6 January 2021).
56. Recognition and Management of Pesticide Poisonings: Sixth Edition: 2013: Chapter 21 Chronic effects (epa.gov). Available online: https://www.epa.gov/sites/production/files/documents/rmpp_6thed_ch21_chroniceffects.pdf (accessed on 6 January 2021).
57. Dassanayake, T.; Weerasinghe, V.; Dangahadeniya, U.; Kularatne, K.; Dawson, A.; Karalliedde, L. Cognitive processing of visual stimuli in patients with organophosphate insecticide poisoning. *Neurology* **2007**, *68*, 2027–2030. [CrossRef]
58. Ray, D.E.; Richards, P. The potential for toxic effects of chronic, low-dose exposure to organophosphates. *Toxicol. Lett.* **2001**, *120*, 343–351. [CrossRef]
59. Terry, A.; Beck, W.; Warner, S.; Vandenhuerk, L.; Callahan, P. Chronic impairments in spatial learning and memory in rats previously exposed to chlorpyrfos or diisopropylfluorophosphate. *Neurotoxicol. Teratol.* **2012**, *34*, 1–8. [CrossRef]
60. Dunstan, R.H.; Roberts, T.K.; Donohoe, M.; McGregor, N.R.; Hope, D.; Taylor, W.G.; Watkins, A.J.; Murdoch, R.N.; Butt, H.L. Bioaccumulated chlorinated hydrocarbons and red/white blood cell parameters. *Biochem. Mol. Med.* **1996**, *58*, 77–84. [CrossRef]
61. Dunstan, R.H.; Donohoe, M.; Taylor, W.; Roberts, T.K.; Murdoch, R.N.; Watkins, A.J.; McGregor, N.R. A preliminary investigation of chlorinated hydrocarbons and chronic fatigue syndrome. *Med. J. Aust.* **1995**, *163*, 294–297. [CrossRef] [PubMed]
62. Overstreet, D.H.; Djuric, V. A genetic rat model of cholinergic hypersensitivity: Implications for chemical intolerance, chronic fatigue, and asthma. *Ann. N. Y. Acad. Sci.* **2001**, *933*, 92–102. [CrossRef] [PubMed]
63. Levine, P.H.; Atherton, M.; Fears, T.; Hoover, R. An Approach to Studies of Cancer Subsequent to Clusters of Chronic Fatigue Syndrome: Use of Data from the Nevada State Cancer Registry. *Clin. Infect. Dis.* **1994**, *18*, S49–S53. [CrossRef] [PubMed]
64. Levine, P.H.; Peterson, D.; McNamee, F.L.; O'Brien, K.; Gridley, G.; Hagerty, M.; Brady, J.; Fears, T.; Atherton, M.; Hoover, R. Does chronic fatigue syndrome predispose to non-Hodgkin's lymphoma? *Cancer Res.* **1992**, *52*, 5516s–5518s. [PubMed]
65. Levine, P.H.; Fears, T.R.; Cummings, P.; Hoover, R.N. Cancer and a fatiguing illness in Northern Nevada-A causal hypothesis. *Ann. Epidemiol.* **1998**, *8*, 245–249. [CrossRef]
66. Daugherty, S.A.; Henry, B.E.; Peterson, D.L.; Swarts, R.L.; Bastien, S.; Thomas, R.S. Chronic Fatigue Syndrome in Northern Nevada. *Clin. Infect. Dis.* **1991**, *13*, S39–S44. [CrossRef] [PubMed]
67. Nacul, L.C.; Lacerda, E.M.; Sakellariou, D. Is there an association between exposure to chemicals and chronic fatigue syndrome? Review of the evidence. *Bulletin IACFS/ME* **2009**, *17*, 4.
68. Brooks, S.K.; Chalder, T.; Rimes, K.A. Chronic Fatigue Syndrome: Cognitive, Behavioural and Emotional Processing Vulnerability Factors. *Behav. Cogn. Psychother.* **2017**, *45*, 156–169. [CrossRef]
69. Saez-Francas, N.; Calvo, N.; Alegre, J.; Castro-Marrero, J.; Ramirez, N.; Hernandez-Vara, J.; Casas, M. Childhood trauma in Chronic Fatigue Syndrome: Focus on personality disorders and psychopathology. *Compr. Psychiatry* **2015**, *62*, 13–19. [CrossRef] [PubMed]
70. Warren, J.W.; Langenberg, P.; Clauw, D.J. The number of existing functional somatic syndromes (FSSs) is an important risk factor for new, different FSSs. *J. Psychosom. Res.* **2013**, *74*, 12–17. [CrossRef]
71. Tofoli, L.F.; Andrade, L.H.; Fortes, S. Somatization in Latin America: A review of the classification of somatoform disorders, functional syndromes and medically unexplained symptoms. *Rev. Bras. Psiquiatr.* **2011**, *33* (Suppl. 1), S59–S80.

72. Van Oudenhove, L.; Vandenberghe, J.; Vos, R.; Holvoet, L.; Tack, J. Factors associated with co-morbid irritable bowel syndrome and chronic fatigue-like symptoms in functional dyspepsia. *Neurogastroenterol. Motil.* **2011**, *23*, 202–524. [CrossRef] [PubMed]
73. Wong, W.S.; Fielding, R. Prevalence of chronic fatigue among Chinese adults in Hong Kong: A population-based study. *J. Affect. Disord.* **2010**, *127*, 248–256. [CrossRef]
74. Nater, U.M.; Jones, J.F.; Lin, J.-M.S.; Maloney, E.; Reeves, W.C.; Heim, C. Personality Features and Personality Disorders in Chronic Fatigue Syndrome: A Population-Based Study. *Psychother. Psychosom.* **2010**, *79*, 312–318. [CrossRef]
75. Kato, K.; Sullivan, P.F.; Evengård, B.; Pedersen, N.L. Premorbid Predictors of Chronic Fatigue. *Arch. Gen. Psychiatry* **2006**, *63*, 1267–1272. [CrossRef] [PubMed]
76. Moss-Morris, R.; Spence, M. To "Lump" or to "Split" the Functional Somatic Syndromes: Can Infectious and Emotional Risk Factors Differentiate Between the Onset of Chronic Fatigue Syndrome and Irritable Bowel Syndrome? *Psychosom. Med.* **2006**, *68*, 463–469. [CrossRef] [PubMed]
77. Fisher, L.; Chalder, T. Childhood experiences of illness and parenting in adults with chronic fatigue syndrome. *J. Psychosom. Res.* **2003**, *54*, 439–443. [CrossRef]
78. Heim, C.; Nater, U.M.; Maloney, E.; Boneva, R.; Jones, J.F.; Reeves, W.C. Childhood trauma and risk for chronic fatigue syndrome: Association with neuroendocrine dysfunction. *Arch. Gen. Psychiatry* **2009**, *66*, 72–80. [CrossRef]
79. Heim, C.; Wagner, D.; Maloney, E.; Papanicolaou, D.A.; Solomon, L.; Jones, J.F.; Unger, E.R.; Reeves, W.C. Early adverse experience and risk for chronic fatigue syndrome: Results from a population-based study. *Arch. Gen. Psychiatry* **2006**, *63*, 1258–1266. [CrossRef]
80. Bhui, K.S.; Dinos, S.; Ashby, D.; Nazroo, J.; Wessely, S.; White, P.D. Chronic fatigue syndrome in an ethnically diverse population: The influence of psychosocial adversity and physical inactivity. *BMC Med.* **2011**, *9*, 26. [CrossRef] [PubMed]
81. Harvey, S.B.; Wadsworth, M.; Wessely, S.; Hotopf, M. The relationship between prior psychiatric disorder and chronic fatigue: Evidence from a national birth cohort study. *Psychol. Med.* **2007**, *38*, 933–940. [CrossRef] [PubMed]
82. Collin, S.M.; Norris, T.; Nuevo, R.; Tilling, K.; Joinson, C.; Sterne, J.A.; Crawley, E. Chronic Fatigue Syndrome at Age 16 Years. *Pediatry* **2016**, *137*, 1–10. [CrossRef]
83. Collin, S.M.; Tilling, K.; Joinson, C.; Rimes, K.A.; Pearson, R.M.; Hughes, R.A.; Sterne, J.A.; Crawley, E. Maternal and Childhood Psychological Factors Predict Chronic Disabling Fatigue at Age 13 Years. *J. Adolesc. Health* **2015**, *56*, 181–187. [CrossRef]
84. Crawley, E. The epidemiology of chronic fatigue syndrome/myalgic encephalitis in children. *Arch. Dis. Child.* **2014**, *99*, 171–174. [CrossRef]
85. Ter Wolbeek, M.; Van Doornen, L.J.; Kavelaars, A.; Tersteeg-Kamperman, M.D.; Heijnen, C.J. Fatigue, depressive symptoms, and anxiety from adolescence up to young adulthood: A longitudinal study. *Brain Behav. Immun.* **2011**, *25*, 1249–1255. [CrossRef]
86. Vangeel, E.; Van Den Eede, F.; Hompes, T.; Izzi, B.; Del Favero, J.; Moorkens, G.; Lambrechts, D.; Freson, K.; Claes, S. Chronic Fatigue Syndrome and DNA Hypomethylation of the Glucocorticoid Receptor Gene Promoter 1F Region: Associations with HPA Axis Hypofunction and Childhood Trauma. *Psychosom. Med.* **2015**, *77*, 853–862. [CrossRef] [PubMed]
87. Hempel, S.; Chambers, D.; Bagnall, A.-M.; Forbes, C. Risk factors for chronic fatigue syndrome/myalgic encephalomyelitis: A systematic scoping review of multiple predictor studies. *Psychol. Med.* **2007**, *38*, 915–926. [CrossRef] [PubMed]
88. Viner, R.; Hotopf, M. Childhood predictors of self reported chronic fatigue syndrome/myalgic encephalomyelitis in adults: National birth cohort study. *BMJ* **2004**, *329*, 941. [CrossRef] [PubMed]
89. Jason, L.A.; Porter, N.; Hunnell, J.; Rademaker, A.; Richman, J.A. CFS prevalence and risk factors over time. *J. Health Psychol.* **2010**, *16*, 445–456. [CrossRef] [PubMed]
90. Hickie, I.; Lloyd, A.; Wakefield, D.; Parker, G. The Psychiatric Status of Patients with the Chronic Fatigue Syndrome. *Br. J. Psychiatry* **1990**, *156*, 534–540. [CrossRef]
91. Underhill, R.; O'Gorman, R. Prevalence of Chronic Fatigue Syndrome and Chronic Fatigue Within Families of CFS Patients. *J. Chronic Fatigue Syndr.* **2006**, *13*, 3–13. [CrossRef]
92. Underhill, R. Myalgic encephalomyelitis, chronic fatigue syndrome: An infectious disease. *Med. Hypotheses* **2015**, *85*, 765–773. [CrossRef]
93. Rusu, C.; Gee, M.E.; Lagace, C.; Parlor, M. Chronic fatigue syndrome and fibromyalgia in Canada: Prevalence and associations with six health status indicators. *Health Promot. Chronic Dis. Prev. Can.* **2015**, *35*, 3–11. [CrossRef]
94. Muller, A.E.; Tveito, K.; Bakken, I.J.; Flottorp, S.A.; Mjaaland, S.; Larun, L. Potential causal factors of CFS/ME: A concise and systematic scoping review of factors researched. *J. Transl. Med.* **2020**, *18*, 1–7. [CrossRef]
95. Boneva, R.S.; Maloney, E.M.; Lin, J.-M.; Jones, J.F.; Wieser, F.; Nater, U.M.; Heim, C.M.; Reeves, W.C. Gynecological History in Chronic Fatigue Syndrome: A Population-Based Case-Control Study. *J. Women Health* **2011**, *20*, 21–28. [CrossRef]
96. Dinos, S.; Khoshaba, B.; Ashby, D.; White, P.D.; Nazroo, J.; Wessely, S.; Bhui, K.S. A systematic review of chronic fatigue, its syndromes and ethnicity: Prevalence, severity, co-morbidity and coping. *Int. J. Epidemiol.* **2009**, *38*, 1554–1570. [CrossRef]
97. Ter Wolbeek, M.; Van Doornen, L.J.; Kavelaars, A.; Heijnen, C.J. Severe Fatigue in Adolescents: A Common Phenomenon? *Pediatry* **2006**, *117*, e1078–e1086. [CrossRef]

98. Huibers, M.J.H.; Kant, I.J.; Knottnerus, J.A.; Bleijenberg, G.; Swaen, G.M.H.; Kasl, S.V. Development of the chronic fatigue syndrome in severely fatigued employees: Predictors of outcome in the Maastricht cohort study. *J. Epidemiol. Community Health* **2004**, *58*, 877–882. [CrossRef]
99. Kennedy, G.; Spence, V.A.; McLaren, M.; Hill, A.; Underwood, C.; Belch, J.J. Oxidative stress levels are raised in chronic fatigue syndrome and are associated with clinical symptoms. *Free Radic. Biol. Med.* **2005**, *39*, 584–589. [CrossRef] [PubMed]
100. Gaab, J.; Engert, V.; Heitz, V.; Schad, T.; Schürmeyer, T.H.; Ehlert, U. Associations between neuroendocrine responses to the Insulin Tolerance Test and patient characteristics in chronic fatigue syndrome. *J. Psychosom. Res.* **2004**, *56*, 419–424. [CrossRef]
101. Jain, V.; Arunkumar, A.; Kingdon, C.; Lacerda, E.; Nacul, L. Prevalence of and risk factors for severe cognitive and sleep symptoms in ME/CFS and MS. *BMC Neurol.* **2017**, *17*, 1–10. [CrossRef]
102. Lacerda, E.M.; Geraghty, K.; Kingdon, C.C.; Palla, L.; Nacul, L.; Kingdon, C. A logistic regression analysis of risk factors in ME/CFS pathogenesis. *BMC Neurol.* **2019**, *19*, 275. [CrossRef]
103. Joyce, J.; Hotopf, M.; Wessely, S. The prognosis of chronic fatigue and chronic fatigue syndrome: A systematic review. *Int. J. Med.* **1997**, *90*, 223–233. [CrossRef] [PubMed]
104. Skapinakis, P.; Lewis, G.; Mavreas, V. One-year outcome of unexplained fatigue syndromes in primary care: Results from an international study. *Psychol. Med.* **2003**, *33*, 857–866. [CrossRef]
105. van Geelen, S.M.; Bakker, R.J.; Kuis, W.; van de Putte, E.M. Adolescent chronic fatigue syndrome: A follow-up study. *Arch. Pediatrics Adolesc. Med.* **2010**, *164*, 810–814. [CrossRef] [PubMed]
106. Maes, M.; Mihaylova, I.; Kubera, M.; Uytterhoeven, M.; Vrydags, N.; Bosmans, E. Increased 8-hydroxy-deoxyguanosine, a marker of oxidative damage to DNA, in major depression and myalgic encephalomyelitis / chronic fatigue syndrome. *Neuroendocrinol. Lett.* **2009**, *30*, 15–22.
107. Maes, M.; Mihaylova, I.; Kubera, M.; Uytterhoeven, M.; Vrydags, N.; Bosmans, E. Coenzyme Q10 deficiency in myalgic encephalomyelitis/chronic fatigue syndrome (ME/CFS) is related to fatigue, autonomic and neurocognitive symptoms and is another risk factor explaining the early mortality in ME/CFS due to cardiovascular disorder. *Neuro Endocrinol. Lett.* **2009**, *30*, 470–476.
108. Bell, K.M.; Cookfair, D.; Bell, D.S.; Reese, P.; Cooper, L. Risk Factors Associated with Chronic Fatigue Syndrome in a Cluster of Pediatric Cases. *Clin. Infect. Dis.* **1991**, *13*, S32–S38. [CrossRef]
109. Ortega-Hernandez, O.; Shoenfeld, Y. Infection, Vaccination, and Autoantibodies in Chronic Fatigue Syndrome, Cause or Coincidence? *Ann. N. Y. Acad. Sci.* **2009**, *1173*, 600–609. [CrossRef]
110. Levine, P.H. Epidemiologic advances in chronic fatigue syndrome. *J. Psychiatr. Res.* **1997**, *31*, 7–18. [CrossRef]
111. Pheby, D.; Saffron, L. Risk factors for severe ME/CFS. *Biol. Med.* **2009**, *1*, 50–74.
112. Nisenbaum, R.; Jones, J.F.; Unger, E.R.; Reyes, M.; Reeves, W.C. A population-based study of the clinical course of chronic fatigue syndrome. *Health Qual. Life Outcomes* **2003**, *1*, 49. [CrossRef]
113. Lin, J.-M.S.; Brimmer, D.J.; Boneva, R.S.; Jones, J.F.; Reeves, W.C. Barriers to healthcare utilization in fatiguing illness: A population-based study in Georgia. *BMC Health Serv. Res.* **2009**, *9*, 13. [CrossRef] [PubMed]
114. Pheby, D.; Araja, D.; Berkis, U.; Brenna, E.; Cullinan, J.; de Korwin, J.-D.; Gitto, L.; Hughes, D.; Hunter, R.; Trepel, D.; et al. A Literature Review of GP Knowledge and Understanding of ME/CFS: A Report from the Socioeconomic Working Group of the European Network on ME/CFS (EUROMENE). *Medicina* **2020**, *57*, 7. [CrossRef] [PubMed]
115. Cullinan, J.; Pheby, D.; Araja, D.; Berkis, U.; Brenna, E.; de Korwin, J.-D.; Gitto, L.; Hughes, D.; Hunter, R.; Trepel, D.; et al. Perceptions of European ME/CFS Experts Concerning Knowledge and Understanding of ME/CFS among Primary Care Physicians in Europe: A Report from the European ME/CFS Research Network (EUROMENE). *Medicina* **2021**, *57*, 208. [CrossRef]
116. Vink, M.; Vink-Niese, F. Work Rehabilitation and Medical Retirement for Myalgic Encephalomyelitis/Chronic Fatigue Syndrome Patients. A Review and Appraisal of Diagnostic Strategies. *Diagnose* **2019**, *9*, 124. [CrossRef] [PubMed]
117. Kingdon, C.; Giotas, D.; Nacul, L.; Lacerda, E. Health Care Responsibility and Compassion-Visiting the Housebound Patient Severely Affected by ME/CFS. *Healthcare* **2020**, *8*, 197. [CrossRef]
118. Cullinan, J.; Ni Chomrai, O.; Kindlon, T.; Black, L.; Casey, B. Understanding the economic impact of myalgic encephalomyelitis/chronic fatigue syndrome (ME/CFS) in Ireland: A qualitative study. *HRB Open Res.* **2020**, *3*, 88. [CrossRef]
119. Ardino, R.B.; Lorusso, L. La sindrome da affaticamento cronico/encefalomielite mialgica: Le caratteristiche della malattia e il ruolo dell'Associazione malati CFS [Myalgic encephalomyelitis/chronic fatigue syndrome: Characteristics of the disease and the role of the CFS patients' association]. *Politiche Sanit.* **2018**, *19*, 91–95.
120. Miwa, K.; Fujita, M. Cardiovascular Dysfunction with Low Cardiac Output Due to a Small Heart in Patients with Chronic Fatigue Syndrome. *Intern. Med.* **2009**, *48*, 1849–1854. [CrossRef] [PubMed]
121. Miwa, K. *Small Heart as a Constitutive Factor Predisposing to Chronic Fatigue Syndrome*; InTech: Rijeka, Croatia, 2012. ISBN 978-953-51-0072-0.
122. Hurwitz, B.E.; Coryell, V.T.; Parker, M.; Martin, P.; LaPerriere, A.; Klimas, N.G.; Sfakianakis, G.N.; Bilsker, M.S. Chronic fatigue syndrome: Illness severity, sedentary lifestyle, blood volume and evidence of diminished cardiac function. *Clin. Sci.* **2009**, *118*, 125–135. [CrossRef] [PubMed]
123. Miwa, K.; Fujita, M. Small Heart Syndrome in Patients with Chronic Fatigue Syndrome. *Clin. Cardiol.* **2008**, *31*, 328–333. [CrossRef]

124. Miwa, K.; Fujita, M. Small heart with low cardiac output for orthostatic intolerance in patients with chronic fatigue syndrome. *Clin. Cardiol.* **2011**, *34*, 782–786. [CrossRef]
125. Costigan, A.; Elliott, C.; McDonald, C.; Newton, J.L. Orthostatic symptoms predict functional capacity in chronic fatigue syndrome: Implications for management. *Int. J. Med.* **2010**, *103*, 589–595. [CrossRef] [PubMed]
126. Centres for Disease Control. Treating the Most Disruptive Symptoms First and Preventing Worsening of Symptoms | Clinical Care of Patients | Healthcare Providers | Myalgic Encephalomyelitis/Chronic Fatigue Syndrome (ME/CFS). Available online: https://www.cdc.gov/me-cfs/healthcare-providers/clinical-care-patients-mecfs/treating-most-disruptive-symtoms.html (accessed on 6 April 2021).
127. Medications for Postural Orthostatic Tachycardia Syndrome. Available online: https://www.drugs.com/condition/postural-orthostatic-tachycardia-syndrome.html (accessed on 6 April 2021).
128. The European Human Biomonitoring Initiative (part of the H2020 Programme of the European Union). Available online: https://cordis.europa.eu/programme/id/H2020_SC1-PM-05-2016 (accessed on 9 January 2021).

MDPI
St. Alban-Anlage 66
4052 Basel
Switzerland
Tel. +41 61 683 77 34
Fax +41 61 302 89 18
www.mdpi.com

Medicina Editorial Office
E-mail: medicina@mdpi.com
www.mdpi.com/journal/medicina

www.ingramcontent.com/pod-product-compliance
Lightning Source LLC
LaVergne TN
LVHW070439100526
838202LV00014B/1624